Without Whose Aid

NURSING AND THE CLEVELAND CLINIC

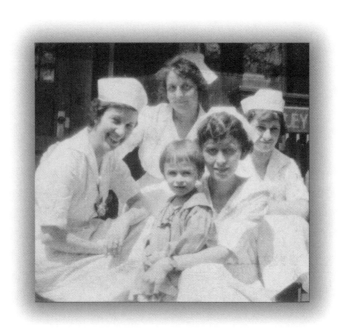

Without Whose Aid

NURSING AND THE CLEVELAND CLINIC

by Diane Ewart Grabowski

THE
CLEVELAND CLINIC
FOUNDATION

Overleaf: *Madeleine Bebout with Nurses*

Published by
The Cleveland Clinic Foundation
9500 Euclid Avenue
Cleveland, Ohio 44195

ISBN 0-9615424-2-X
Printed and bound in the United States of America

Dedicated to

the Nurses and Nursing Personnel

of the Cleveland Clinic,

Past, Present, and Future.

Table of Contents

Foreword

This profession has provided it all....to leave the world a bit better
because someone's pain was diminished, someone's sorrow comforted,
someone's choice restored, someone's child did not die alone.
Leah L. Curtin,
in *Nursing Management* 19 (July 1988): 10

The reason for this book is found in the following passage from Anne Morrow Lindbergh's *Gift from the Sea* (quoted by Leah Curtin, in *Nursing Management* 19 [July 1988]: 9): "When one is a stranger to oneself then one is estranged from others, too. If one is out of touch with oneself, then one cannot touch others."

Nurses have been and continue to be integral to the mission of The Cleveland Clinic Foundation: Better care of the sick, investigation of their problems and further education of those who serve. This great institution is physician-led, but from its very beginnings, nurses and the staff who support them have played a major role, so much so that its very mission would go unfulfilled without them.

In recognition of the Foundation's 75th anniversary, this book highlights those countless contributions and inspires a renewed appreciation for the importance of nursing work.

Separate and distinct professions, medicine and nursing are nevertheless interdependent upon each other, so much so that one cannot think of one without the other. Recent advances in medical science and technology have blurred some of their professional distinctions, yet the primary focus of medicine remains the curing of disease, while the heart of nursing is the promotion and restoration of health and wellness. Perhaps it is for this reason that Florence Nightingale wrote (in a letter to Sir Henry Acland in 1869, excerpted in Monica Baly, ed., *As Miss Nightingale Said: Florence Nightingale Through Her Sayings — A Victorian Perspective* [London: Scutari Press, 1991], 68): "Experience teaches me that nursing and medicine must never be mixed up. It spoils both."

While the essence and intent of nursing is readily understood, the definition of nursing is not. Saddled by the constraints of traditional women's work during the early feminist movement of the 1960s, nurses themselves have undervalued their work and contributions.

At some time or another, virtually every nurse has responded to a question about his/her profession with "I'm **just** a nurse." Physicians, lawyers, teachers, and ministers almost universally never respond to similar questioning with "I'm just a ...." Reinforcing the notion of "less than" are well-meaning people who will, from time to time, comment, "You are so **bright,** why didn't you become a doctor?" Asking that person if they would choose to be cared for by a dull nurse quickly underscores the need for bright and well-educated nurses.

So, in small part, the undertaking of this book is a passion to right this wrong. I couldn't agree more with Annie W. Goodrich, a former dean of the Army School of Nursing, that there is an "ethical significance of nursing."

While Effie J. Taylor, in 1933, defined nursing as "adapting prescribed therapy and preventive treatment to the specific physical and psychic needs of the individual," she also said that "the real depths of nursing can only be made known through ideals, love, sympathy, knowledge, and culture, expressed through the practice of artistic procedures and relationships" (quoted in Virginia A. Henderson, *The Nature of Nursing: Reflections After Twenty-five Years* [New York: National League for Nursing Press, 1991], 2). This definition of nursing is as appropriate today as it was 60 years ago.

Virginia Henderson's definition of nursing has stood the test of time and guides my own thinking about the nurse's role, especially in a care system which focuses as much upon achieving health as it does eradicating disease. "The unique function of the nurse is to assist the individual, sick or well, in the performance of those activities contributing to health or its recovery (or to peaceful death) that he would perform unaided if he had the necessary strength, will or knowledge. And to do this in such a way as to help him gain independence as rapidly as possible" (ibid., 21).

At first glance, her definition of a nurse as a substitute for what a patient lacks within himself seems rather simplistic. But upon more thoughtful reflection, one sees the complexity of this definition of nursing practice. In her book, *The Nature of Nursing: Reflections After Twenty-five Years* (ibid., 22), she writes, "Think how rare is 'completeness,' or 'wholeness,' of mind and body: to what extent good health is a matter of heredity, to what extent it is acquired, is controversial, but it is generally admitted that intelligence and education tend to parallel health status. If then each man finds 'good health' a difficult goal, how much more difficult is it for the nurse to help him reach it: she must, in a sense, get 'inside the skin' of each of her patients in order to know what he needs. She is temporarily the consciousness of the unconscious, the love of life for the suicidal, the leg of the amputee, the eyes of the newly blind, a means of locomotion for the infant, knowledge and confidence for the young mother, the 'mouthpiece' for those too weak or withdrawn to speak."

Leah Curtin, the editor of *Nursing Management*, through her editorials, has, for me, restored a reverent perspective on the magnificent artistry of nursing. Recently she wrote that mankind has always had a "need to help and to be helped" (in *Nursing Management* 19 [July 1988]: 9). A paradox of our society is to undervalue the worth of nurturing while highly respecting and revering selfless motherhood. Unanimously, we would agree with Leah Curtin that "gentleness is preferable to violence." She has so eloquently reminded us that "Nursing's traditions are humanitarian in the fully philanthropic meaning of that term 'love of mankind'....to anticipate charity by preventing suffering, by teaching our neighbors to care for themselves, by rendering them independent" (ibid.).

Virtually no other discipline, save for nursing, is allowed to touch others in their most private and vulnerable moments, to see them in their hopelessness and helplessness. It is this uniqueness of nursing which needs to be told, for it is an exquisite profession.

The Cleveland Clinic nurses exemplify the best of nursing practice. Working with them I have seen firsthand how they have given of themselves and how through their daily work these definitions of nursing have come alive for the patients for whom they care. It is for them this book was written.

But, no matter how good the idea, without someone to execute it, it has little value. And so tremendous appreciation must be given to the Nursing History Task Force led by Foundation staff nurse Sue Horn, R.N. This book, quite simply, would never have been written without their enthusiasm, dedication, and their unwavering belief in the importance of this work. We were so fortunate to find a talented and sensitive writer, Diane Grabowski, who spent countless hours with this task force going through numerous oral histories and thousands of archival records and conducting interviews with current and retired nurses and nursing personnel.

In this book, the work and accomplishments of nurses are placed within the context of the historical time in which they occurred. I came to realize the importance of this when I would hear nurses speak disparagingly about Florence Nightingale's "militaristic" approach to nursing education. Not understanding that Victorian England differentiated women from ladies, they failed to see what she required of "her" nurses was really society's requirements to be a lady — thus, respected, above reproach, and to be taken seriously. Her insistence that nurses carry charts for the physicians was not meant to place them in a subservient role, but rather to give them a reason to be at the physician's side so that they could insist he wash his hands between patients. That simple measure reduced mortality in the Crimean War by over 50 percent and contributed to the acceptance of the germ theory postulated by Pasteur.

As we rapidly approach the year 2000 the health care system as we know it today will cease to exist. Dissatisfaction with the performance of the current system, tremendous cost pressures arising from within both the government and private business sectors, the wizardry of space age technology and a belief in one's personal responsibility for health are causing the dismantling and rebuilding of our medical organizations. Hospitals, today's cornerstone of health care, will remain only for those whose care cannot be provided for otherwise. The tools of medicine and nursing are changing; lasers are replacing scalpels, magnetic resonance is replacing X-ray, medical records are becoming paperless, and various technologies are delivering care previously done only by nurses.

Observing these changes one marvels at the foresight of Florence Nightingale when she said, "Hospitals are only an intermediate stage of civilization" (quoted in Henderson, *The Nature of Nursing*, 13). And, Virginia Henderson's observation of 25 years ago that hospital regimens "often failed to change the patient's way of living that sent him to the hospital in the first place" (ibid., 14) runs parallel to the contemporary wisdom of today.

These times of uncertainty and unprecedented change are disturbing to nurses whose only frame of reference is nursing within a hospital. But mankind's soul and body will always need to be helped, to be refreshed, and to be cared for. Nurses and nursing are vital in a world that is struggling to over-come loneliness, poverty, domestic violence, stressful lifestyles, and many other social ills that weaken our resistance to disease. The setting for nursing care and the tools of nursing are changing, but the need for nurses continues.

This book is truly a celebration of the first 75 years of Cleveland Clinic nursing and those nurses, past and present, who created it. It is also a legacy to future nurses, for in knowing their heritage, they will be in touch with them-selves and will continue to touch the lives of others.

SHARON J. COULTER
Chairman, Division of Patient Care Operations

Preface

In 1989, at the request of Chairman Sharon J. Coulter, the Division of Nursing of The Cleveland Clinic Foundation set up a Nursing History Task Force. Its primary mission was to "research Nursing's strong contribution to the Foundation's formation and growth"; one of its goals was the publication of a book-length history of Cleveland Clinic nursing in 1996, the 75th anniversary of the institution's founding.

By the time I became involved with the project as author/editor in 1993, work on the proposed history was already well underway. The members of the Task Force had done preliminary research, started an oral history program, determined the scope of the book's content, and had begun discussing design specifications. At the same time, Ms. Coulter, and the Task Force members, were prepared to give the author wide latitude in writing the manuscript. The general requirements laid down were inclusive rather than exclusive: the book should include nurses who had worked with the Clinic's founding physicians before the Clinic itself opened; it should include nurses working in all divisions and departments of the institution, not just the Division of Nursing; and, it should include all nursing personnel, not only registered nurses.

I was fortunate in being presented with a subject that fell in with my own interests as a historical writer: the work of women in a traditional "women's profession." We look, quite properly, with pride at the advances women have made in professions like law and medicine; but at the same time we often unintentionally belittle women who are "only teachers" or "only nurses." Nurses and teachers, female and male, deserve a great deal of recognition and credit. There is nothing "only" about educating our children, or helping us to regain and keep our most precious possession — our health. While I do not think I have given an unreasonably rosy picture of nursing or Cleveland Clinic nursing personnel, I have certainly chosen to focus on their collective accomplishments.

My greatest problem was doing justice to everyone. There are, at present, more than 3,000 nursing employees at The Cleveland Clinic Foundation. Thousands more have worked there in the past 75 years. Each person has a story worth telling, a story that can add to the collective picture of nursing at the Cleveland Clinic. The Task Force members hope it may be possible, in the not-too-distant future, to publish an expanded version of this history. Anyone who has information, whether documents, photographs, or memories, in their heads or on paper, that could be used to revise or add to this volume is urged to get in touch with the Task Force via The Cleveland Clinic Foundation Archives (P22, The Cleveland Clinic Foundation, 9500 Euclid Avenue, Cleveland, Ohio 44195; telephone 216-444-2929).

I do wish to direct attention to the endpapers of the book, which contain the signatures of 468 Cleveland Clinic nursing personnel. Again, the Task Force members are to be credited with the idea, which gave each person who was on roll at the time when the signatures were gathered (late 1994 to early 1995) the chance to say, "I was here, caring for the patients of The Cleveland Clinic Foundation."

A few notes on usage and methodology need to be added. Because this is a nursing history, the word "care" is generally used to mean *nursing* care. To avoid the awkwardness of "she/he" and "her/him," the feminine pronouns are used when referring to nurses in the collective. Since "Miss" and "Mrs." were the standard titles of address during most of the period covered by the study, they are used throughout the first four chapters; in the last chapter, "Ms." is used.

Ohio had no provision for the registration of nurses until 1916, and did not make registration mandatory until much later. It was not possible to determine exactly which of the nurses active in the earlier periods were registered, and which were not. Only nurses who are designated in documentary sources as "R.N." are referred to as such in the text. However, the absence of this abbreviation beside a name does *not* mean that the individual in question was not a registered nurse; in fact, it is likely that most, if not all, of the nurses referred to by name in this text were actually registered. Likewise, academic degrees are specified upon the first mention of an individual's name when possible, but there are undoubtedly instances in the text where a nurse has a degree or degrees which are not indicated. With the exception of some advanced practice areas, abbreviations designating specialty certification are not used. No degree or other abbreviations are used after names in photo captions and sidebars.

The use of the word "Clinic" varies according to context, and can mean either the entire institution or its ambulatory practice area only. The inpatient area is referred to as the Clinic Hospital, or simply "the Hospital." Where clarification seemed necessary, I have prefaced the word Clinic with "ambulatory" or "outpatient"; or, on the other hand, used the fuller version "Cleveland Clinic" to indicate the institution as a whole.

I have attempted, in a limited way, to put the history of nursing at The Cleveland Clinic Foundation into the broader contexts of Cleveland, nursing, and social history. However, I see this book primarily as a case study, a single piece of mosaic that I hope scholars in the field of nursing history and related areas will be able to incorporate into their own grander designs.

Most of the unpublished documentary sources consulted during the research process are in the holdings of The Cleveland Clinic Foundation Archives; others are at the Western Reserve Historical Society, the Stanley A. Ferguson Archives of University Hospitals of Cleveland, the Historical Division of the Allen Memorial Medical Library, and the *Cleveland Press* Collection, housed in the Cleveland State University Archives. Most of the hard facts contained in the narrative came from these sources. Interviews and observation were used to flesh out this basic information.

Where possible, nurses' own words, or the words of co-workers and patients, have been used to tell their story. All direct quotes, as well as background information provided by specific secondary sources, are given complete citations in the endnotes. The only exceptions are the blanket citations "personal communication/oral history" and "response to 'oral' history questionnaire" used to identify material from oral histories, interviews, and conversations (see p. xvii). This was done because some people were modest about furnishing information that could be attributed to them as individuals. Although this is a departure from standard historical scholarship, I hope it can be excused in this instance.

I cannot praise the members of the Task Force itself too highly. As noted above, they began work on this history long before I did. Collectively, they planned, organized, brainstormed, evaluated, promoted, explained, and did just about everything that needed to be done to bring the project from idea to reality. They selected all photographs and determined their placement within the book. They supported, encouraged, and assisted me at all times. Susan Horn, staff nurse on nursing unit G81, Chairman of the Task Force, coordinated the entire process, arranging for everything from meeting agendas to the signatures on the endpapers, and devoted enormous amounts of her time and energy to moving the project forward. Corinne Hofstetter, retired Supervisor of Clinic Nursing and currently a supervisor with Patient Pride[SM], implemented the oral history portion of the project, served as our link with the large corps of retired nursing personnel, and shared her extensive knowledge with unfailing kindness and generosity. Frederick Lautzenheiser, the Clinic's Associate Archivist, guided me through the documentary sources held by the Archives, arranged for photographic reproduction, and also took responsibility for the important task of indexing the volume. Sandra Shumway, Assistant to the Chairman, Division of Patient Care Operations, provided administrative liaison, and handled innumerable details with grace and tact. JoAnne Porras, Graphic Designer, single-handedly transformed a typescript into camera-ready art. She designed the book, from dust jacket to cover to text, in its entirety. Together, she and Carol Ann Stroia of Lorain Printing furnished all necessary information about the intricacies of book design and the printing process to the Task Force, which had responsibility for making all choices regarding the production and final appearance of the book.

On behalf of the Task Force members, as well as myself, I would like to thank, first and foremost, Sharon Coulter, who provided the original impetus for the project. Without her aid, and continuing support, the idea would never have become a reality.

Carol Tomer, Cleveland Clinic Archivist, generously provided support and space for the Task Force's work. Much of the information in the book is based on records assembled and organized under her leadership. Both she and Fred gave advice and answered questions on all matters relating to Clinic history. Without their work, documentary evidence on the Clinic's past would be neither available nor accessible. Nancy C. Erdey, Archivist, Stanley A. Ferguson Archives of University Hospitals of Cleveland, gave much valuable help and was particularly generous in assisting with the reproduction of photographs from the UHC collections. Several other area archival repositories also provided important resources, and thanks are due the following individuals and institutions: Glen Jenkins, Ingrid Ebner, and Jennifer Kane, Historical Division of Allen Memorial Medical Library; William Becker, Cleveland State University Archives; and, the entire reference room staff of the Western Reserve Historical Society.

We are also most grateful to the following individuals for sharing their expertise and advice: internal reviewer Dr. Shattuck Hartwell, Jr.; external reviewers Dr. Barbara Brodie, University of Virginia, and Dr. Eleanor Crowder, Pennsylvania State University; and our excellent copy editor, Lynn Novelli.

Photographs in this volume were provided courtesy of the repositories mentioned above, and also through the generosity of the following individuals and organizations: Karen Bourquin; Chandler Everett and Shirley Wittine of the Central School of Practical Nursing; Sharon Coulter; Helga Sandburg Crile; Adelle Dulas; Bill Graber and the family of Elizabeth Graber; Paul Hamilton; Elizabeth Hartman; Corinne Hofstetter; Susan Horn; Alexa McCubbin; Susan Richards; Sandra Shumway; Linda Solar; Karen Westmeyer; and Dolores Wiemels. Thanks also to Tom Merce and Tony Buck of the Clinic's Division of Marketing and Managed Care, and Don Gerda and others of the Clinic's Department of Photography, whose photographs appear in the volume.

The following individuals supported and assisted the production of the book in ways too numerous to mention: Ginger Ranallo and the staff of Graphic Services, especially Jayma DiSiena and Mark Allie; Division of Patient Care Operations administrative secretaries, especially Marcia Pecjak, Brenda Liggins-Morgan, and Jennifer Outler; executive secretary Dorothy Dwosh; Elaine Clayton; Ann Dugan; Nancy Fierle; Lucinda Mitchin; Steve Szilagyi; Mary Slattery; and Cecily Lawless of Laurel School.

Special thanks are due to Linda Solar, who did a fantastic job of organizing two group interviews with operating room nurses, and hosted my day-long visit to the operating room itself. She, and her colleagues on the ENT and other operating room services, kindly shared information and gave insight, both serious and humorous, into their work. Mary Johnson, Director of Ambulatory Nursing, provided information about her department's recent past, present status, and future outlook; arranged for access to recent documentary material with the assistance of secretary Laverne Cowgill; and developed an itinerary for my visit to various Clinic departments. For that visit, I was fortunate enough to have the perfect guide, float nurse Madeline Soupios, whose personal perspective on Cleveland Clinic nursing made the time doubly worthwhile. For my in-depth tour and visit to Hospital nursing unit G81 I wish to thank, again, Sue Horn, as well as her co-workers, and especially Nurse Manager Debbie Mastri, for her help in this instance and also for her general support of the project.

So many people were kind enough to give of their time and their memories, or their perspective on the present. They served as sources for the writing of this book, and they deserve a listing of their own. These individuals provided information in a number of ways. Some participated in group discussions; some gave interviews on a one-to-one basis; some filled out an oral history questionnaire developed by the Task Force; some spoke to me at length during the days I spent observing the work of Cleveland Clinic Foundation nursing personnel. On behalf of myself, and the Nursing History Book Task Force, I would like to thank all of them, and also the numerous other people I encountered in the course of my visits to the Cleveland Clinic campus, who helped me to learn more about nursing there.

Betty Ambrose	Paula Habzda	Susan Richards
Diane Anderson	Elizabeth Hartman	Florence Rindchen
Kathleen Baccus	Corinne Hofstetter	Cynthia Schisano
Michelle Balsamo	Susan Horn	Donald Sinclair
Judith S. Becker	Joyce Janisek	Linda Solar
Stephanie Blatnik	Dori Janka	Patricia Sommer
Lois Bock	Florence Johns	Madeline Soupios
Hella Bolz	Mary Johnson	Irene Spada
Bonnie Borac	Helen Judge	Kay Stelmach
Dee Brescia	Faye Kleinbaum	Margaret Tampson
Sue Buzby	Linda Kraus	Vae Lucile Van Derwyst
Olive Cannon	Mary Lippert	Maureen Walsh
Linda Carlone	Alexa McCubbin	Irene Werley
Trana Daniels	Kathleen McWeeny	Harriet Witherspoon
Dorothy Devorak	Joanne Madeline	Mary Alice Yurick
Margaret Fisher	Dianna Malek	Esther Zeitz
Shirley Gullo	Debbie Mastri	Maria Zickuhr
Betty Gurney	Ursula Menart	
	Edith Metz	
	Lorraine Mion	
	Annette Pirozek	

Introduction

The year 1996 marks The Cleveland Clinic Foundation's 75th anniversary. Major anniversaries are a time to look back, and remember. To celebrate someone's birthday, or wedding or employment anniversary, friends, family, and co-workers gather together, and perhaps assemble a scrapbook or a video. Businesses, associations, or organizations often take advantage of the occasion to compile a corporate history. In the case of the Cleveland Clinic, histories have already been written. The first one, titled simply *The Cleveland Clinic Foundation*, was published privately in 1938, only 17 years after the Clinic was founded. The standard history, *To Act As A Unit*, was published in 1971 to commemorate the institution's 50th anniversary. It focused on the development of the administrative structure of the Cleveland Clinic, and on the accomplishments of its medical staff. It was updated in 1985, and is being updated again for the 75th anniversary.

Without Whose Aid: Nursing and the Cleveland Clinic joins these books, not as a sequel or a supplement, but as a look at the same history from a different perspective. History is, at its heart, a story. Its richness lies in the fact that it is not a single story, but many stories, of many people. Historians, like storytellers, must choose a point of view, or focus. The focus for *Without Whose Aid* was chosen by nurses, who saw that the Clinic had many stories yet to be told. These stories documented their own profession's past contribution to the organization's primary mission, "better care of the sick."

There is, of course, some overlap between *To Act As A Unit* and *Without Whose Aid*. It is impossible to begin the story of the Clinic without reference to the four physicians always referred to as "the founders," who agreed to associate in this not-for-profit medical practice. The title itself comes from a passage in a talk given by one of the Clinic's founding physicians in the 1920s, in which on behalf of himself and his patients he expressed a sense of obligation to nurses, "without whose aid I am sure such success as I have had would not be possible." If he could return to speak to the Clinic's nursing personnel today,

1

the wording might be a little different, but the meaning would be the same: "We couldn't have done it without you."

The Cleveland Clinic opened its doors in 1921, and it might be expected that its nursing history would begin at that point. However, just as a biography may begin with its subject's ancestry, the history of an institution may begin by tracing its origins in what went before. The history of the Clinic is really the history of its mission, rather than its bricks and mortar. According to the authors of *To Act As A Unit*, it was during the First World War that "an idea was born that led to the founding of The Cleveland Clinic."

Three of the founders served with the Lakeside Unit. This military hospital unit, with many of its members from Cleveland's Lakeside Hospital, was stationed in Rouen, France, as Base Hospital No. 4 of the American Expeditionary Force. Physicians, nurses, and enlisted men worked together in an organization that combined specialized medical practice with a spirit of teamwork. The Lakeside Unit, and its dedicated personnel, served as both model and inspiration for the future Cleveland Clinic. On this basis, the first chapter of *Without Whose Aid* opens in 1917, with the arrival of the Lakeside Unit nurses in France, and goes on to examine their role in the organization that gave birth to the Cleveland Clinic. It seems particularly appropriate to begin the story of the Clinic's nurses here, since, like the Clinic, the modern profession of nursing was born of war.

The second chapter starts with a retrospective look at earlier settings in which the Clinic founders worked with nurses: Lakeside Hospital, where the founders served on the visiting staff and admitted patients; and "the Office," as the founders called the private practice in which three of them were associated. Lakeside Hospital had special significance because many, perhaps most, of the nurses on the staff of the Clinic in its early years had worked there or attended its Training School for Nurses. A nursing "school" at this time was not only an educational facility. It was a whole attitude, or culture, which students absorbed and carried on with them into their subsequent careers, just as they continued to wear their own schools' pins and caps. The close association of nursing leader Isabel Hampton Robb with the Lakeside school meant that Cleveland Clinic nurses were strongly influenced by her ideals of professional nursing.

The remainder of Chapter Two resumes the chronological story with the opening of the brand-new Cleveland Clinic in 1921; Chapters Three through Five continue the narrative up into the 1990s. If the Clinic was a child of the First World War, it came of age during the Second, and settled into its maturity during the 1950s. Here, at the point where rapid institutional growth began, the likeness to an individual life cycle fades, perhaps because the historical perspective is still too close. As of this period the story also leaves behind, for the most part, focus on individual personalities, and looks primarily at the collective activities of Cleveland Clinic nursing personnel.

The word "collective" needs some qualification. Nursing at The Cleveland Clinic Foundation has never had a unitary structure. Historically, the institution's nursing personnel have cared for patients in three main areas: the Clinic, or outpatient area, which housed the offices of the institution's staff physicians; the Cleveland Clinic Hospital nursing floors, or units, where these physicians admitted their patients; and the operating rooms where they performed surgery. Ambulatory Nursing, often referred to as "Clinic Nursing," was made up of the nurses and support staff who worked in the Clinic medical offices. It was separate from the institution's Department of Nursing, which was made up of the nursing personnel who cared for inpatients in the Hospital. Operating Room Nursing was at different time periods a part of the Department of Nursing, or an independent Hospital department. In either case, it also tended to maintain a separate identity.

The main plot of this story concerns the Hospital Department of Nursing, which became the Division of Nursing in 1987. (At The Cleveland Clinic Foundation, a division is higher on the organization chart than a department — that is, divisions are larger, and are made up of departments.) Although there is no such thing as a "typical" Cleveland Clinic nurse, more nurses have always worked on the Hospital inpatient units than in any other area, and their activities have been better documented over time. Ambulatory Nursing and Operating Room Nursing play supporting roles in the narrative, but are equally important in the actual work of the Cleveland Clinic. Together, the three areas form a complete cycle of care, and without the work of nursing personnel in each area, the cycle would be broken.

Advanced practice nurses have also had a place at the institution from the time of its founding. For example, nurse anesthetists gave all anesthetics during the first phase of the Cleveland Clinic's history, and remained an integral part of the Department of Anesthesiology even after the Second World War, when many hospitals went over to all-physician anesthesiology departments. Nurse anesthetists associated with the Clinic's founders helped to develop nurse anesthesia as a profession in the United States.

Another group of nurses, who were not Cleveland Clinic employees, also played an important role in caring for inpatients there from the 1920s to the 1950s. Private duty nurses, working as independent contractors, were hired to care for individual patients on a case-by-case basis. These nurses were paid directly by the patients, but the Hospital nursing office usually made the arrangements to call them in. The substantial number of calls for private duty nurses from the Cleveland Clinic Hospital made it possible for a large number of Cleveland nurses to make a living in this field. Their numerical strength influenced the policies of the Greater Cleveland Nurses' Association, the local affiliate of the Ohio State Nurses' Association and the American Nurses' Association.

"Nursing" in the context of this study includes the work of all members of the various nursing departments — R.N.s, L.P.N.s, nursing assistants, operating room technicians, patient care technicians, unit secretaries, and others — under the various names by which they have been known over the years. Again, because one group, the registered nurses, was over time the largest and its activities the best documented, it provides the focus for the narrative. But in this case, too, all nursing personnel worked together to complete the cycle of care — from preparing a patient for examination to preparing the operating room for surgery, from giving baths to giving medications to giving home-going instructions — and are included in the story.

Over the years, most differences between nursing at the Cleveland Clinic and at other institutions seem to have been more in degree than in kind. It goes almost without saying that, working in an advanced, internationally known referral center, Cleveland Clinic nurses are responsible for the care of a large number of critically ill patients with a wide variety of unusual conditions, and are necessarily true experts in nursing practice. They have often gained familiarity with new or complex technical procedures earlier than employees of the average hospital or physician's office, and so have been able to serve as a resource to other nurses.

The importance and relative independence of the Operating Room and Ambulatory Nursing Departments were also a distinctive feature. The large proportion of surgical cases in the patient population meant that the Cleveland Clinic had a particularly large and skilled staff of operating room nurses who were, by the 1950s, assigned full-time to the various specialized surgical services. Since the Clinic Hospital was originally an adjunct to the outpatient Clinic, rather than vice versa, ambulatory nurses had, from the very beginning, a central role in giving nursing care to the institution's patients.

Finally, the fact that the Cleveland Clinic never had its own nursing school differentiated it from many academic medical centers and from other large Cleveland hospitals. The presence of an all-graduate nurse staff in the 1920s established a high standard of patient care and nursing practice as a precedent for later generations of Cleveland Clinic nurses. The absence of resident nursing students meant that the Clinic Hospital had to find alternative ways of filling its staffing needs.

Despite these special characteristics, the overall outline of events is a familiar one to students of nursing history. It represents the common experience of nurses, and this gives the story a wider significance. The history of Cleveland Clinic nursing is more a mirror for the profession, reflecting the general course of American nursing in the twentieth century, than an exception or an oddity. It is a story in which nursing personnel everywhere will be able to see themselves, and one in which they all can take pride.

1

Fortunes of War

Au bruit de la guerre
J'ai reçu le jour!

Amid the chaos of battle
I first saw the light of day!
— Marie, the "daughter of the regiment,"
in *La Fille du Régiment*, by Gaetano Donizetti

It was in a military hospital, amid the tumult of battle,
in the great Crimean War, that the modern system of nursing
found its birthplace. Here came into existence a force born to
do battle forevermore in the never-ceasing struggle for life.
— Isabel Hampton Robb, at the dedication
exercises for Lakeside Hospital, 1898

The First Over There

Rouen, France. May 25, 1917. World War I, the "war to end all wars," was in
its third year. As this clear, warm, late spring day drew to a close, the hospital
ship *Western Australia* — actually a converted yacht — docked at the city's stone
quay. The *Western Australia* was a familiar sight in Rouen. It picked up convoys
of wounded soldiers for transport to England. But this evening, it was the
passengers about to disembark who attracted a crowd. Shouts of "Vive les
Américains!" mingled with the music of a drum and bugle corps playing on
board ship. People poured out onto the quayside from the nearby hotels,
cafes and streets, "wild to see the first American soldiers."[1]

For this was the first contingent of the U.S. Army to arrive in France, the
vanguard of two million more Americans who would arrive in Europe over the
next year and a half, to serve in the First World War. Though a military unit,
these first Americans did not come to do battle; they came to heal. On board
the *Western Australia* were the 27 medical officers, 155 enlisted men, 4 civilian
personnel, and 64 nurses of Base Hospital No. 4 —informally known as the
Lakeside Unit — of the U.S. Army Reserve Medical Corps. Many of them were
Clevelanders; most of the medical officers and nurses worked at, or had
trained at, Cleveland's Lakeside Hospital; a number of the enlisted men were
students at Cleveland-area colleges.

On the shore to greet them all was Major George W. Crile, who had arrived
in Rouen ahead of the rest of the unit. A well-known Cleveland surgeon and
chief of surgery at Lakeside Hospital, he would in a few years, with three
colleagues, found the Cleveland Clinic. In many ways, the Lakeside Unit —
also a brainchild of Crile's — served as the prototype for the Clinic. The phrase
"to act as a unit," which Dr. Crile used in a 1918 diary entry to characterize his
long-time relationship with Lakeside Unit surgeons (and future Clinic
co-founders) Frank E. Bunts and William Edgar Lower, would later be used to
describe the Cleveland Clinic's ideal: everyone working together to advance
patient care. The Lakeside Unit nurses were, in a sense, the vanguard of
Cleveland Clinic nursing: like the Clinic's future nursing staff, all were

5

graduate nurses, many had trained at Lakeside Hospital, and all were motivated by the stresses of battlefront nursing to "act as a unit."

The medical officers and enlisted men who disembarked from the ship wore the khaki uniforms of the U.S. Army. The nurses did not; over ankle-length dresses they wore three-quarter length, dark blue capes lined with scarlet and marked on the left side with a plain red cross; their wide-brimmed hats were made of black velours. As Reserve Nurses of the American Army Nurse Corps, the Lakeside Unit nurses received their "commissions" through the American Red Cross (A.R.C.). The Red Cross loaned them capes, hats, and also blankets, along with $50 each to complete their outfits of duty uniforms and bedding.

The Commandant of the Port and the British and American consuls were standing by with Major Crile to greet the Unit, but little time was spent in dockside ceremony. Immediately after setting foot on French soil, the Unit proceeded to what would be its base for the better part of the next two years, General Hospital No. 9 of the British Expeditionary Force, a few miles outside the city.

> When we disembarked we drew up in regular formation; first the officers then the drum corps, the nurses and the enlisted men. We marched thru the streets to beyond the first barrier where the officers and nurses took hospital vans and the men marched the rest of the way.[2]

Not only residents of Rouen, but also soldiers of the Allied forces lined the cobblestone streets that May evening.

> Uniformed men from the corners of the British world shouted to us in a tongue that we knew, and the blue-clad French cheered us in words we could not always understand.[3]

Rouen was a river port and a cathedral city. During the First World War it hosted one of the largest British bases in France. And it was the city where, in 1431, the young peasant woman Jeanne d'Arc, or Joan of Arc, the military folk heroine of France, had been burned alive as a heretic. A stone slab and an iron grille in the old marketplace marked the spot.

But on that first march through the city, the Lakeside nurses were probably thinking not of historic markers, but of home. Instead of the noisy crowds of welcoming strangers, they were perhaps seeing with the mind's eye the familiar faces of those who had gathered to say good-bye, quietly, at Cleveland's Union Station on May 6, only a few weeks back.

> There were a few flowers, a few tears, the cheers and "Godspeeds" of relatives and close friends, but no bands, no flapping of banners, no official review to mark the departure of the first contingent recruited for active service in Europe under the Stars and Stripes .... the unit had assembled and slipped away in the drizzling rain almost before the city realized that Cleveland was sending its initial draft to swell the ranks of the allies in the fighting zone.[4]

Constance Hanna, a Unit nurse, in later years recalled it thus:

> The train was held at the station for two hours....I was one of the youngest members of the unit. I remember hearing one of the older nurses sob. I turned to my sister and said, 'I guess I'd better not cry.'[5]

THE LAKESIDE UNIT

The Unit's official name was Base Hospital No. 4 of the American Expeditionary Force. Organized by Dr. George Crile, it was the first American military unit to arrive in Europe during the First World War.

Many of the Unit's nurses and physicians came from the staff of Lakeside Hospital, where Dr. Crile was chief of surgery. A few years after the end of the war, Dr. Crile left Lakeside Hospital to found the Cleveland Clinic. (Lakeside Hospital joined with other medical institutions to form University Hospitals of Cleveland.)

The dedication and team spirit displayed by Lakeside Unit personnel in caring for the casualties of war greatly impressed Dr. Crile and his colleagues, Dr. William Edgar Lower and Dr. Frank Bunts. In founding the Cleveland Clinic, they hoped to bring the same spirit to civilian health care.

The Unit's Nurses

Swathed in their blue capes, faces shaded by the black velours hats, the 64 nurses of the unit looked very much alike. During the long sea voyage, even their steps had been drilled to uniformity; enlisted men, medical officers, nurses, and the 4 civilian members of the Unit had had frequent drill practice on the deck of the *Orduna*, the ship that carried them across the Atlantic. And of course the nurses in some ways were alike — they had their profession and their gender in common. Most of them were relatively young, and all but a few had never been married.

This was typical for nurses, as well as for women in occupations like teaching and clerical work, during the early part of the twentieth century. Most nurses were white, native-(or Canadian-)born women. According to popular belief, the ideal background for a nurse was a rural upbringing, in which a young girl would grow up accustomed to discipline and hard work.[6] The Lakeside Unit nurses, by and large, fit into this pattern. All were white, and they were mainly of British, German, or Irish descent, even though Cleveland's first and second generation immigrant population, including substantial numbers of eastern and southern Europeans, was at this time reaching peak levels. Many Unit nurses had rural or small-town roots. But despite the similarities, each woman had her own story.

Grace E. Allison was the Unit's Chief Nurse. In civilian life, as superintendent of the Lakeside Hospital Training School for Nurses, she held the highest nursing position at Lakeside Hospital. Assistant Chief Nurse Harriet Leete might have seemed an odd candidate for military nursing, since her expertise was in working with mothers and children. However, as superintendent of nurses at Cleveland's Babies Dispensary and at the city health department's Bureau of Child Hygiene, she was accustomed to working independently, making decisions, and giving advice. Elizabeth Folckemer, Edith Morgan, and Austa Engel likewise had public health experience, but went overseas as rank and file nurses, not in positions of command.

Austa White Engel, Marie Shields, Elsie Brower, and Minnie Bowman were the only Unit nurses listed as "Mrs." in 1917. Constance Hanna, the "baby" of the Unit, was in her early twenties. Lillian Grundies, several years older, had not worked or trained at Lakeside Hospital, but was connected to the Unit directly through Dr. Crile and his partner (and second cousin) Dr. Lower, having worked in their private practice as the nurse in charge of surgery. Like several other Unit members, Miss Grundies was a child of German immigrant parents. Canadian-born Arvilla Walkinshaw had been Mrs. Crile's private duty nurse when the couple's last baby was born. Mary Jane Roche and Josephine Cunningham, who had trained as nurse anesthetists at Lakeside Hospital under Agatha Hodgins, possessed skills that were crucial to the performance of the "shockless surgery" Dr. Crile advocated.

Clara Illig of Ilion, New York, now lived and worked in Cleveland; so did Caroline Smith of Northfield, Minnesota, and Mollie McKenney of Yale, Michigan. Minnie Victoria Strobel from Massillon, Edith Morgan from Youngstown, Inez McKee of Sandusky, Margaret Lane of Toledo, Betty Connelly of Cambridge, Ina Starr of Litchfield, Mabel Allyn of Chardon, Helen Briggs of North Olmsted, Nettie Eisenhard of Greenspring, and Mabel Horn of Bellevue, all born or bred in Ohio's towns and cities, answered the call of national service and joined the Unit.

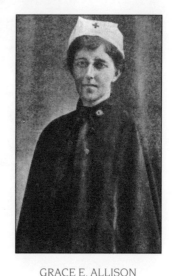

GRACE E. ALLISON
Miss Allison served as Chief Nurse of the Lakeside Unit from 1917 through the summer of 1918. A native of Michigan, she had graduated from the Lakeside Hospital Training School for Nurses in 1908, and subsequently received a B.S. degree from the nursing program at Teachers College of Columbia University. She held the position of Superintendent of Lakeside's school for 10 years (including her military service), until 1923. She then spent 14 years as Superintendent of Samaritan Hospital in Troy, New York, retiring at the end of 1938. Active in a number of professional organizations, her interests outside nursing included training and showing thoroughbred horses.

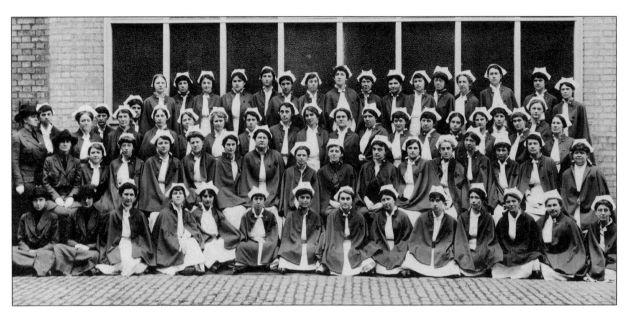

Miss Horn was from a medical family; her sister was a physician in Bellevue. Miss Allyn's father and brother both practiced as homeopathic doctors. Two pairs of sisters served with the Lakeside Unit: Helen and Mary Lois Van Meter of Chillicothe, and Augusta and Martha Militz of Cincinnati.

The Reason Why

By the time of the First World War, nursing was established as a women's profession. Since warfare was similarly reserved for men, and since nursing aimed to preserve life and health while warfare caused death and destruction, the two were strangely, but intimately, linked.

Many historians have pointed out the importance of war in the development of nursing. Modern nursing had its birth in the barracks at Üsküdar (Scutari), where Florence Nightingale and her band of nurses tended the miserable, neglected soldiers of the Crimean War. Just as she was credited with founding modern nursing, so the Civil War — along with the American publication of Miss Nightingale's *Notes on Nursing* in 1860 — was credited with giving the initial impetus to nursing as a profession in the United States.[7]

Moreover, nurses and soldiers had experiences in common. The uniforms, the regulations, the training, the regimentation — all were characteristically worn, or obeyed, or undergone, by both nurses and soldiers. But most importantly, the nurse was a powerful ally on the battlefield. American nurses had demonstrated this during the Spanish-American War, less than a generation earlier. Margaret Lane, Austa Engel, Lillian Grundies, Elizabeth Folckemer, and all their companions were carrying on this tradition of military nursing, as they arrived in Rouen to take their part in caring for the casualties of the great conflict of their own day.

The United States had entered World War I late. The European nations and their empires had been at war since August 1914. By the time President Woodrow Wilson signed the American declaration of war on April 6, 1917, many Americans had already taken sides. They had seen the stories in the newspapers: Germany had run over "little Belgium"; had sunk passenger liners like the *Lusitania*; had executed British nurse Edith Cavell as a spy. While all these things were true, the roots of the conflict were much more complicated. An intricate web of alliances and treaties had so entangled the powers of Europe, that a few shots from an assassin's gun could start a full-scale war lasting more than four years. But with France, Britain, and the other Allies struggling to hold their own, many Americans believed it was time for the United States to enter the war against Germany and the Central powers.

On April 28, 22 days after the American declaration of war, Dr. Crile had received a telegram from U.S. Surgeon General William C. Gorgas, calling the Lakeside Unit to active service. Within two weeks, on May 8, 1917, the Lakeside Unit had left New York harbor on board the *Orduna*. It was the day after the second anniversary of the sinking of the *Lusitania*. The Unit's members must have remembered the *Lusitania*, and wondered if the *Orduna* would cross safely or meet a similar end. The danger was a real one, and preparations were made accordingly, as one medical officer later recounted:

> Each day there was lifeboat drill. The ship's siren would blow a long blast as a warning. Everybody on the ship had to go to his berth, put on a life belt and then go as quickly as possible to his place at a lifeboat. When the siren blew you never knew whether it was the real thing or just another drill. The last day or two of the journey our Commanding Officer through his Quartermaster, issued to every officer a large Colt pistol. I am sure that the doctors did not know what this was all about. [Dr. Arthur Eisenbrey] and I agreed that the only use that it would be was to sink us all the faster if the submarines should dump us into the water.[8]

In the end, the *Orduna* reached Liverpool, England, on May 18, with no firing of pistols and no incident beyond a false alarm when the American ship sent to escort them in could not be immediately recognized as a friendly vessel. The British greeted the Lakeside Unit with great enthusiasm as the first contingent of the American forces coming to assist the faltering Allied cause; King George V and Queen Mary formally received the medical officers and nurses at Buckingham Palace, after the nurses had been introduced individually to the Queen at a private audience.

The hospital reserve units had been the first American units called up because they were needed to help staff British military hospitals, overwhelmed by the heavy casualties of trench warfare. Eventually, more than two million Americans would serve in the American Expeditionary Force overseas. But when the Lakeside Unit disembarked at Rouen on May 25, and began work at the British military General Hospital No. 9 a few days later, they were indeed the first American unit "over there."

A ROYAL WELCOME
The arrival of the Lakeside Unit in England marked the beginning of American participation in the Allied cause. Before the Unit continued on to France, King George V and Queen Mary received the medical officers and nurses at Buckingham Palace. Nurses also attended a private audience at Marlborough House, where each one had the opportunity to shake hands with the Queen. "The procedure was to curtsey as we advanced, again as we took her hand and again as we withdrew."

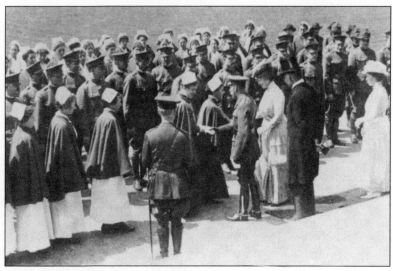

The Unit from Lakeside

It was no accident that a unit from Cleveland gained this honor. U.S. Secretary of War Newton D. Baker was a prominent Cleveland lawyer and politician. The head of the American Red Cross, Mabel Boardman, was the daughter of a Cleveland businessman; some members of her family still lived in the area. But the most important Cleveland connection was Myron T. Herrick, a wealthy Cleveland businessman and the American Ambassador to France in 1914 when the war began. Through him, Dr. Crile had gone with a team of surgeons and

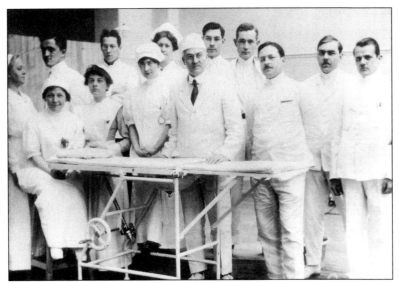

nurses to serve at the civilian American Ambulance Hospital in Paris for three months in 1915, where they amazed the French and British with the efficacy of their nitrous oxide anesthesia and blood transfusions. Dr. Crile's experience there prompted him to propose the base hospital form of organization to the U.S. Surgeon General; and, eventually, the experience of Drs. Crile, Lower, and Bunts with the Lakeside Unit base hospital would lead to the establishment of The Cleveland Clinic Foundation.

Officially, all of the nurses, medical officers, enlisted men, and civilians of the Lakeside Unit were volunteers. They had volunteered to serve together in one of the university-based reserve hospital units assembled by the U. S. Army, in concert with the American Red Cross, on the basis of Dr. Crile's organization plan. "The personnel of 'the university-based unit would be' composed of individuals who have had similar training and who know each other well, and the nursing staff would also be composed of nurses familiar with the methods of these surgeons." The emphasis on surgical method was not surprising, coming from Dr. Crile, a man who had the reputation of "tying the best and quickest knot of any one in the profession."[9]

The idea of carrying over familiarity or team spirit from civilian to military life was not a new one; in fact, many British soldiers had been permitted or encouraged to join up in just this way, in "pals battalions," as hometown comrades, as members of a sports team, as employees of a business. But it was a new way for the U.S. Army to organize its hospitals, particularly in its inclusion of nurses, as well as medical men, as part of a cohesive team to deal with the casualties of war.

Lakeside Hospital, the primary teaching hospital of the Western Reserve University School of Medicine, was the focus of the Cleveland unit. Dr. Crile, as chief of surgery at the hospital and the medical school, as well as the moving spirit behind the whole base hospital enterprise, was the Unit's highest ranking clinical medical officer and surgeon. His partner Dr. Lower, in charge of genitourinary surgery at Lakeside, was the surgeon next in the chain of command. Several of the junior medical officers were in training at Lakeside as residents or fellows; most of the other medical men of the unit also practiced in

PARIS, 1915

Before the official entry of the United States into World War I, the American Ambulance Hospital had been set up in a Paris suburb to help care for casualties, mainly French. It was a fashionable cause, supported by the rich and famous of several countries, some of whom volunteered to serve as auxiliary nurses, orderlies, and ambulance drivers. Surgeons and nurses also volunteered. Dr. Crile (center) and his 12-member team spent three months at the hospital. Members included Amy Rowland (far left) as research assistant, nurse anesthetists Agatha Hodgins and Mabel Littleton (2d and 4th from left), and operating room nurses Iva Davidson (back row) and Ruth Roberts (3d from left).

Cleveland, and a number of them had Lakeside or Western Reserve University affiliations. Forty-three of the 64 nurses were Lakeside graduates. Most of the other nurses resided in Cleveland or the surrounding area.

The unit's commanding officer, Major Harry L. Gilchrist, a graduate of the Western Reserve University School of Medicine and a career army physician, was assigned to handle the Unit's administrative affairs. He was assisted by adjutant Captain Arnold D. Tuttle, likewise an army doctor. Major Gilchrist had recruited the Unit's enlisted men from area colleges — Western Reserve University, Baldwin University, and Wallace College in greater Cleveland, and Allegheny College in Meadville, Pennsylvania — and from area businesses as well. Their ages ranged from 17 to 35, but most were between 19 and 24. These young men served as orderlies and also did much of the general work around the hospital and camp.

War fever, patriotism, and a desire to fight perceived oppression motivated the Unit's enlisted men, who joined a hospital unit only because it offered the first opportunity to go "over there." A number of them eventually transferred to other units, often with officers' commissions; but as long as they stayed at Rouen, their work (if not their tractability) earned high praise from the nurses and medical officers.

The desire to serve their country and humanity inspired the nurses and physicians as well. They had to be powerfully motivated to sacrifice comfort and certainty, leave their families, and risk their lives. Moreover, as healers, they were committed to the care of the suffering. Yet, their situation was not quite so simple. Since several of the medical officers had been junior staff physicians or residents at Lakeside, Dr. Crile, Dr. Charles F. Hoover, the Unit's chief of medicine, or other senior Unit physicians had been their chiefs of service. Dr. Crile had declared Chief Nurse Grace Allison indispensable to his base hospital concept: "The Lakeside Unit with a nursing directress other than the present head of the Training School, would nullify at the start the efficiency desired."[10] In civilian life, several of the Unit's nurses held head nurse or other positions at Lakeside Hospital. Nurse anesthetists Mary Roche and Josephine Cunningham were crucially important to the Unit's surgical work, as were Lakeside operating room nurses Inez McKee and Helen Briggs. Whether Dr. Crile and Miss Allison only made a general plea for volunteers, or whether they also may have made specific requests to nurses they felt especially suited for the Unit's work is not known. Perhaps Miss Allison's joining up was an incentive to nurses who worked under her or who had trained under her; perhaps Dr. Crile asked nurses he knew well, like Lillian Grundies and Arvilla Walkinshaw, to come with him; perhaps his undoubted charisma was request enough. Or maybe the patriotic cause did speak for itself. For whatever reason, and fortunately for the base hospital concept, a core of nurses and physicians familiar with the Lakeside methods signed up to serve with the Unit.

B.E.F. General Hospital No. 9

The first American hospital units were stationed at British base hospitals and began work in France long before American combat units arrived in force. Consequently, the patients they cared for were from Britain or its Empire. Six units, including the Lakeside Unit, had been "loaned" to the British government and at first functioned entirely under British orders. Although the Lake-

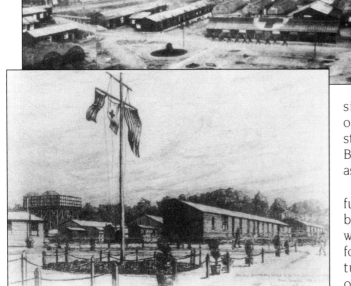

GENERAL HOSPITAL NO. 9
The Lakeside Unit, Base Hospital Unit No. 4 of the American Expeditionary Force, arrived to staff British-built General Hospital No. 9 (aerial view, above) in May 1917. The etching (below) shows the first American flag to fly with that of an Allied European power during the war. Initially, nearly all of the Unit's patients were British, since American troops had not yet arrived in any force. As of September, a few U.S. troops had been admitted to No. 9, but the Lakeside Unit did not care for many American battle casualties until the spring of 1918. By April, there were enough U.S. soldiers at No. 9 to fill an "all-American" ward, but British patients still outnumbered them.

side Unit was officially Base Hospital Unit No. 4 of the American Expeditionary Force (A.E.F.), it was stationed at Rouen at General Hospital No. 9 of the British Expeditionary Force (B.E.F.), and became known as "No. 9" to everyone except A.E.F. headquarters.

The Unit began its service in a fully constructed, fully operating hospital. Its plan, with many small buildings housing different functions and wards, was typical of military hospitals built to care for combatant forces. "Huts," small wooden structures with corrugated metal roofs, housed most of No. 9.

Each hut consists of forty-one patients and under our own organization they are divided into five surgical units, each unit being in charge of two ward huts and a corresponding number of tent huts. The surgical ward huts consist of a large hut in one end of which is the sisters' [nurses'] office and a special room for dressings or extremely sick cases, a splint room, a bath-room, a stretcher room, linen room. They are well provided with light and in the middle is a door on each side opening into the grounds, where the patients may be rolled out into the open air. The beds are very comfortable....There are two officers to each section. The operating theatre is in the operating hut with a sterilizing room, a wash room, a splint room and the X-ray department. It is possible to have two operating tables in use at the same time.[11]

There were 20 ward huts altogether, and 14 tent huts in addition. The tent huts also accommodated 40 or more beds each, but most of these beds were used only during periods of high occupancy. Half of the ward huts were devoted to surgical cases, half to medical cases.

The camp was built on high, well-drained ground, so mud was not a problem. Typically British were the well-kept grounds, with flower beds planted between the huts. Besides separate quarters for officers, enlisted men, and women, there were individual buildings for the usual auxiliary hospital functions — administration, laboratory, morgue, supply rooms, kitchen — plus camp facilities such as mess huts, a bathhouse, latrines, and outdoor water tanks, which supplied the base's running water.

Rouen was about 60 to 80 miles behind the front lines, and did not, in normal times, take in casualties directly from the battlefield. Field ambulances (hospitals) located at the front served this function; they stabilized patients and sent them on to the Casualty Clearing Stations (C.C.S.s), also at the front but about 7 to 10 miles behind the actual line of battle, where surgeons performed operations that could not be done at the field ambulances. The C.C.S.s also kept and nursed the worst cases, both medical and surgical.

Once patients were able to travel, they were evacuated in convoys, usually by railway, to the base hospitals, where surgery was also performed, and patients were nursed. Some men who lived long enough to reach the base hospitals died there, but most survived. The medical officers at the base hospitals then had the responsibility of determining the fate of the remaining patients: a soldier could be deemed fit for active service, and returned to the front; if his recovery would take longer than three weeks, he would be sent to a convalescent hospital, from which, most likely, he would also ultimately be returned to active service; or, if indefinitely unfit for further service, he would be sent home. Members of the Lakeside Unit soon came to know when a major Allied offensive was imminent. First, word would come to No. 9 to evacuate as many patients as possible. Then, large convoys would arrive from the C.C.S.s, so that the latter would be cleared of patients as far as possible and ready to take in fresh casualties from the battlefield, who would in turn be transferred to the base hospitals as soon as practicable.

Instituted almost immediately upon the Unit's arrival in Rouen was the meeting of the "Professional Council," at which the administrative heads met to discuss issues concerning the hospital's operation and the Unit members' activities. It met frequently in the early days of the Unit's service at Rouen; later, when the Unit had settled into its new home, fewer meetings were necessary. Commanding Officer Gilchrist, Adjutant Tuttle, Clinical Director Crile, Chief of Surgery Lower, Chief of Medicine Hoover, Director of Laboratories Howard Karsner, Chief Nurse Allison, and Dr. Crile's longtime secretary and research assistant Amy Rowland (one of the Unit's civilians) were the usual attendees. One of the first matters the Council had to deal with was the transition from British to American staffing at General Hospital No. 9.

> Miss Tawler [the British matron, or chief nurse] said we could not possibly take over the nursing in less than 3 weeks. Miss Allison felt we could take it over sooner, and said her nurses had found many ways of conserving

UNIT PERSONNEL
This group photograph of the Unit's enlisted men (top rows), medical officers, and nurses seated in front of the administration building, General Hospital No. 9, also shows the neat grounds and garden plots laid out by the British military.

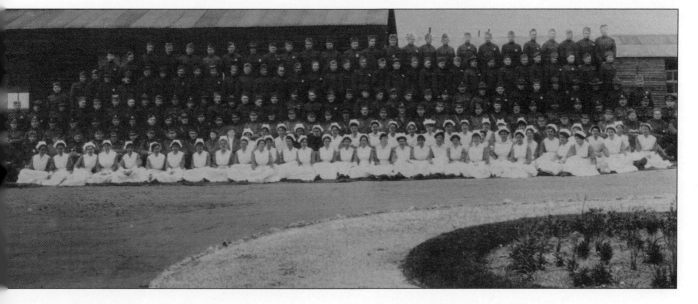

effort and time already. 'I believe there are only 7 |British| ward nurses left. When they find that our nurses really know something about nursing, I think they will change their minds.'....She said her nurses were under an executive board of nurses, comprised of the various heads. This board will take up all problems related to the nursing side of the work.[12]

At the June 4 meeting Miss Allison reported that she and her nurses, having been on duty on the wards for a week, were ready to take over entire responsibility for the nursing of No. 9's patients "with the aid of the extra V.A.D.'s."[13]

Volunteer Aide or Professional Nurse?

The V.A.D.s — for Voluntary Aid Detachment — serving in British hospitals were women between the ages of 20 and 45 who had completed basic first aid or home nursing courses, plus at least a few months of hospital training. They corresponded more or less to the Red Cross volunteer aides being trained in the United States, although they received pay (at a very low rate). In theory they worked as aides under the direction of fully trained professional nurses, or "sisters," as they were known in Britain. In practice, the V.A.D.s sometimes assumed responsibility for entire hospital wards, for there were not enough sisters to fill the vast need for wartime nursing care. The British Matron-in-Chief for France had offered 31 V.A.D.s to work under Miss Allison's direction at No. 9 until additional nurses could arrive from the United States to fully staff the hospital. All present at the June 4 Council meeting favored accepting the V.A.D.s, especially Dr. Crile, who had "made inquiries regarding the efficiency of the British V.A.D. and |found| they are very useful, having the equivalent grade of a nurse who has completed the second year in the training school."[14]

However, the proposal for V.A.D.s brought up a number of issues. Accepting them as temporary workers avoided the most significant one, that of professionalism. No volunteer aides from Cleveland had gone overseas with the Unit, although, according to a newspaper article, some local women had taken "special training" for the work. The issue of bringing aides over did come up in a Council meeting. Dr. Crile voiced the opinion that aides would sooner or later be a necessity, and that it would be better to have Cleveland women than strangers; Miss Allison skeptically observed that, based on her experience at Lakeside Hospital, many of "those who could afford to come without salary, would not be good workers," but expressed herself willing "to make a try at them."[15]

In the end, only one American Red Cross aide was eventually assigned to the Unit, to do clerical work. But the debate over volunteer aides was not a trivial one, mirroring as it did a nationwide discussion that came to a head in Cleveland at the same time as the Unit was carrying on with its work in Europe. As the nation committed more and more troops overseas, the demand for nurses at home and abroad outstripped the number of trained, practical, and student nurses in the labor force. How the shortfall should be made up was the main topic of debate.

Nursing leaders like Annie Goodrich and Adelaide Nutting favored an Army school of nurses, to provide professional training for more women; others, including officials of the Red Cross and some hospital superintendents, notably Dr. S. S. Goldwater of Mt. Sinai Hospital in New York, favored the use of volunteer aides. In May 1918, in Cleveland, at the joint annual meeting of the American Nurses' Association, the National League of Nursing Education, and the National Organization for Public Health Nursing, proponents of both plans argued the issue. As one historian has pointed out, the "fervor of nearly half a century of the struggle to have nursing defined as skilled work needing more than womanly sympathy to achieve results" animated the will of the nursing leaders to carry their point. When the general staff of the War Department rejected the plan for the Army school of nursing, nursing leaders and advocates, including Frances Payne Bolton of Cleveland, went to Washington to ask Secretary of War Baker to intervene on their behalf. He approved the plan for the Army school, which was duly established with Miss Goodrich as dean.

However, the general issue of the solution to the nursing shortage problem continued under discussion. Samuel Mather, president of the Lakeside Hospital board of trustees, wrote to Dr. Crile in September that he had just attended the annual hospital convention in Atlantic City and "heard some very interesting discussions - between Miss Goodrich and Miss Nutting, on the one hand, Dr. Goldwater and Mr. Borden, on the other," on the subject.[16]

Although the Lakeside Unit never had to import large numbers of American aides, it did have to depend on the British V.A.D.s until more nurses could arrive, and even here, tensions existed between volunteer and professional. The V.A.D.s were experienced in the care of war casualties but not educated as nurses; the American women were graduate nurses but new to the war. Awkwardness was also present between the American nurses and the British sisters they were replacing. The Lakeside Unit was, in a sense, pushing the British staff off their home turf, albeit at the request of the British government. On the day the Lakeside Unit arrived at No. 9, wrote Amy Rowland, "the nurses greeted us cordially although we learned afterward that they felt rather bitter, some of them, to be 'turned out' of their hospital. But they were certainly nice enough on this day, and gave us a dainty lunch with claret cup which was a grateful drink after our hot march."[17]

More practical was the matter of the differing sets of rules for the British and American women. "Miss Tawler says the new V.A.D.s will not come in under the rigid rules now in force in the Unit. It was decided to allow them to come in under the British rules."[18] This brought up the question of rules for the Unit's nurses. For the men of the Unit, no such problem existed. They were "in the Army now" and were subject to Army regulations. The position of the nurses was less clear, as symbolized by their lack of Army uniform. They were members of the Army Nurse Corps Reserves but had been enrolled through the Red Cross, and were also outfitted, to a limited extent, through the Red Cross. (The Lakeside Unit nurses had had to have their duty uniforms made after arriving in England.) They had no military rank but were not civilian employees. The nurses of the reserve base hospital units naturally identified more with their home hospitals than with the Army, at least to begin with. The Army Nurse Corps, created in 1901 and now on the threshold of its first real battle, had a future before it, but only the shortest of traditions behind it.

"What is Really Best for the Nurses"

Whatever rules and regulations did not come ready-made from the Army, the Professional Council of No. 9 quickly set out to manufacture for itself. The Council discussed all sorts of issues relating to camp life and patient care, but issues related to nurses' behavior provoked the most lively interchanges.

Duty assignment, a non-controversial topic, was decided first, so that the actual work of the Unit could begin. On May 28, the memorandum of nurses' assignments, signed by Chief Nurse Allison and effective immediately, was posted.

With duty assignments made, the Professional Council turned its attention to the nurses' off-duty activities. An order signed by Major Gilchrist on June 1 stated:

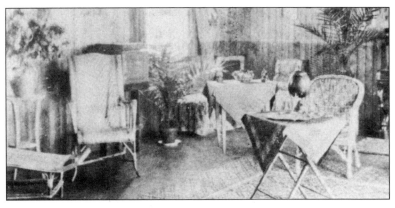

NURSES' LIVING ROOM
Long wooden huts roofed with corrugated iron housed most of the facilities at General Hospital No. 9, including the nurses' quarters. Nurses lived two to a room in eight-room dormitory huts heated by oil stoves. A separate building contained a living room and a dining room. Although long hours on duty, early curfews, and "officer-nurse regulations" restricted social life, Unit personnel did their best. "On Wednesday evenings, our Nurses' Mess is open for callers, and for the past three weeks our officers have been dropping in for bridge."

Upon the recommendation of the Chief Nurse, each Nurse will be granted permission to be absent from Camp Limits one half-day per week as far as conditions in the hospital will permit. During this period of absence she is at liberty to select such diversion as she knows to be of unquestionable character. Dining at Hotels and Cafes is strictly forbidden.

At other hours off duty for purposes of recreation, nurses will be permitted the use of surrounding parks, but within the limits of the general military encampment grounds only.[19]

The Council wanted to make sure that in case of an emergency a sufficient number of nurses would be near at hand to be called back to the wards. As a result, only nurses on half-day holiday were permitted to leave the encampment.

Only a few days later, when it was decided to let the V.A.D.s in under British rules, rules for the Unit nurses had to be discussed again. "Major Crile said that what they wished to arrive at is - what is really best for the nurses." Majors Lower and Tuttle favored more relaxed rules; Miss Allison suggested more "mental diversion," in which she liberally included holding dances in the nurses' quarters.[20]

A few weeks later, the crux of the matter of nurses' off-duty rules finally came under specific and lengthy discussion: relations between the sexes, in this case, between the Unit's nurses and officers.

Miss Allison next brought up the question of the association of the nurses and officers, which was followed by a lengthy discussion. She stated that the English felt from our ruling now in force, that our nurses cannot be trusted. Dr. Crile felt....the question is, 'What will be the effect if there should come attachments?' For this reason, he felt that going out by two's would be objectionable. Dr. Hoover felt that in many cases it would be impossible for the nurses to take excursions, even in groups, unless escorted by officers. He felt more freedom should be permitted. Miss Allison stated that all the nurses were of mature years, and were a sensible lot, and that at Lakeside, graduate nurses were not restricted in any way....Captain Tuttle said that the seclusion of both officers and nurses was unnatural, and that for his own part he felt it was rather dangerous to make it necessary for the officers to go to the city for companionship other than among themselves. Major Crile said his stony heart had been softened by each succeeding plea of Capt. Tuttle....Major Gilchrist objected to one officer and one nurse being seen together constantly. Major Crile felt everything should be left to Miss Allison's judgment, but she felt the ruling, affected the officers as much as the nurses. Major Gilchrist and

Capt. Tuttle both told of experiences in previous service, where nurses were always permitted to go out with the officers.

The final ruling of Major Crile was that the officers may come to call, to tea or to any social events — in fact that no restrictions whatever were to be made. However he urged that all give as little occasion for comment as possible — to keep on the safe side. He felt that all should encourage social intercourse as far as possible, but discourage single couples going out together. Groups are all right.[21]

Amy Rowland, whose status as a civilian employee and immediate assistant to Dr. Crile gave her a unique position within the Unit, was quartered with the nurses, and had definite ideas about the regulations constraining their off-duty activities.

Social life is interfered with by the much-discussed officer-nurse regulations. There is not enough 'amusement' within our own encampment, but I hope some definite plans will be made for the long winter evenings. I spoke with Miss A some time ago about it; and have said all that is wise since....The Nurses' Mess is closed every night after the last dinner. It should be open until whatever is decided upon as the proper closing time. Some of the nurses are fond of cards. The piano should be used more; and the gramaphone would be if there were more opportunity. It should not be improper for the nurses to push back the furniture and dance with each other if the spirit moves to the gramaphone or piano. Our own doctors and the nurses' friends from other units should be allowed to call on certain evenings. When if desirable some one or more could act as official hostesses or chaperons.[22]

"Officer-nurse regulations" were probably inevitable when occupational groups defined by gender worked and lived in such proximity, and in an age when the idea that women were weak creatures who needed protection from men and from their own sexuality was generally accepted. However, given the constant contact between nurses and officers, they could not ignore each other as men and women. A medical officer called Mary Roche's silk-stockinged legs "the one cheerful sight at the C.C.S." The nurses had their opinions, too. "Dr. Shawan is the smartest looking thing in his uniform - everybody is quite crazy about him," stated Arvilla Walkinshaw.[23]

The most important regulation on fraternization between the sexes came direct from Army headquarters and was communicated to the personnel of No. 9 on September 28, 1918. "Any member of the Army Nurse Corps who marries while on active service in France will be returned immediately to the United States for duty and will not be discharged in France." This ruling came a little late, as stenographer Ida Preston, another of the Unit's civilian members, remarked. "Since the order is not retrospective, it does not affect our two brides, but for a day or two they were both pretty excited."[24]

NURSES' DINING ROOM
Nurses, medical officers, and enlisted men all had separate dining areas. Nurses rotated through duty assignments in the nurses' quarters and mess as well as on the wards. During the spring of 1918, Nettie Eisenhard took her turn at supervising the mess. "Miss Eisenhard in the Mess is splendid....She certainly got up a fine Easter dinner, and occasionally she goes into the kitchen herself and makes a pie or cake for the whole crowd."

THE LAKESIDE
SLUICILEERS
The Unit's enlisted men served
as orderlies, assisting nurses on
the wards and meeting incoming
convoys of wounded. They also
carried messages (there were
no call bells), scrubbed floors,
and did the heavy work around the
base. Most were in their early
twenties, and had no experience
whatsoever in hospital work.
They pitched in with a will,
nonetheless, and the high spirits
that sometimes earned them a
reprimand from the head nurse
or commanding officer also
cheered up the patients. They
nicknamed themselves the
Lakeside "Sluicileers," referring
to their work with the bedpans.

Less exciting, but more generally applicable and relevant to everyday life, were regulations on uniform and dress. Nurses were required to wear uniforms "at all times outside the nurses' enclosure, whether in wards, at concerts, in the woods or in the city." This was an about-face from stateside rules, noted a British nursing publication, "for at Lakeside (their training school) it is considered a crime to go out wearing the slightest sign of uniform!"[25] As the weather grew cold, nurses were ordered to take precautions against chilblains. On the other hand, they were forbidden to wear cardigans, apparently because it detracted from uniformity.

Women in nursing became accustomed to leading regulated lives during their training school days. Even after graduation they still had to live up to certain unwritten expectations, both on- and off-duty, in order to maintain the respect of other nurses, physicians, and the community in general. Nurses employed by hospitals often lived in hospital residences; private duty nurses staying in patients' homes were under observation 24 hours a day. The rules, although perhaps excessive, were based on sound reasoning. At this time, the first training schools in the United States were only 40 years old; the first training school in Cleveland, at Huron Road Hospital, had opened in 1884. Nursing was still fighting for recognition as a skilled profession and could not afford to have revived the old image of the nurse as an ignorant servant or drunken inmate revived. In civilian life, nurses themselves were often the most zealous enforcers of the codes regulating not only nursing practice, but personal conduct as well.

"Mighty Fine Boys"

At No. 9, the Unit nurses were not alone in being subject to many rules. The enlisted men, too, came in for their share, over and above general Army regulations. For instance, they were required to take baths at least once a week — not a pleasant pastime in the winter months — with their name and date of bath being recorded in a "bath record." Contrary to British practice, they were forbidden the use of alcohol in their mess. No evidence exists of regulations for nurses regarding baths and alcohol. (Also, the Unit's women had the privilege of drawing off hot water from the kitchen supply for their baths.)

Nurses' relationships with enlisted men were strictly professional. There were no regulations on social relations corresponding to the "nurse-officer regulations," because social relations between nurses and enlisted men were not recognized. This was, most likely, due in part to traditional ideas about social class (however inappropriate they were in view of the mixed social origins of all ranks of Unit members) and, more importantly, to the exigencies of discipline. Although enlisted men were assigned to a variety of tasks in the hospital and the camp, their most important duty was to serve as orderlies on the wards, under the direction of the head nurses. Too much familiarity might damage the nurse's ability to maintain order on her ward. In any case, most of the nurses of the Unit were at least a few years older than most of the enlisted men, and tended to adopt a maternal attitude toward them. If discipline suffered, motherly indulgence toward "our boys," rather than a sweetheart's tenderness, was more likely to blame.

Fundamentally, however, the anomalous, unranked position of the Army nurse had much to do with creating whatever problems existed. As early as

June 4, 1917, the Council realized the matter had to be clarified. "It was decided that the orderlies are under the supervision of the head nurse on the wards — just as they are in a civil hospital, and if any question arises which calls for additional authority — the matter should be referred to the medical or surgical officer in charge of the ward."[26] Of course, this chain of command was identical to that used in American hospitals of the era, but the enlisted men came from outside the hospital culture and so did not fall into their places as automatically as the physicians and nurses. Arvilla Walkinshaw wrote about the situation in a letter to her former patient, Mrs. Crile.

> The work is rather difficult for us, having untrained orderlies - and as we have no rank it is rather awkward to deal with them. They have a lemon tree in their mess, and if we give an order or insist on any ward routine, we - that is our names - are placed on the lemon tree. I expect my name is on every branch as I have the reputation of being the 'strictest head nurse.' We have a number of mighty fine boys who will make good officers and never good orderlies.[27]

Not until October were orders from the Secretary of War regarding the status of members of the Army Nurse Corps and Army Nurse Corps Reserve, U.S. Army, published in the daily orders at No. 9:

> As regards medical and sanitary matters and work in connection with the sick, members of the Army Nurse Corps and Army Nurse Corps Reserve are to be regarded as having authority in matters pertaining to their professional duties (the care of the sick and wounded) in and about military hospitals next after the officers of the Medical Department, and are at all times to be obeyed accordingly and to receive the respect due to their position.[28]

The perceptive Amy Rowland had already made some notes in her diary, "for discussion at some future time," on the relationship of nurses to enlisted men, and also to medical officers.

> Nurses in Canadian Army have rank of 2nd Lieut. which makes relations with orderlies easier. Our orderlies especially the sergeants consider themselves superior officers to nurses and are upheld by some of the M.O.'s Position of nurse often almost unendurable in a civil hospital; even more in an army hospital. Discourtesy of younger M.O.'s.[29]

Dr. Crile, on the other hand, felt that even once the regulation was in force, and the head nurse fully responsible for the ward, "the chief difficulty...lies...in the reluctance of the head nurse to report any laxity in the conduct of the orderlies. I may add, however, that in general, the result [of the regulation] is most satisfactory."[30]

At times, nurses were considered too indulgent with patients as well. Only a month after the Unit took over the staffing of No. 9, the Professional Council was discussing the matter.

> Major Crile felt very strongly that nurses should not supply flowers on the wards. In the discussion it was brought out that nurses were also furnishing fruit and milk for patients, and that doctors were also feeding patients. Major Crile felt that such things should not be done because 1) it is not the function of the nurse; 2) it is too apt to cause a bid for rivalry; 3) and it establishes a dangerous precedence [sic] — the end result is not good. Major Gilchrist was asked to draft an order, in which while expressing an appreciation of the splendid spirit of the nurse, such furnishing of supplies for patients should be forbidden.[31]

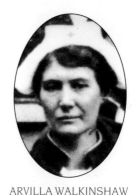

ARVILLA WALKINSHAW
Many Canadian-born women came to the United States to practice nursing. They included leaders like Isabel Hampton Robb and Agatha Hodgins, and rank-and-file nurses like Miss Walkinshaw. A graduate of the Children's Hospital in Toronto, Miss Walkinshaw joined the staff of Lakeside Hospital as head nurse of its children's ward in 1905. She resigned to work as a private duty nurse. She cared for Dr. Crile's wife, Grace, when the couple's youngest child was born. Her wartime letters to her former patient were observant, honest, and humorous. After the war, Miss Walkinshaw married Dr. Samuel Webster of Cleveland, and settled permanently on the city's west side.

The Unit at Work

As the Unit settled into its routine, a modus vivendi was reached. The Professional Council's meetings grew fewer and farther between until it apparently withered away entirely. At any rate, everyone grew too busy with the tasks at hand to have much time for meetings. Major Crile's research mission, and even more his energies, carried him off to C.C.S's, to field hospitals, to conferences in Paris, and eventually detached him from the Unit he had spawned, although he continued to return to No. 9 at intervals and considered it one of his "three homes" in France. At his request, he was detached and named director of his own research unit rather than take over the administrative duties of No. 9 when Colonel Gilchrist was transferred to another post. But by this time No. 9 was running smoothly, its personnel "acting as a unit" in Dr. Crile's absence as well as in his presence.

Around the time the Lakeside Unit arrived, the patient census was relatively low — about 500 to 600 patients, in a hospital with a capacity for 800, and through the use of tents, an expansion capacity of 1,650. The first convoy, a small one of 45 patients with mostly slight injuries, came in on June 1. Within a few weeks, more numerous convoys of up to 150 patients each, some with more severe wounds, were arriving from the attack at Messines Ridge. The bugle call announcing "convoy in" — often in the middle of the night — meant heavy work for the enlisted men and the nurses, especially those on night duty. Men detailed for convoy duty would report to the convoy tent opposite the administration building, where the ambulances with wounded men arrived. Cases were divided into "sitting" and "stretcher" cases, with the former able to travel sitting up and to walk from the ambulance to the wards.

STERILIZING ROOM
Equipment similar to this was used to sterilize the instruments used in the operating room and dressing tent of General Hospital No. 9. Here, nurses Edith Carman, Inez McKee, and Helen Briggs pose in the sterilizing room set up in a tent during the Lakeside Unit's trial mobilization at a site near Philadelphia in 1916.

Our boys have learned to handle the incoming men splendidly. Each ambulance usually brings four lying cases; the men are summoned by a bugle and line up at the side of the road, and without confusion, the ambulances are quickly unloaded. Each man has his field card, which tells the nature of his wound and the treatment already received…. Ambulance after ambulance drives up, is unloaded, the men carried through the receiving tent and away to the designated ward with hardly a pause in the procession. Duplicate sets of stretchers are kept so that as the ambulance drives on after being unloaded it is met at the other end of the tent by orderlies who replace the stretchers which have just been taken off with the men, and the ambulances go for the next load. The orderlies all like convoy duty for it gives them a chance to get first hand stories from the Front.[32]

The nurses then assumed care of the patients, as Marie Shields recounted in an article submitted to a hometown newspaper.

We work at top speed. Already we have been busy for hours, sterilizing instruments and preparing bandages.

Many of the wounded are brought in on stretchers. Some are only parts of men. Bandages, stiff with blood, hide, or

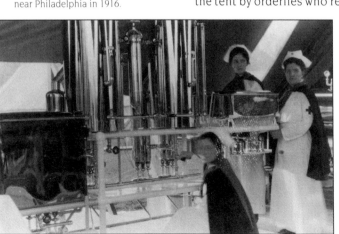

20

partly hide, gaping wounds. Other men walk, hobbling in spite of their injuries, and trying to help each other. To see them, in their desperate attempts at cheeriness, is most heartrending....

The least wounded are given baths, probably the first they have had in many days. But many must have their wounds dressed first, and there are others who must be hurried direct to the operating tables.

The physical strain on the nurses while all this is going on is terrific. Often I have wished for many pairs of hands.[33]

On July 4, Miss Allison reported that under a new arrangement for taking care of convoys, "last night the walking cases which came in on the convoys were sent at once to the wards, in one instance 11 patients being sent to one ward. At night there is but one nurse to each two wards, and this meant that the nurse had to bathe and clean each patient before he could be put to bed, because it would not do to put dirty patients into a clean ward without cleaning them up."[34] The chiefs of service agreed that perhaps it was better to go back to the old system and put the walking patients to bed in a tent ward for the night, and then clean them up and assign them to the appropriate wards the next morning.

Surgical cases included:

> severely infected wounds, compound, comminuted fractures of the extremities and a considerable percentage involving the joints, especially the knee and elbow. Most of these arrive here two or three days after the receipt of the injury....There is nothing particularly new in the treatment of wounds, all manner and form of antiseptics having been tried.[35]

"The wounds...are all badly infected. Wound infection is the problem of the war, so far as it is related to the medical profession," stated Dr. Lower.[36] Worst were the gas gangrene cases, which carried a high mortality rate.

WARD FOR THE
SEVERELY WOUNDED

The wards of General Hospital No. 9 were housed in tents or narrow wooden huts, with beds lined up along two walls. Low iron frames supported the mattresses on which the patients lay, so that nurses and orderlies had to do a great deal of bending and stooping. When the census was very high, two beds were pushed together to be shared by three men, and straw ticks placed on the floor in addition. A special room for critically ill patients at one end of the building, next to the nurses' station, functioned somewhat like an early form of intensive care unit.

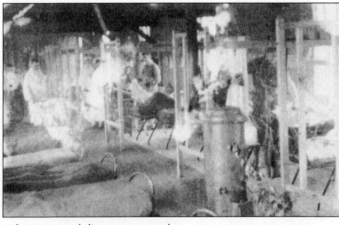

Medical cases included men with respiratory infections and diseases spread in the poor sanitary conditions at the front, such as influenza, pneumonia, bronchitis, and dysentery, as well as victims of the war's most dreaded weapon: gas. "The gasses used were chlorine, mustard gas, and phosgene. Mustard gas was a vesicant causing serious pulmonary reaction and huge blisters when applied to the skin." On July 24, nurse Edith Morgan reported that "many of her men had been gassed, and that these men were all of them quite deaf as a consequence."[37] Men who had been gassed were sometimes cyanotic, gasping for breath, or they might have burns all over their skin and their eyes. Many soldiers feared gas far more than they feared bullets or shells.

Two huts of 41 beds each made up a ward, with one or two medical officers assigned to each ward. The huts numbered up through 10, plus 12 of 14 tents, were designated as medical wards. Surgical cases were assigned to huts 11 through 20 by type of injury, according to body location: knee and hip joint injuries, to Nos. 11 and 12; fractures of thighs and legs, to Nos. 13 and 14;

fractures of upper extremities to Nos. 15 and 16; head and chest injuries to Nos. 17 and 18; elbow and shoulder joints to Nos. 19 and 20. To begin with, four nurses and six or seven orderlies were assigned to each pair of huts during the day shift. The ward's head nurse and an assistant nurse worked in one hut, a senior and a junior nurse in the other. Although the Lakeside Unit nurses were all graduates, this nomenclature reflected the staffing pattern at Lakeside Hospital, where graduate head nurses supervised the work of probationer, junior and senior students.

No. 9 also initially had two nurses assigned to the outpatient department and four nurses assigned to duty in the nurses' quarters. At night, the nursing staff consisted of a general surgical supervisor, a general medical supervisor, and one nurse for every two huts.

Miss Allison's first memorandum on nurses' duties included the following assignments: Nettie Eisenhard and Helen O'Brien as head and senior nurse, respectively, in hut Nos. 11 and 12, the surgical ward for knee and hip cases. The ward's assistant nurse was Margaret Lane, with Lillian Grundies as junior. Minnie Strobel was head nurse in hut No. 13, and Austa Engel senior nurse in hut No. 14. Edith Morgan, as head nurse in hut No. 15, was in charge of the ward caring for fractures of upper extremities; Elizabeth Folckemer served as junior nurse in hut No. 16.

On the medical side, Betty Connelly was in charge of hut Nos. 7 and 8, with Caroline Smith as the senior nurse; Ina Starr and Mary Ellen Schultz held the corresponding positions in the ward comprised of hut Nos. 9 and 10. Mabel Horn and Constance Hanna were junior nurses in hut Nos. 3 and 4. Arvilla Walkinshaw was the first night surgical supervisor, Isabel Bishop the medical supervisor; Marie Shields served as night nurse for the thigh and leg fracture ward in hut Nos. 13 and 14.

During the daytime, each hut had several enlisted men, typically three or four, serving as orderlies. This meant that two nurses and three orderlies could be responsible for the care of 40 patients, some of them in critical condition. Fortunately, when the Unit first arrived, the wards were not full, and the V.A.D.s served as a complement to the American staff.

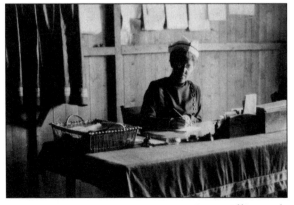

MATRON'S OFFICE
Chief Nurse Allison, shown here at the desk (actually a cloth-covered table) in her office, was usually referred to as the "Matron" of General Hospital No. 9, in accordance with British usage.

Nursing Organization at No. 9

Staff scheduling and all other routine administrative matters relating to nursing were handled in the office of the Chief Nurse, or Matron. The Chief Nurse also gave nursing a voice at meetings of the Professional Council. On the one hand, she was recognized as a professional, serving as an equal member (the only other woman who attended, Amy Rowland, did so primarily as a recording secretary and had no voice); on the other, the medical officers had four representatives and administration had two (the two career army physicians), compared to the nurses' one.

Grace Allison, the Unit's first Chief Nurse, was a competent, if not charismatic leader. In her civilian post at Lakeside Hospital, she headed a nursing staff made up largely of students. The Lakeside Unit, made up entirely of graduate nurses like the rest of the Army Nurse Corps and Nurse Corps Reserve, was a window on the future of nursing rather than a reflection of its own time. Used to dealing with young, inexperienced students, Grace Allison appears, from the evidence of her letters and reports, to have developed a formal and distant style. Some of the Unit's women civilian workers did not get along well with her. She was not, however, an authoritarian — she met with a council of head nurses on "all problems related to the nursing side of the work." And the entire nursing staff of the Unit met at least once as a group to discuss and vote on matters concerning them. Miss Allison was well aware that the graduate nurses of the Unit were responsible adults, and made that point to the Professional Council whenever she had occasion to do so.

According to all accounts, crises or misfortunes brought out Miss Allison's best side. During the first great rush of work at No. 9, in July 1917, Ida Preston remarked that both Miss Allison and the medical officer serving as acting clinical director had "'arisen to the occasion'" and made themselves "immensely respected." The following March, Miss Preston declared that "no one could have been nicer to me when I was sick than [Miss Allison] was, and all who have been ill since the first of the year say the same thing." Dr. Crile also wrote that spring that Miss Allison was "proving out splendidly."[38]

In the summer of 1918, the Lakeside Hospital trustees, informed from overseas that although she had "done the work very well," it had been "a big strain upon her," and she needed "some change and let-up," called her back to her position in Cleveland where, Dr. Crile noted, she would be of great help in preparing more nurses for overseas service, if necessary.[39] Settling matters via transatlantic mail took some time, but on September 10 Miss Allison was able to step down from her post. Elizabeth Folckemer, who had started as junior nurse of Ward 16, succeeded her. Perhaps being promoted from the ranks gave Miss Folckemer increased insight into the daily lives of the Unit's nurses; perhaps she simply possessed that rare gift, an indefinable flair for leadership.

"Miss Folckemer is certainly a wonder, and everyone adores her. There has never been such a good feeling and such co-operation since we landed, as there is right now." The good feeling persisted past the armistice in November. "Miss Folckemer is certainly making good in Miss Allison's place. She has judgment, tact, the ability to put herself in another's place, is fair, impartial, and commands the respect of everyone in the Unit - officers, nurses and men alike."[40]

A few other nurses assisted the Chief Nurse in her administrative duties. Harriet Leete, the Unit's first Assistant Matron, left Rouen within a few months of her arrival to assume a position with the American Red Cross in Paris, as head of a child health and welfare project. Red Cross officials had informed Dr. Crile that they needed a nurse for this position, and he, familiar with Miss Leete's background in the field, apparently asked her to go. She wrote to him from Paris:

> As I seem to be separated from the Unit, may I express to you my great appreciation for having been a part of it for the first few months. My loyalty to and interest in the Lakeside Unit prevented me from becoming interested in this new big constructive piece of work which is so greatly needed.
>
> I shall, of course, endeavor to be of service here, but it can never lessen my loyalty to the Lakeside Unit.[41]

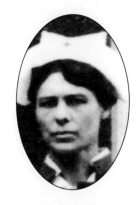

ELIZABETH FOLCKEMER
The Unit's second Chief Nurse, she took over from Miss Allison in September 1918. Miss Folckemer, from Springfield, Ohio, attended nursing school at Lakeside Hospital, graduating in 1911. She went on to a distinguished career in public health nursing. At the time she joined the Lakeside Unit, she was assistant director of Cleveland's Visiting Nurse Association. Described by a journalist as a "tiny dynamo," she led the VNA as director for more than three decades following her return from France in 1919.

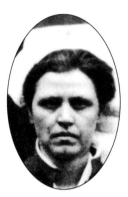

NETTIE EISENHARD

Miss Eisenhard, a Lakeside Hospital graduate (1911), was one of the nurses sent forward from General Hospital No. 9 to serve at a casualty clearing station near the front line of battle. For her bravery in remaining at work in the operating room under shell fire, she received the Royal Red Cross medal from the British crown. After her return from France, she was appointed a head nurse at Lakeside Hospital, resigned that position to take a public health job with Cleveland's Federal Reserve Bank, and then left nursing for marriage to Charles Buescher and a home in Lakewood, Ohio.

Later in the month, the Red Cross requested more nurses with training in social service work — Miss Leete had suggested the names of Edith Morgan and Austa Engel. Dr. Crile "felt that the game of the babies upon whom the future of France depends should certainly be played," but when he spoke to the two nurses, they preferred to remain with the Unit.[42] The Council decided that all nurses originally attached to the Unit should remain if they wished, so Miss Morgan and Mrs. Engel stayed, the latter eventually assuming the position of Assistant Matron under Miss Folckemer. In the meantime, Minnie Strobel succeeded Harriet Leete as Miss Allison's assistant.

Besides the Chief Nurse, the woman with the most administrative responsibility in the Unit was probably the nurse in charge of the operating theater, Clara Illig. Her abilities became evident during times when great numbers of casualties came in for surgery.

"On Saturday we began to get the first fruits of the new push, and some of the worst cases we have ever received came in, several bad gas gangrenes among them. There were thirty-one operations and Major Lower is loud in his praises of Miss Illig's organization. Everything moved by clockwork, there seemed to be no hitches and everyone was exuberant."[43] On the following day, nine operations were done in less than an hour.

Miss Illig and her colleagues had also assisted Dr. Crile with plans for work at casualty clearing stations. In July 1917 he wrote in his diary: "At present I am spending all of my time in research and organization. The group of operating room nurses took some rough sketches of mine and have elaborated on them until I believe we have a good plan for a whole series of operations, in the advanced hospitals."[44]

Except for the chief nurse, her assistants, the nurse anesthetists, and, to an extent, the operating room nurses, little permanent hierarchy or specialization existed in the organization of nursing at No. 9. The wards had a nurse in charge and a senior nurse, and there were night supervisors, but nurses rotated among these positions and among the wards, for stints of days or weeks, seemingly almost at random. For instance, Austa Engel worked in hut No. 14, a surgical ward, then took charge of hut No.13 for less than two weeks, was transferred to the Surgical Dressing Tent, where she apparently worked from October through January, and then, after a week's absence, was assigned to hut No. 10, a medical ward. About six weeks later she went to night duty in hut No. 17; in June she was given charge of hut No. 8, and in September 1918 became Assistant Matron of the Unit. Nettie Eisenhard began as the head nurse of hut #11, and then was detached for duty as an operating room nurse at a casualty clearing station in September. She returned to the base on Christmas Eve, and spent a short time working in a medical ward, before being assigned to supervise the running of the nurses' quarters and mess. Edith Morgan worked in at least five different wards, both medical and surgical, and had charge of some, in addition to serving as a night supervisor and taking a turn in the nurses' mess. Margaret Lane also worked in several different wards, sometimes as the nurse in charge, before training as a nurse anesthetist and finally going to the front with the Unit's Mobile Hospital No. 5.

But even with the continual changes in duties and the long shifts; even with the debate over social proprieties and ward discipline; even with all the orders and notices and bulletins, many of the Unit nurses seemed to feel they enjoyed greater liberty as Army nurses abroad than as civilian nurses at home. "Our discipline is not like that in the civil hospitals at home. Doctors, nurses and patients are all on the most friendly and informal terms. There are no rigid rules," commented Marie Shields. The way Caroline Smith remembered her service days, 20 years later, provides a key to understanding the seeming contradictions in how the Unit nurses felt about life at Rouen. "I guess the excitement kept us all going....we had so much more responsibility than nurses at home have."[45] Despite all of the rules governing the behavior and duties of World War I-era Army nurses, despite — and even because of — the difficult conditions and pressures under which they worked and lived, the Unit nurses had confidence in their own abilities to deal with the task at hand. As long as the convoys of stretchers continued to pour into the hospital grounds, they could not forget how great was the need for the skills they had gained through education and experience.

"A Full and Busy Day"

Saturday, July 21, 1917, began with the arrival of a convoy of 125 patients. Convoys of a similar size had been received during the previous day as well, so that No. 9 was handling an unaccustomed number of patients and surgeries. Fortunately, additional nurses for the Unit arrived as well.

> At four o'clock the eighteen American nurses arrived, the ones we had been looking for for several days. They were not Lakeside nurses, or even Ohio nurses, about half of them being from Texas, and several from Johns Hopkins....They were in the blue uniforms [of the Army Nurse Corps], and our nurses were very keen over the insignia which they were wearing on their collars — the U.S. such as our officers have, and the caduceus with the gold letters.[46]

By this time, good feeling had grown up between the Lakeside Unit nurses and the V.A.D.s working with them. The arrival of the second group of American nurses meant the departure of the British women, and the Unit nurses had planned a farewell party for that very evening, in which the newcomers joined. The party was

> an informal masquerade for ladies only. It was very interesting to see the original costumes which some of the girls worked up with just what limited materials were on hand.... During the height of the celebration, two neat-looking V.A.D.'s appeared, who had not been seen before. They started to dance,

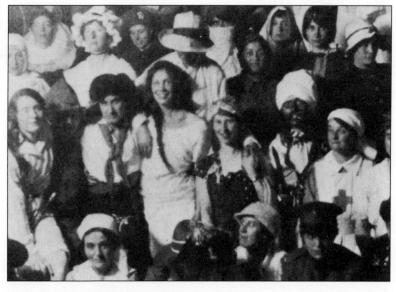

one American sister claiming the right of a dance immediately. However, after circling the room once or twice, and finding it rather difficult to lead, she asked the British sister if she would not lead for a round or two. Whereupon a deep masculine voice replied, "Yes, I will!" Soon merry shouts proved that the "cat was out of the bag" and the two V.A.D.'s were

MASQUERADE PARTY
As a farewell to the British V.A.D. workers who had assisted them until more American nurses could arrive, the Unit nurses put on a "ladies only" masquerade party in July 1917. Guests came dressed as: "a stunning Pierrot," "a very handsome cavalier," and "an Indian Sikh," as well as Joan of Arc, "Devils, Priests, Nuns," "Scotch 'kilties,' Blighty patients, convalescent patients, bathing girls, summer girls, and so forth." Costumes offered men a way to join in the fun: disguised as V.A.D.s, two officers crashed the party.

Colonel Gilchrist and Major Tuttle. Major Hoover and Major Crile were then taken over to visit the party, and last of all Major Lower appeared. As he entered our sitting room, one of the V.A.D.'s made a flying leap from across the room, threw "her" arms around his neck, and kissed him on both cheeks in true French fashion. Poor Major Lower was exceedingly embarrassed. He took the arms from around his neck, and with his back against the wall, held his cane in front of him to ward off any further demonstrations of affection. And it was not for some minutes that he realized that the ardent V.A.D. was his fellow officer, Major Tuttle, Adjutant.

This all sounds interesting, but the most interesting event of the day was the order received about five-thirty in the afternoon for three teams to leave at eight the following morning - Sunday - for Casualty Clearing Stations at the front.[47]

In fact, as Amy Rowland noted, she and Dr. Crile's other assistants ended up having to spend the evening at work in preparation for his departure and could only run over to the party for a few minutes to admire the costumes. "Major Gilchrist had lent me his full dress uniform, sword and all, which I passed on to Miss Lane, who was so stunning in it, that I was very glad of the chance that passed it on."[48] Miss Rowland and the others worked until after 1 a.m., so that despite the short notice, the 12 Unit members were ready to leave as ordered.

Early the next morning, nine ambulances carrying surgical teams left Rouen on a hot, dusty ride to the casualty clearing stations in Belgium. The first "Flying Squadron, for emergency at the Front," had been chosen only a month after the Unit's arrival in France. Dr. Lower as surgeon, Lillian Grundies (accustomed to working with Dr. Lower in civilian life) as operating room nurse, Mary Roche as anesthetist, and Private John Harbaugh as orderly, prepared for going to a C.C.S. by attending "Gas School" on June 29, 1917, along with British soldiers on their way to the front. This involved attending lectures on the effects of gas, being fitted with gas masks, and finally "spending five minutes in a gas chamber being gassed." Dr. Lower stated in his diary that nurses Grundies and Roche "were the first American nurses to receive gas instructions, and as far as the instructor knew, the first women to be given the gas test....with two English, one Australian, and one American nurse from the St. Louis Unit."[49]

In addition to Dr. Lower's team, No. 9 had hurriedly assembled two other teams, led by Dr. Crile — who had arranged to have himself ordered to take a team — and Dr. Harold Shawan. Nurses Helen Briggs and Inez McKee had been assigned to these teams as operating room nurses. Extra physicians went along to give anesthetics, since No. 9 had only one remaining nurse anesthetist, who could not be spared.

No sooner had the C.C.S. teams departed than a large convoy of new patients began to come in. The British were preparing an offensive, and were clearing the front line medical facilities by sending patients "down the line" to the base hospitals. The summoning of the additional surgery teams for the C.C.S.s was also part of the preparation.

The Casualty Clearing Stations

The ambulances reached Belgium that evening. On the way, their passengers had seen large numbers of trucks, some observation balloons, and airplanes, which were being attacked by anti-aircraft guns. By the time they

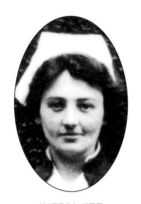

INEZ McKEE

Nurses Inez McKee and Helen Briggs, both Lakeside nursing school graduates, served together at a casualty clearing station and received commendations from British Field Marshal Douglas Haig. Miss McKee worked as an operating room nurse at Lakeside Hospital before joining the Unit. After the war, she married Charles Schoepfle, a professor of chemistry at the University of Michigan. Miss Briggs also married but remained in the Cleveland area. She and her husband, Reuben Elliott, had five children; their oldest daughter entered nursing school at Mt. Sinai Hospital during the Second World War.

arrived at the C.C.S.s "the canonading [had become] more intense," but the exhausted new arrivals went to bed anyway. "At ten-thirty the earth was quaking and a great variety of shooting was going on, of the rapid firing anti-air craft as well as of the heavier guns. About eleven there was a terrific explosion, four or five in succession, then a response by heavier guns. Our cots shook and a poor patient in the next tent groaned loudly."[50] Already the masquerade party of the night before must have seemed a distant memory. In the morning, pieces of shell were found near the tent nurses Grundies and Roche had occupied. (Since the areas where some of the C.C.S.s were located were also the sites of munitions dumps, aerodromes, transport vehicle pools, and the like, they were targets of German bombing raids.)

Dr. Lower's team was scheduled for the night shift. On July 25, they went on duty at 9:30 p.m."amidst a terrific bombardment," and except for a meal break, remained at the operating table until 8 a.m. the next morning.[51] They had done 18 cases during the night, including three amputations.

Four days later, on July 30, Dr. Lower noted in his diary that "'we go over the top' at dawn tomorrow." Personnel at the C.C.S.s had spent the day preparing supplies, overhauling instruments and sharpening knives "in great abundance, for cutting is quite the order of the day when work begins."[52] The third battle of Ypres — known to those who fought it as "Passchendaele" — was about to begin.

C.C.S. No. 10, where Dr. Lower's team was stationed, was about eight miles from the front line. On the morning of July 31, it had eight teams and eight tables, ready and waiting.

> The first cases began arriving at about 7 a.m. and continued to come in steady streams, and by the scores until at the end of 24 hours over 2000 had been taken in. Operations began at 8 and went on continuously for 24 hours at all tables. At the end of that time we had done 224 operations, but only a part of the whole number had been operated. Cases arriving in the morning could not be reached until late in the afternoon or night. Then the delayed cases kept coming, cases that could not be reached by the stretcher bearers or were lost in shell holes. Trains were arriving and leaving, taking their load on to the Base Hospitals....The flood of arrivals was too great for the surgical teams to grind out and at the end of the day (24 hours) only a part of the work had been done. The acute cases were now chronic — legs and arms that could have been saved 12 hours ago were now necessarily amputated, or many that were still saved became gangrenous (gas gangrene) on the second and third days and were then amputated. The comparatively clean cut surgery of the first 12 hours now became a stinking putrid mess of cutting and slashing.[53]

On this first day, Lower, Roche, Grundies, and Harbaugh worked for 22 consecutive hours — 39 operations performed, on one table, with one crew.

"I was genuinely proud of these, my children," wrote Dr. Crile after hearing about it. "I threw them on their own resources and found they surpassed all my expectations." Later, he called them the "star team."[54]

After six hours of rest, they went back to work. That day too, and the following days, brought rain, mud, wounded, and more wounded. Some Scottish soldiers came in walking, their kilts "stiff with mud."[55] Enemy soldiers made up part of the caseload; on August 2, Dr. Lower operated on seven Germans. By that time, the great rush of cases was beginning to slow.

CASUALTIES OF WAR
The first great rush of casualties encountered by Lakeside Unit members, in the summer of 1917, came from the Ypres salient, and consisted of shell and shrapnel wounds, "all badly infected." In late November, General Hospital No. 9 began receiving cases from the Cambrai front, which were cleaner: "Many of the wounds have needed nothing more than a re-dressing." One of the great tragedies of the First World War was the use of poisonous gas. Nurses found the care of gassed men, with damaged respiratory systems and skin burns, especially challenging. Respiratory treatment was "symptomatic and supportive," including inhalations, alkaline gargles, and administration of oxygen. Treatment of burns to the eyes and nasal passages consisted of sodium bicarbonate solution douches, followed by sterile albonine. Orderlies had to sprinkle dampened sawdust on the floors before sweeping, so that irritating dust would not be raised.

A week later, Dr. Crile arranged for Dr. Lower and his team to be transferred from C.C.S. No. 10 to No. 17, where he himself was working. Here, too, work went on against all odds. On the night of August 17, a German bombing raid repeatedly interrupted surgery. In the operating theater the instruments on the tables, the windows in their frames, the earth itself shook. The lights were cut; patients who could move got off the tables in the dark and lay down on the floor with the medical officers and nurses.

But the first days of Passchendaele at No. 10 could never be forgotten. "Of all gruesome things, I have seen none to equal these blood-besmeared wrecks of humanity lying all about — cheerless, drawn faces — silent, suffering human beings, looking more like so much scrappage of inanimate material than anything which we are wont to call human beings."[56]

The Base Hospital

The patients who lived went on from the C.C.S.s to the base hospitals. Every once in a while, Lakeside Unit personnel at No. 9 would discover from a man's field tag that he had been operated on by one of their own surgeons at a C.C.S. Some patients underwent additional surgery at No. 9; some needed nursing and medical care on the wards; some "walking wounded" could be cared for at the Surgical Dressing Tent. The tent, staffed by three nurses, one officer, and two orderlies, was an innovation instituted at No. 9 by the Lakeside Unit to care for the large number of slightly wounded cases received there.

> The cases are paraded to the dressing tent....The infected cases are treated for such a time — generally only a few days — until the wounds are sufficiently clean to admit of excision and suture. Excision of the wound, or revision of the edges, as may seem best, is done under local anesthesia or N2O - O, in the small operating hut, and the wound is then sutured, primary union resulting in more than 95 per cent of the cases.[57]

Other cases received at No.9 were much more severe. Even though anti-tetanus serum was given as soon as a wounded man reached a field ambulance, some patients still developed tetanus. One man who came into No. 9 had had his entire elbow shot away. Although his wound was doing nicely, some twitching in his leg was noted, and later in the day, his jaws became locked. He was given 4500 units of serum subcutaneously in the early evening, and 5000 units into the spine during the night. "At morning rounds Captain Sanford gave orders that the serum was to be pressed....Miss Dunlap was detailed as a special nurse. She said there was no great arching of the back, partially because of the inability to use his leg, but at any noise or jar he did so slightly. She gave morphine every half hour....No attempt was made to push nasal feeding."[58] Despite these efforts, the man died.

As Dr. Lower had noted, infection was perhaps the greatest surgical problem of the war. Surgeons faced with infected wounds, as well as medical men fighting respiratory, gastrointestinal, and other infections, had no antibiotics to help them. Since no clearly effective way of dealing with infected wounds was available, Dr. Crile instituted a trial of five of the various methods being employed by the British and French medical services. Three of them involved the use of Dakin's solution (an antiseptic containing sodium hypochlorite); the others used salt or B.I.P. (bismuth, iodoform and paraffin). Initially, Eusol (a form of Dakin's solution) and B.I.P., or Bipp, seemed to be the most effective

QUIET, PLEASE
Excessive noise, especially at night, has always been a problem on hospital wards. At General Hospital No. 9, administrators ordered night nurses and orderlies to "move quietly about the wards, avoiding the noisy heavy stepping which so often occurs. Doors and stoves must be opened and closed quietly and loud talking absolutely prohibited." However, ward staff could not care for severely wounded patients and incoming convoys in total silence. Nurses satirized their own efforts to enforce quiet: "Nurses should severely deal with all patients who disturb the night shift between the hours of 9:00 and 6:00 a.m. Orderlies coming on the wards for convoy patients in the night add a gay and festive air by singing. It is also suggested that a clog step would be appreciated by the long-suffering patients."

at No. 9, but Dr. Lower was of the opinion that "the antiseptic plays a minor part, and that free drainage and the resistance of the patient largely solves the problem. All ragged wounds, where possible, are excised....All foreign bodies, where feasible, are removed early....The nest in which the foreign body is found is then excised, leaving no area of infection present."[59] Nursing care — attention to dressings, to drains, to supporting and increasing "the resistance of the patient" — became a crucial factor in recovery.

One of the methods under trial, the Carrel-Dakin treatment, had shown great promise elsewhere. Developed by French surgeon and Nobel laureate Alexis Carrel, along with chemist Henry Drysdale Dakin, it consisted of irrigating wounds with Dakin's solution at regular intervals. However, it was not at first effective at No. 9, and was on the point of being given up there when Katherine Lilly came to visit. Miss Lilly, a former Lakeside Hospital nurse, was now in France working with Dr. Carrel. During her stay she was able to supply "detailed instructions as to preparing and titrating the solution," and she also

> kindly consented to oversee the work during the few days that she will be here. Of course, one of the main objections to the method is that it takes so much time on the part of the nurse, and they have obviated that at Compiegne.... At stated intervals, the electric clock starts irrigation automatically in all the wards, and all the nurses have to do is to change the dressings once a day and flush the tubes and replace them.[60]

No. 9 did not have sufficient electric power to operate an automatic system, but it was decided to proceed with the use of Carrel-Dakin anyway; one of the medical officers was interested in the technique, and Nettie Eisenhard, the head nurse on his ward, was experienced in its use at Lakeside.

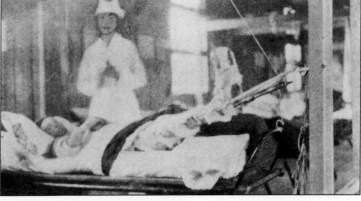

Other treatments being tried at No. 9 were: for infected joints, marsupialization, incision and drainage, or extensive lavage of joints; for compound fractures, Blake's system or the Thomas splint; and, for anesthesia, ether, chloroform, or nitrous oxide. "From the surgical side, each day emphasizes more and more that the greatest asset our Unit has at the present time, is the use of Nitrous Oxid anesthesia," declared Dr. Lower.[61]

THOMAS SPLINT
Dr. Crile, an indefatigable researcher, was active in investigating the effectiveness of various wound and other treatments. Nurses played a key role in administering treatments (for instance, irrigating wounds with specified solutions) and observing patients' progress. The Thomas splint was one of the methods used for the numerous compound fracture cases. Dr. Lower declared that the splint's "rebirth" during the war had "brought about a most striking improvement in the treatment of fractures of the femur."

Nitrous oxide anesthesia, administered by nurse anesthetists, was key to Dr. Crile's trademark "shockless surgery." The pioneer nurse anesthetist, Agatha Hodgins, had been a key member of the Lakeside Hospital team working at the American Ambulance Hospital in 1915; there, too, nitrous oxide anesthesia was a marvel to visiting physicians and patients alike, and training under Miss Hodgins a greatly coveted privilege. The Lakeside Unit anesthetists, Mary Roche and Josephine Cunningham, had learned from her at Lakeside Hospital and now, in their turn, began helping to train another generation of nurse anesthetists. Emily Colquhoun, Betty Connelly, Margaret Lane, Hester MacFarland, Mabel Allyn, Helen O'Brien, and Carrie Crites all received instruction through the nurse anesthetist training course instituted by the Unit early in 1918.

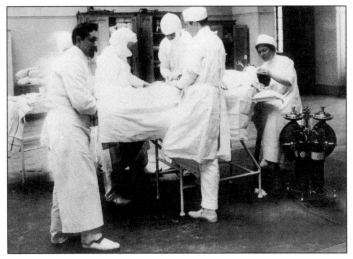

NITROUS OXIDE ANESTHESIA

Dr. Crile had long championed the use of nitrous oxide anesthesia, and preferred nurses as anesthetists. The photograph above shows Agatha Hodgins giving anesthesia at the American Ambulance Hospital in 1915; below, operating room nurses Iva Davidson and Ruth Roberts stand between an anesthesia machine and a liquid gas cylinder. American Ambulance patients who had previously undergone ether anesthesia testified to the superiority of nitrous oxide, saying they woke up more quickly and experienced no nausea. Nurse anesthetist Mabel Littleton heard one French soldier sing the Marseillaise "from beginning to end in very clear and distinct tones" while still anesthetized.

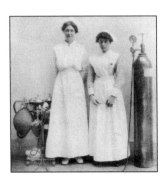

Nurses who specialized in administering anesthesia and assisting in the operating room were still relatively rare in the United States, and, of course, not all could go overseas and deprive the hospitals at home of their skills. In addition to providing anesthesia training, the operating theater at No. 9 served as a teaching center for nurses chosen for duty at the C.C.S.s. Out of the generalized pool of nurses who rotated from ward to ward at No. 9, a cadre of nurse specialists began to develop, who would add to the numbers available for hospital-based nursing after the war.

Eventful Arrival

On September 17 a third group of nurses for the Unit arrived. These reinforcements did come from the Cleveland area; 7 of them were Lakeside Hospital graduates, including 3 who were working as head nurses there. They had been a month on the way, and had had a close encounter with a U-boat on their last day at sea. "While the nurses were at dinner, there was a great jolt, the life boat signal blew, and everyone was rushed into life belts and found their places on the upper deck beside the life boats, where the young aviators sang "Pack up your troubles in your old kit bag and Smile, Smile, Smile."[62] The ship did reach port safely, despite sustaining damage in the form of "a hole as large as a man" (possibly caused by an American destroyer firing at the submarine). The 17 women, led by Lakeside head nurse Gertrude Schnaitter, reached Rouen, where they were assigned to duty the following day.

But they were not home safe yet. They had crossed the Atlantic by ship because that was the only way to travel. Airplanes were still very much of a novelty at this time — fragile things, they had wings of wood covered with fabric, and open cockpits. Although their use in freight and passenger transportation was negligible, airplanes were coming into their own as instruments of war. Air raids both terrified and fascinated people, at least at first. Having survived the U-boats, the 17 nurses next had to face the airplanes.

Only a night or two after their arrival, the bugle call that announced an air raid shrilled through the camp. Strangely enough, exactly the same thing had happened just after the arrival of the first members of the Unit in May. The second air raid warning at No. 9, like the first, sounded near midnight, as Ida Preston related.

> In the evening as we came from the Con Camp concert we noticed that the search lights were busy. At 11:30 we were all aroused by the Air Raid alarm. This means that we must all get up and dress in the dark, that no lights must be lit....Miss Allison in curl papers and felt slippers went to the administration building, where she reported to the C.O. Major Lower was out in pajamas, rubber boots, and steel helmet. The order to dress was just as carefully followed by the rest of the Unit, except the men, who are used to getting up at night for convoys and can dress quickly.[63]

Amy Rowland continued the story.

> A motley crew gathered around the huts awaiting orders. The medical officers at such times must report to their wards, nurses hold themselves in readiness for orders....After a little over an hour Colonel Gilchrist said we might lie down, but be ready to be called The safety signal did not come until three o'clock, just before a convoy came in....Miss McKee when she came back from the C.C.S. told us that when there was an air-raid there she put on her steel helmet, tied a wash basin over her abdomen, and crawled under the bed. So we told the [new] girls that Colonel Gilchrist had said they could go to bed, but if a later alarm came to put pails over their heads, hold wash basins over their abdomens and crawl under the huts and I have been told that some of the girls began a search for extra pails and basins, as only one of each is supplied to a hut. There was no excitement. Everyone was ready for anything. A good deal of quiet fun and complete good humor.[64]

With the eventful arrival of the additional Lakeside women, the No. 9 nursing staff reached its full complement of just over one hundred, although some nurses from other units were later assigned to the hospital on a temporary basis.

The nursing staff was divided into two shifts, day and night — day nurses came on duty at 7:30 a.m., night nurses at 7:30 p.m. When the caseload was light to normal, a 3-hour break was allowed during the shift, so that although nurses were not actually working 12-hour days, they were, for all practical purposes, working split shifts. Nurses also had a half-day off each week, plus "unassigned" days at intervals and two or three weeks of leave per year. However, during the many periods of heavy work when the census was high, especially before, during, and after major battles, shifts were extended, leaves canceled, and 16-hour days not unusual.

Off-Duty

During their off-duty hours, the nurses could go to Rouen, form sightseeing parties to local attractions, take walks in the woods, and attend concerts and theatrical entertainments at the British base's convalescent camp. In their quarters, they could write letters or read, talk, or play cards. Once in a while, the Unit held a dance. Unit members received invitations to parties, sporting events, and other amusements from the other American hospital units at Rouen as well as from the British. Although the nurses attended sports mostly as spectators, they occasionally participated as well.

> Not content with baseball honors won by the Cleveland Base Hospital Unit No. 4 team now on duty in France, Miss Mabel Allyn, nurse with the unit, has brought fame to the feminine members of the Sixth City Squad....While 3,000 nurses, officers, and privates of other bases witnessed and cheered events on the British Royal Engineers' sport program, Miss Allyn won an auto driving contest, outstripping a field of fourteen male members.[65]

Every week the nurses held a tea for officers. Tea, and conversation with American women, were sure draws for British guests; the Unit's own officers attended less frequently, or for different reasons. "I am always there in a front seat, largely because I get something to eat," Captain Henry Sanford said bluntly.[66]

AT RISK

Infectious disease generally posed a greater threat than enemy fire to wartime medical workers. Lakeside Unit nurses suffered from colds, influenza, and erysipelas — a skin infection more common as well as more serious in the days before antibiotics. Surgeons and operating theater nurses were especially susceptible to infections of the hands and fingers. By today's standards, preventive measures were haphazard. Chief Nurse Allison had to make a special request that "gowns and gloves be provided for the wards for the bad dressings." Overall, the Unit was fortunate in that no deaths occurred among its members while overseas. Diseases including meningitis, pneumonia, and influenza claimed the lives of other health workers stationed at Rouen base hospitals, including a nurse temporarily attached to the Unit.

NURSING NEWS
The Unit's night nurses put together a comic newsletter, which they called "Hot Dressings." In it, they lamented the difficulty of sleeping in the daytime — "In passing the Night Sisters' Hut, never speak to your slightly deaf friends unless they are at least fifty yards distant" — and made fun of their uniforms. "The prevailing color for the coming season... is dove grey. Skirts are to be worn not more than six inches below the knee...and white overdress not more than ten miles below the hem of skirt." The "Want Column" included an ad for: "A few high speed nurses for night work, with ten pairs of hands, a dozen pairs of feet, all rubber heeled, patience of Job, a low, sweet voice. It is quite essential that they enjoy admitting and discharging at least 30 patients on both wards at the same time, with a dozen or so operations gratis, on the side."

In general, Unit members declared their food adequate enough, if somewhat monotonous. Nurses, medical officers, and enlisted men all had separate messes, but similar menus. Staples of canned "bully beef" and beans were occasionally varied by fresh meat and vegetables. By the end of the war, supplies were growing scarce, and some rations, notably bread, were cut down. Sugar, not plentiful to begin with, became a much-coveted luxury. The loss in transit of a promised box from home containing candy and shoes was a great disappointment to stenographer Ida Preston. "Personally, I could cry if anyone looked at me. I have been living for weeks in the hope of having a taste of candy again, and its loss is nearly as keen as that of the shoes, even though it is impossible to buy shoes over here."[67]

The nurses' mess and living room was a separate building in the center of the section of the camp containing the nurses' and civilian women's quarters.

> We live in wooden huts. A long hall runs down one side from which eight rooms open, so that each hut houses sixteen nurses. A few of us are fortunate to room alone....We are fortunate to have cold running water in the huts and if one is up early she may get hot water at a faucet outside the kitchen hut, but the supply is quickly exhausted. There is a bathtub in each hut, where cold baths are easily obtained.[68]

Some, like Miss Preston, enjoyed the companionship of roommates and neighbors just down the hall. "We are all very nicely settled by this time. Miss Barney and I were given single iron beds with springs and mattresses, and that is all in the way of furniture." Having obtained or made a few other furnishings, they had "quite cozy quarters....it is pretty hard to find a time when there is not something interesting to do. In fact, it is just like college dormitory days again." Arvilla Walkinshaw felt less enthusiasm but accepted her lot with good humor, as she expressed in a letter: "This is being written in a very spasmodic way - some prisoners are building a duck pond and chicken yard outside my window, my room-mate is making coffee on an oil stove at my elbow, and my neighbor is discussing French lessons."[69]

The wooden huts, roofed with corrugated iron — "which affords much pleasure to those who especially enjoy the sound of a downpour of rain," noted Miss Allison — gave adequate shelter during mild weather. But as the days shortened, and winter drew near, comfort grew as scarce as sugar. The first sign of things to come was strict rationing of the oil for the stoves used to heat the nurses' rooms. Sociability gained practical value as nurses took turns visiting each other in the evenings, and conserving their rations of oil, while enjoying the warm stove in a friend's room, or the coal fire in the mess, where they could now stay until bedtime. "However, we are all warm and cozy at night for we all have plenty of bedding, warm gowns and a fine woolly sleeping bag, the latter being given us by the London Chapter of the American Red Cross."[70] But then, there was morning.

> I wonder if you don't hear our groans over there when the six o'clock bugle blows and we have to roll out into this cold, cold world. The water pipes are all frozen and many bursting and if a few more floors are flooded we will soon have a skating rink. Try to use the wash cloth, and it is frozen stiff—try to clean your teeth, tooth paste frozen—go to put on your shoes, feet so swollen with chilblains you can't get into them. For over a week I had to wear my bedroom slippers with a large pair of arctics which another girl loaned me, but I got there just the same. But, again I say, we are all well and want to stay here. This is a wonderful experience for all of us.

We are being taught many things—the chief of which is to economize, and how to get along happily with what we have and be thankful we have it. We are all wearing two pairs of woollen stockings, the night nurses wear three pairs, and we wear two sweaters under our heavy capes or coats, and when we get ready for bed we put on everything we can get our hands on except the stove and the lamp. Our extra oil arrived today from Paris, and now we are happy because we can have one pint of oil a day instead of every other day.

Here's a new remedy for bursting water pipes: Yesterday one of the nurses was clever enough to chew up some gum and plugged one of the pipes with it until she could find somebody to turn the water off. I tell you, necessity is the mother of invention in the army.[71]

Once on duty, nurses found no relief from the cold. Tents and wooden huts of the same type housed the hospital's patients. In January 1918, Miss Allison wrote: "Water is cut off for three days again, and fuel is scarce at present. Air, especially around the freezing point is plentiful. Our huts are built similar to rough summer buildings and ours especially is up two feet from the ground, making the floors very cold. Our wards have registered 32 and 36 F. during the warmest hours of the day, and with fires."[72]

Even under these conditions, the patients had few complaints. "Some of them have not had any sleep for days and nights, and occasionally we get a man who has lain out wounded in a shell hole for periods varying from one to four days, often without food or water and perfectly helpless." For such men, the baths, the clean white sheets, the hot food, and the professional care and the kindness they received from nurses, doctors, and orderlies alike, made No. 9 seem like heaven, at least compared to where they had been. "Oh, my God!" was the reaction of one new patient when he saw the cocoa and toast a nurse had made for him.[73]

Taking Care of Tommy

Over and over, the Lakeside Unit nurses and physicians expressed affection and admiration for the British soldier.

> Our patients here are all English Tommies and they are without doubt the most absolutely wonderful set of men I ever handled.... instead of complaining, you have to pry their troubles out of them. When I make my morning rounds and ask them how they are feeling, they give me a bright smile and say, 'Champion,' or 'Not too bad,' or 'In the pink,' no matter if they are peppered with wounds and running a high fever.[74]

wrote Dr. Sanford. Minnie Strobel said exactly the same. "Oh, they are the nicest things, and in the morning when we go in and ask them how they are feeling they won't complain, but will say, 'Not too bad, sister,' and at the same time we know they must be suffering like the dickens. Some say, 'Well, sister, I'm all right within myself, but my arm or leg, etc., is a bit painful.'"[75]

For most members of the Unit, this was their first trip overseas and their first extended contact with citizens of another nation. In 1917 there were no passenger airlines, no transatlantic telephone lines, no television, and not even commercial radio broadcasts. The only way to hear the speech and learn the everyday habits of other peoples was through face-to-face encounters. Unit members spent a great deal of time with their "cousins" from Britain and

LANGUAGE BARRIER
Working in a British hospital, Lakeside Unit nurses had to learn British English, as well as the current slang of the battlefield. British soldiers were "Tommies," nurses were "Sisters," and the chief nurse was called "Matron." Customs also differed. Chief operating room nurse Clara Illig was at first astonished to find that for one-half hour every afternoon "even in our most strenuous times...we forget our work in the relaxation of a cup of tea." A Unit nurse and medical officer, greatly concerned about the "inflamed condition" of a patient's knees, finally discovered that he belonged to a Scottish regiment and wore a kilt into battle. The mysterious condition was only a sunburn.

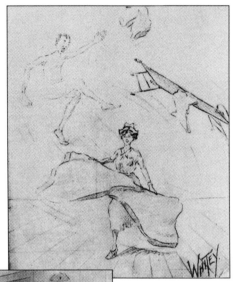

AS OUR BRITISH PATIENTS SAW US.

THE LIGHTER SIDE
Lakeside Unit nurses and physicians continually marveled at the plucky spirit shown by their British patients, many of whom had gone through horrifying experiences in the trenches. Some of the bedridden men made sketches to while away the time, including these comic pictures of a nurse making a bed and passing medications.

its Empire. They also learned something of the ways of their host country, France; they even met German prisoners of war. However, getting acquainted with the British was the easiest because just enough of a barrier existed, in vocabulary, pronunciation, and customs, to make things interesting without seriously hampering communication.

Lakeside women quickly became accustomed to being called "Sister" rather than "Nurse," by "Tommy." Members of the first contingent of nurses eventually learned enough British slang to be amused when a newly arrived nurse responded to a patient's plaintive remark, "Sister, I feel chatty," with the words, "I'm sorry, but I'm very busy this morning!"[76] For the British soldier, being "chatty" meant "having lice."

The single most important word, though, was "Blighty." "Blighty" meant England; it meant home and family. "Getting a Blighty" — being wounded badly enough to gain passage home — meant leaving the killing fields that the farms of France and Belgium had become, with their barbed wire, shell holes, and trenches, where the ground trembled underfoot for hours during artillery barrages, and men literally sank and drowned in a sea of mud. It meant no more "going over the top," no more killing, no more fear, no more death. By 1917, some of the troops had served for nearly three years, perhaps been wounded more than once, recovered, and returned to the front again. No one knew when the end of the war would release them. And among the new recruits and conscripts were very young men, in their teens, who might never been far from home before, certainly not under conditions like this. No wonder the longing for Blighty so deeply impressed, and at times shocked in its intensity, the women and men of the Lakeside Unit.

As they were brought in minus a leg or an arm, severely wounded, and we were wondering whether they would "make it," they would look up at us and say, "Sister, do you think it is bad enough that I'll get a 'Blighty?'[77]

The great song you hear here is 'Take Me Back to Dear Old Blighty,' and when we make our rounds in the hospital and mark a man's temperature chart with a big 'B' it means that he is well enough to travel and is going home. The patients soon learn all the symbols we use, and watch us like cats to see what we put on the charts. The look that comes over their faces when they see the 'B' is something that money couldn't buy.[78]

A big "B," for "blighty," means the man is so seriously wounded that he must be sent home for a while at least. And Tommy longs to see that "B." It must be a temptation to the doctors to put it there, just to see what we call the "blighty smile."

A "C" means the patient is ready to go to the 'con camp,' and that he'll be sent back to the trenches without a bit of "blighty."[79]

The purpose of the military hospital, though, was not to send Tommy back to "dear old Blighty." Dr. Crile assented to this; he also saw the inherent irony.

"Now the problem - surgical problem - is how can we get the men back? We must see that the lightly wounded get quick and good attention so they may return quickly into the line; and be wounded again; back again until they are finished."[80] American hospital units had been "lent" to the British to bolster their war effort until American troops and supplies could arrive in force. Dr. Lower expressed it thus:

> The position of the military surgeon is entirely different from that of the civilian surgeon. His object is to have empty rather than occupied beds. Line officers must furnish ammunition and materiel equipment; the surgeon's duty is to keep patching up and resupplying as rapidly as possible - men.[81]

Extraordinary Bond

However, keeping this longer, dispassionate view in sight could be very difficult when the faces of the men were so much closer. "There was always this extraordinary feeling of attraction between a wounded man and his nurse. I've never known anything like it. It was quite impersonal, but there was a sense of sympathy and understanding that was indescribable," declared a British nurse.[82] Spending days or even weeks not only watching, but nurturing, a man's physical recovery — and beyond that, talking to him, writing letters for him, admiring crumpled photographs of his family — the nurse could not but hope her

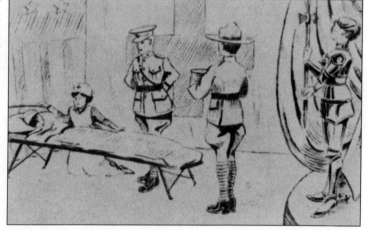

"boy" would get a "B." At least one Lakeside nurse decided to take matters into her own hands.

> The nurses were always fond of the Scotch soldiers. Their stories and the way they told them always held an appeal, and when they told the nurses of the wife they married just before they left, and of the babies or of the sick mother they had always supported, the nurses always wanted the lads chalked up "red" for Blighty, instead of "blue" for C.C. (Convalescent Camp) which eventually meant back to the Front.
>
> One day Major Lower, realizing the nurses' sympathies were with the lads, came in and talked to them, telling them their patients were soldiers, not civilians, and while cautioning them not to be emotional, but factual, in their judgment, he also reminded them that for every English or Scotch boy that went to Blighty, an American went to the Front to take his place.
>
> However, one day when he came in with his blue and red pencil to chalk up for C.C. or Blighty one of the nurses, Miss Autro White Engel [Mrs. Austa White Engel], knowing a little Scotch lad she had as a patient would never pass Major Lower for Blighty, hid him in the cupboard. As luck would have it, that day Major Lower, in inspection, opened that very cupboard and out sprawled the Scotch lad at his feet. He, of course, saw the humor of the situation. Although the boy did not get his blue mark that day, he did later, but after that Major Lower never went to a ward to chalk up again that he did not open all the cupboards and even the drawers.[83]

SERVICE
Another British soldier contributed a more serious view. While Unit personnel admired the courage and cheerfulness of their patients, patients appreciated the devoted care they received from the Americans. In this sketch, an enlisted man stands ready to take orders, while a medical officer evaluates the patient's condition, and a nurse kneels down beside the bed. The artist called the sketch "The Keynote of the American Hospital, Rouen: Service," and added a figure of the French heroine Joan of Arc at the right-hand side of the picture, possibly to represent the idea of service.

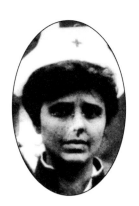

AUSTA WHITE ENGEL
Mrs. Engel, who tried to save
one of her patients from being
sent back to the front by hiding
him in a cupboard, was one of the
few nurses in the Unit who had
been married. From Warren, Ohio,
she was a 1904 graduate of the
Lakeside Hospital nursing school.
She returned to Warren to work as
a private duty nurse. After a short
first marriage she resumed her
career, as a public health nurse
in Cleveland. Following the war,
she remarried and moved to
Cranford, New Jersey.

This episode, more than any other, illustrates the paradox of the nurse at war, as well as the limitations of her role as the "physician's hand." It also shows that individual nurses were, upon occasion, prepared to go beyond those limits. The Unit's physicians themselves struggled with the same issues. Medical officer Arthur Eisenbrey went to the forward line of battle, partly at his own request, to make some observations and obtain some research material for Dr. Crile. After the younger man returned from the expedition, Dr. Crile found him "stretched out on a cot. His first words were: 'I had no idea it was like that.'" His friend and fellow officer Marion Blankenhorn explained Dr. Eisenbrey's mood thus: "I think he realized the uselessness of most of what we were doing and the uselessness of war itself."[84]

The nurses were fortunate in not having the responsibility of deciding whether to "chalk up" a man for Blighty or send him back to the front. Their differing responsibilities had the effect of bringing them closer to the patients. "In no case is the physician or surgeon always there," Florence Nightingale had observed.[85] The constant attendance of the nurse, in her role as the physician's hand, brought with it, in a very natural, unselfconscious way, another role — that of patient advocate. On occasion, as in the case of the little Scotch lad, these two roles came into conflict.

Most cases did not involve such dilemmas. One very young British soldier came to No. 9 with a badly infected gunshot wound in his left hip, with joint involvement. Since he had not "been up" at the line for long yet, his skin was still fair, not bronzed like that of most soldiers, and his youth made him "the admiration of everyone." But his condition continued to deteriorate. Edith Morgan, the nurse in charge of his ward, suggested that seeing his parents might help him more than anything else, so Dr. Lower "said he might be visited. On the 14th his mother and father came over to see him and it was soon quite apparent that their presence gave him renewed hope and he [became] more cheerful and looked better than ever before."[86]

The nurses of the era understood very well that caring for the patient involved attention to his status not only as an individual or a soldier, but also as a member of a family. "We write letters for our patients, read letters that have arrived or talk with them about their loved ones." Responsibility extended to the end of life, and beyond. "I have five more letters to answer, but they are sad ones and I dread to write them, but it is a part of our duty and must be done. Yesterday I wrote seventeen letters to families whose husband, son or brother had either died or was about to."[87]

Short of hiding them in cupboards, the Lakeside Unit nurses still went above and beyond the call of duty, and occasionally outside the bounds of the regulations, in taking care of their "boys." Often this involved getting special "treats" for them — usually edible. The Professional Council's regulation against giving extra food to patients was disobeyed almost as soon as issued. The Council's minutes for July 30 recorded that "Major Gilchrist said he had again found the nurses furnishing food for the patients, speaking particularly of Miss Strobel, who had provided sardines for her ward the day before."[88]

Elizabeth Bidwell, a Lakeside graduate who had come at the end of the summer with the second group of reinforcements, risked the wrath of the commanding officers to obtain an ordinary potato.

She had as a patient a very ill little Scotch lad, who above everything else wanted a "spud." He so yearned for a "spud," and since he was not going to get well anyway, Miss Bidwell thought he might as well as not have a bit of happiness. So in the dark of evening she went out and pulled up a row of "spuds" [from the vegetable gardens planted between the huts] and kept them for the little Scotch lad, giving him one of those stolen potatoes a day.

Major Lower who as C.O. had the reputation of knowing everything and being infallible so far as being fooled was concerned, noticed the empty row. For several days that empty row was a subject of much conversation, but Miss Bidwell said she was not going to confess - and the Scotch laddie had his wish fulfilled.[89]

The nurses were careful to cater to British tastes, as Mabel Horn recalled in later years.

I came from Bellevue, Ohio, and my sister, Dr. Dora Horn, was practicing medicine there. One of her English patients always brought her English fruit cakes at Christmas. So early in November I wrote my sister and said "if I could just have one of Mae's fruit cakes for my boys." At that time I did not know that my letters home were being published in the "Bellevue Gazette." When that letter came out, the town responded.[90]

The parcels sent contained 50 pounds of fruitcake, 50 pounds of sugar, cookies, candy, games and a gramophone. Miss Horn and her colleagues also realized that their patients might like liquid refreshments even better than fruitcakes, and planned ahead for Christmas. "The patients were all very fond of stout, the English version of Canadian Ale, but the supply was limited to only the very sick and had to be requisitioned from headquarters. Little by little, the nurses ordered more than they needed until they had a bottle for every man in the hospital."[91]

In the end, it seems, the Professional Council gave up, and admired.

The work of the nurses is beyond praise. They have given lavishly of their skill and energy; they have given all their thought, and despite all that could be done to the contrary, they have given much of their money for individual things they wished to do for their patients; they have earned the unstinted praise given them by their patients; they have been dignified in their bearing, and wherever seen, have been universally respected by soldiers and civilians.[92]

Christmas, 1917

Holidays, especially Christmas, drew all people at No. 9 — nurses, patients, enlisted men, and medical officers — into a unit. They all had learned what war could do to the mind and body, a knowledge that outsiders, even their own families, did not share. During the day's festivities, at least, the hospital became home, and everyone there, family. "We are all convinced that we have never spent as impressive and satisfactory a Christmas as we did yesterday. As for many of us being homesick, none of us had a minute to wish we were home, and every time I thought of you it was with a feeling that I wanted you all here with me," wrote Minnie Strobel to her family in Massillon, Ohio.[93]

Snow began to fall in mid-December 1917. Major Lower, at that time the C.O., worried that the base would not be able to deal with any significant

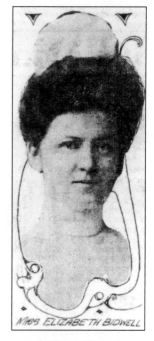

ELIZABETH BIDWELL
Bessie Bidwell, evidently a woman of determination, went out after dark and raided a Unit vegetable garden to satisfy a patient's craving for potatoes. Miss Bidwell graduated from the Lakeside Hospital nursing school in 1905; the above photograph shows her in the round cap worn by the Hospital's nurses at the beginning of the century. She spent her civilian career, which spanned nearly fifty years, in private duty nursing. Many of her cases were Cleveland Clinic Hospital patients. She was one of Dr. Crile's favorite private duty nurses and cared for him during episodes of illness near the end of his life.

winter storm. "But after noting the cheer, exultation and delight of the Sisters and men, I quite changed my mind. They all acted as though this was a message from the States and instead of being in the least depressed or feeling unequal to the task, they enjoyed it as school children do."[94]

The diaries and correspondence of Unit members contain a striking number of references to familial relationships. Just as Dr. Lower compared the "Sisters and men" to children, so the nurses referred to him, and especially to Dr. Crile, as a "father." "Major [Crile] is back and it seems more like home when he is here, although Major Lower makes a splendid father for our family," wrote one nurse. "We were most happy to have Major Crile come back to us, as we are all so very fond of him, and we do feel a real protection when he is about; he is so kind and just to us all," declared another.[95]

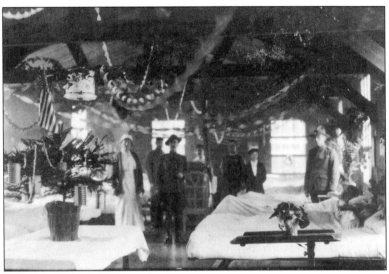

FIRST CHRISTMAS
In 1917, British soldiers lived through their fourth wartime Christmas. For Lakeside Unit personnel, it was the first Christmas spent away from home. Like members of a family, nurses, enlisted men, and patients worked together to decorate their wards. "You can imagine the surprise and exclamations of the patients when the Americans appeared with loads of greens and turned the wards all into a tea garden. The patients...helped every way they could — every man who had two arms and hands helped, and even some with only one arm.... All the bed patients that were able made all kinds of fancy things out of paper and pretty shades for the lights."

To the nurses, the enlisted men and the patients were "our boys." Of course, during World War I as during many other wars, everyone referred to soldiers as boys. But the everyday use of the expression, along with the British designation of the nurse as "sister," tended to promote the notion of hospital as family; and at Christmas, when real families were absent, the little fiction almost seemed to come true. On top of their regular tasks, nurses devoted much time and effort to providing decorations, sweets, Christmas stockings, and small presents for the soldiers in the hospital.

On Christmas Eve, a group of orderlies, nurses, and officers, accompanied by a small organ and two violins, sang Christmas carols in each ward. The patients "sang with us as hard as they could sing. The men's voices are wonderful, and on every ward, when we were about to leave they would say, 'Oh, please just one more.' By the time we finished nobody had much voice left. We had 200 new patients come in during the night, but we were prepared for any emergency."[96] On Christmas morning, in addition to the stockings, the patients enjoyed a special breakfast of sausage, eggs, and fruit.

Then the rest of the morning had to be spent as usual, attending their dressings, etc., and getting ready for the big tea in the afternoon [which] was the most satisfactory performance of all our festivities. The nurses on each ward carried out their own plans. We sent to London and purchased sixty pounds of fruit cake and some smaller cakes, then a lot of nurses from America were fortunate enough to have a box or two come through from America which contained fruit cake, and one nurse had flour and sugar sent to her with which she made delicious doughnuts. Besides the patients, each ward took in a number of our enlisted boys for the tea....The refreshments on each ward varied somewhat according to the different nurses' ideas, but consisted chiefly of ham sandwiches, cold beefloaf, cake, fruits, nuts, tea and coffee, all they could eat....For one whole afternoon everybody forgot there was ever a war....With the weather so cold and water pipes bursting everywhere, we didn't have a drop of water on the grounds fit to use, and the enlisted boys had to go a distance of nearly half a mile and carry every drop of water for the tea, drinking water, wash water and dish water, but even that didn't make any difference. In one of the tents over 200 men were served....The wards were beautiful — no two alike — and it was such fun going from one to another and seeing the different ideas carried out and it was marvelous what could be done with what we had to do with.[97]

Dr. Lower summed up the day thus:

I have never seen a finer Christmas spirit displayed than was shown here by all of the personnel of this Unit. The Sisters, especially, showed unusual ingenuity and cleverness in converting the crude wards into veritable fairy lands, with holly, ivy and mistletoe, gathered from the woods and fields nearby....

No two wards were alike — each had the individual touch of its keepers — no hired decorators — no expensive gifts — real old-fashioned stockings made by tender hands. Not in many years have I seen this. The old time Christmas of our younger days was once more put on the stage, and I was amazed to find how far the modern Christmas had gotten away from the old time one, how the commercial Christmas had surely covered up and smothered the real Christmas of the individual, and how the dollar had displaced and removed the one great pleasure of Christmas — the giving of one's self.[98]

The Spring Offensive

During the Unit's stay in France, holidays and special occasions often seemed to fall when the hospital was most busy. At the time of the memorable Christmas of 1917, No. 9 was just getting back to normal after a great rush of work at Thanksgiving. Before Easter, in the last weeks of March 1918, the Germans began a huge offensive, driving forward toward Paris. It began with a gas attack; No. 9 took in more than 500 gassed cases.

Then, the wounded began to pour in as never before, not in regular convoys, but continuously. On March 23 four operating teams worked all day long, and two worked all night. Stenographer Ida Preston was assigned to work in the operating theater on a 12-hour shift. Anne Upham, the Unit's dietitian, spent part of her days on Ward 1, making beds. Miss Allison sent her assistant nurses back to the wards and coped with the administrative work alone.

The midnight census, as Easter Sunday (March 31) began, was 1,740 patients, 100 more than No. 9's crisis capacity. During the previous 24 hours, 1,078 cases had come through — this remained the record for the hospital. By April 2, the operating theater had been running continuously for 12 days, averaging 100 patients per day. "We have head wounds, chest wounds, abdominal wounds, cases never seen here primarily. Americans are coming down wounded, some from the 6th Engineers, some from our Aviation companies."[99]

Providentially, a box of supplies arrived during the rush. "The Parker handles and blades I took at once to the theatre, and they were greeted with shouts of joy, for with the heavy work of the past week, the knives were getting very dull."[100]

Minnie Strobel, now the Unit's Assistant Matron, had returned to work on the wards full-time during the crisis. She described the situation in the hospital:

Well, I guess the very greatest battle since the battle of Waterloo is now in progress, and there is a line of ambulances driving into our camps constantly. Our nights now are just like our days, there is no difference. Yesterday — just alone in one day — we admitted and discharged 1,078 patients. I say discharged, this does not mean they are well; it only means they are able to be moved on to another hospital, so we can take in more. They go out on stretchers. We are now away above our capacity and last night any man who had a bed all to himself certainly had a luxury, and he only had it because he was too bad to accommodate anybody else.

We have them packed in like sardines. Two beds were put together so we could put in three patients. Besides this, there were many straw ticks on the floor, and men on the floor just on a blanket. Even this did not do the work. There were [deleted by censor] sitting up here and there all night because there wasn't another space available for them to lie, even on the floor....

They are right from the trenches, in their uniforms. Many that came in yesterday didn't have a bit of nourishment, or a bite to eat, for four or five days, and such wounds you never saw. Many die, and any number with arms, legs, hands and feet off.

We have many mothers, fathers and wives here now and you know what that means, the poor things are only permitted to come when there is no hope for anything but death.[101]

From March 21 to April 3 the "special cases" operated by the Unit were: 39 cases of gas gangrene; 100 amputations; 56 knees; 35 chest cases; 12 hemorrhages; 13 fractured femurs; and 140 other fractures.

An unnamed enlisted man gave a graphic account:

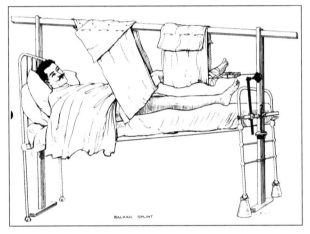

BALKAN SPLINT
This device proved a simple, inexpensive, and effective way to suspend an injured arm or leg. It cost about 23 cents, according to Dr. Crile, who also noted that patients could use it "for light housekeeping," as a clothes rack or hat tree. Remarked stenographer Ida Preston, who accompanied Dr. Crile on rounds, "I was surprised at the way the patients in the big over-bed Balkan splints are able to move about in bed. Some of them can nearly sit up in bed, and all seem to move about quite freely."

I think our fellows never worked so hard in all their lives as they were up most of the night and all of every day carrying stretchers and working in the operating theatre. The theatre with six tables worked day and night for six days without a single rest, the doctors and nurses working on eight hour shifts and the orderlies on twelve. I shall never forget the third night after the offensive began; - after working all day Speck and I carried stretchers until long after midnight and of course we had the opportunity of watching our three best surgeons at work. Talk about a slaughterhouse or butcher shop. Just imagine what it would be like to have a hundred, yes five hundred men, in the wards, out in the yard, everywhere waiting for their turn to get on the table - with wounds of all descriptions in every part of the human anatomy. Imagine men with stinking, gangrenous, dangling arms and legs waiting from three in the afternoon until after midnight for their turn on the table - to hear them shrieking - moaning - begging - dying. But it sure is fascinating to stand in the theatre and watch three doctors and the nurses, and orderlies taking care of six tables all at the same time. It is funny to hear the men going under the anesthetic and coming out. Believe me, you hear the worst swearing and cursing and bits of obscene language ever invented.

Just to give you an idea of what is likely to be taking place at the same time: At the farthest table there will be a man with his intestines shot in two, and the doctor has them out on a table sewing them up; on the next table is a man with his leg shot off and a shrapnel wound in his shoulder; on the next is one with a bullet in his brain and probably a piece of his skull taken out; on the next is one with his lower abdomen and lungs punctured with shrapnel; while on the next table there is a poor devil with a gangrenous leg which smells so badly one can hardly stand it in the room.[102]

On top of the incredible amount of work, in the background was the possibility that the hospital would have to be evacuated if the German offensive came near enough. Early in the offensive, C.O. Major Lower was preparing for this. "As the hospitals had to be evacuated in 1914, we wonder if it may be repeated. I...am instructing all to have light bedding rolls and small haversacks in readiness; to get what rest and sleep we can and be ready for anything that may come along. While it seems a long way to the line in a country we do not know, yet measured in a known country, it is about as if the enemy were at Ashtabula or Sandusky."[103]

As it happened, the German advance was halted before it neared Rouen, and although the number of air raids on the city increased, No. 9 suffered no damage, and the Unit was not evacuated. However, several Unit personnel serving at a C.C.S. very near the front were.

> Dr. Barney, Dr. Brock, and Severn and Willyard returned from the C.C.S. which they had evacuated. They feared Dr. Harrison might have been captured. The following day Miss McKenney and Miss Schultz arrived, neither with any baggage except the bags they could carry, and their shoes slung over their backs. Miss Schultz had to get away in her operating room garb, she left so hurriedly. All her clothes were lost, and she had been separated from Dr. Harrison, and did not know where he was.[104]

"Beyond All Praise"

It was while serving in the C.C.S.s, and in Mobile Hospital No. 5 (organized to accompany the American army as it advanced in the late summer and fall of 1918) that Unit personnel came closest to the front and at greatest risk to their lives. During the time between July 1917, when the first three teams left, and the evacuation of the C.C.S.s in April 1918, a number of teams from the Lakeside Unit had served at the front, generally for periods of a few weeks to a few months. In that time, 12 Unit nurses worked at the C.C.S.s. Mary Roche and Josephine Cunningham, the Unit's two original nurse anesthetists, both took lengthy turns at the front. "I had three months at the Clearing Station and was really very fortunate inasmuch as I was twelve weeks at one end of the line and three weeks at the other end. It was a most interesting experience and while it was a bit too interesting at times, yet I did enjoy it very much. I was giving anesthetics for Dr. Shawan and Captain Graham."[105]

Dr. Crile felt that "the real work" of wartime surgery was being done at the C.C.S.s and that service there was a professional opportunity for the Unit's medical officers. Thus, he tried to make sure that as many of them as possible had this opportunity. "It is intended to give the older men a tour of duty at casualty clearing stations as opportunity affords. Assignments for duty will be made first with reference to the welfare of the unit - secondly with justice to the work - as far as seniority can be followed and these objects gained, seniority in Lakeside graduation will govern."[106] For the nurses, service had to be its own reward. At this time, a nurse had very limited upward career mobility. What mobility existed had little to do with the types of operations at which she

UNDER FIRE

During the German spring offensive of 1918, Lakeside Unit nurse Mary Ellen Schultz and her British nurse roommate, stationed at a C.C.S., awoke to the noise of a shell attack. They dressed and ran outside. "There an appalling sight met our eyes. An operating room not thirty yards away was a mass of kindling wood, while badly wounded men were lying on the ground a hundred or more feet away. Already medical men were carrying them to our operating room on stretchers. We followed after applying first aid dressing to the most seriously wounded.

...I learned that the hospital next to ours had already evacuated while orders for our removal were expected every minute. But there was no thought of packing our belongings....there were over a hundred wounded men to take care of, and we knew these would be followed by hundreds more.

...Our last operation was a transfusion on a chap who had had both legs shattered by a shell. We then set about binding up the wounds of the soldiers and packing them off in ambulances. Lockjaw treatments and some of the most critical dressings were given by everyone, including padres and enlisted men."

had assisted or the types of cases she had nursed; factors like the prestige of the nursing school she had attended were more important.

Occasionally, however, reward in the form of special recognition did come to the Unit's nurses. In June of 1918, during a visit to No. 9, the Matron-in-Chief of the British Nursing Service in France announced that Miss Roche and Miss Eisenhard were to receive the Royal Red Cross, the highest honor given to nurses by the British Crown. The American nurses had not expected the unusual public tribute: "These proved a very great surprise to everyone." The British Matron-in-Chief also told Lillian Grundies that she, too, would be receiving the Red Cross, although for some reason her name had not come through with the others. Miss Eisenhard received her medal for "bravery in remaining at work under shell fire in a casualty clearing station," according to a stateside newspaper. Inez McKee and Helen Briggs — also both casualty clearing station veterans — as well as Chief Nurse Allison and Colonels Gilchrist and Crile, were cited for their service by British Field Marshal Haig. Back home, local newspapers interviewed Miss Briggs' proud parents in North Olmsted, Ohio, and noted that "both girls [McKee and Briggs] are under 25."[107]

Another newspaper article featured the heroism of Mary Ellen Schultz during the evacuation of the C.C.S. to which she had been assigned. It quoted Lakeside Unit medical officer Lieutenant Benjamin Harrison (who did also return safely to the base after having been separated from Miss Schultz) as saying, "'She is the gamest little woman I ever saw.'" Dr. Crile, in a letter home to his daughter, speculated that the heroism of "Miss X" [probably Miss Schultz] kindled the interest of "a splendid looking young officer of the aviation corps...by his voice and manner a southerner" into love. Not finding her in when calling at No. 9 on his way to Paris, the aviator was about to leave when an officer said to him, "'I presume you know Miss X is a heroine. She was under terrible fire and stayed to rescue and help the wounded and had won everyone's praise and admiration.'...Thereupon the gallant officer asked with hesitation if it were possible to have paper to write a note. And thereupon he began writing furiously and getting up even greater speed when I left."[108]

On June 22, 1918, a "patriotic meeting" was held in Cleveland under the auspices of the Council of National Defense to reinforce support for the war effort. The speakers, from the United States, Canada, and England, all connected with the medical phase of the military campaign, gave the Lakeside Unit high praise, not neglecting to mention the nurses. One account of the meeting quoted the words of a Canadian medical officer who had been at the front. "I saw Miss Roche, Miss Briggs, Miss Grundies, Miss McKee at work at the C.C.S. I know from experience that their work is beyond all praise. I don't know what we should ever have done without them; yet they are only examples of your entire personnel."[109]

Mobile Hospital No. 5

No more teams from No. 9 worked at the C.C.S.s after the premature return of Miss Schultz, Lieutenant Harrison, and their colleagues. But in late summer, the A.E.F. began establishing its own mobile hospitals just behind the front lines where American troops were now fighting in large numbers. At Dr. Crile's request, Lakeside Unit personnel were assigned to staff a mobile facility, Mobile Hospital No. 5.

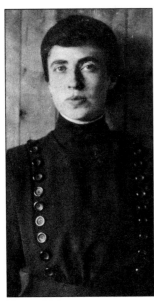

MARY JANE ROCHE
Shown here in uniform, Miss Roche was a highly skilled nurse anesthetist. In later years, Agatha Hodgins called her "one of the best I ever trained. From the first I knew she would be exceptional." Before the war, Miss Roche had worked as an anesthetist at Lakeside and Mt. Sinai Hospitals in Cleveland. After the war, she married naval commander W.L. Stevenson, but according to Miss Hodgins, "something went wrong" with the marriage. Mrs. Stevenson, a native of California, returned to the west coast and her chosen career, "doing a magnificent job" as chief anesthetist of Franklin Hospital in San Francisco.

Just now the excitement is over the formation of the new mobile unit, and the camp is in a ferment to know who are to be included in the personnel. I am glad I have not the job of selecting the twenty nurses, for about 80 are wild to go and some are sure to be sore, it they are not among the fortunate few. The men are not as anxious to go, as to remain behind, for the lure of the Sam Browne [i.e., the chance for an officer's commission and possible transfer to a combat unit; the "Sam Browne" was the belt worn by officers] seems to have most of them in its spell, and they are loath to lose their chance by leaving here.[110]

While at the C.C.S.s Lakeside nurses had worked only in the operating theaters, here some would be assigned to ward duty. Of the 20 nurses selected, Betty Connelly served as the head; Elizabeth Bidwell became the night supervisor; Mabel Horn, Clara Illig, Margaret Lane, and Mary Ellen Schultz were also among "the fortunate few."

In late September, No. 5 was sent to Bois de Placys, five or six miles behind the line — the most advanced hospital, according to Dr. Crile, for the imminent Meuse-Argonne offensive. Dr. Crile, although by this time Senior Consultant in Research for the entire A.E.F., also went with the mobile unit and performed the first surgery there. The site formerly had been a French barracks; existing barracks huts were used for the wards, and trucks equipped to serve as a mobile hospital housed the sterilizing plant, X-ray department, kitchen, and laundry. The bed capacity was 240, but expanded to 700 at its peak. Although reinforcements from other units more than doubled the original number of officers and men to 12 and 85, respectively, the nurse staffing remained constant at only 20. "Ward work was very heavy and depressing because of [the] shortage of nurses and men and lack of equipment," stated the mobile unit's commanding officer.[111]

Everything had to be camouflaged. During the frequent air raids in the vicinity, all lights had to be extinguished. Nurse Caroline Smith remembered this vividly, 20 years later.

> The air raids were bad, and the close bombing. It was particularly terrifying to care for patients in the dark....It was a madhouse caring for all those seriously wounded men without sufficient personnel and equipment.

MOBILE HOSPITAL NO. 5
Going to the front lines with the Unit's mobile detachment was a coveted assignment, although the work was hard and potentially dangerous. Some of its 12 medical officers, 20 nurses, and 85 enlisted men posed for a group photograph. Mobile Hospital No. 5 had 240 beds, but as many as 700 patients could be squeezed in at a pinch. Its personnel coped with air raids, mud, rats, and influenza while caring for the casualties of the Argonne offensive, many of them American.

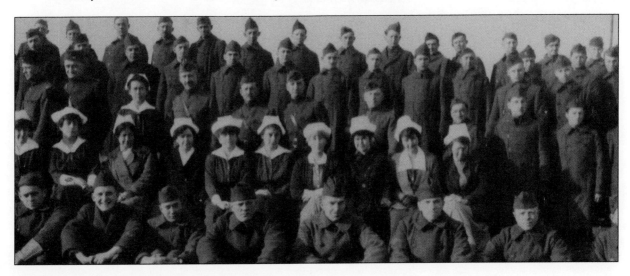

There were so many deaths, and that was the first time our unit had taken care of American soldiers in a large body. We were right next to the anti-aircraft guns, and bombs were dropping all around us.[112]

The hospital's location in a ravine helped protect it, but had two unwelcome consequences: mud and rats. Duck boards provided some solid footing, but everyone had to wear boots. The nurses slept in an old barn, and Elizabeth Bidwell told Dr. Crile that rats would "jump right up onto their beds."[113]

Mobile Hospital No. 5 began receiving casualties on September 25; on October 13 word arrived that the war had ended. It turned out to be false. Allied troops went into battle again the next day and from October 15 to October 21, 600 casualties, American, French, and German, came into No. 5.

"Everything is overflowing with patients. Our divisions are being shot up rapidly; there are many machine gun wounds....There is rain and mud and 'flu' and pneumonia." Even as the end of the war was in sight, the great influenza epidemic of 1918-1919 — less spectacular but more deadly than the war — had begun to claim its victims.

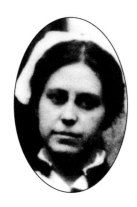

CAROLINE SMITH
Miss Smith lived an interesting and varied life. She was born in Mexico, where her father was a Methodist missionary. A member of the Lakeside Hospital nursing school class of 1911, she devoted much of her postwar career to child health and welfare, heading the Crippled Children's Division of the Cuyahoga County Health and Welfare Board. But her experience of caring for the casualties of war always remained a vivid memory. "There were so many deaths," she said, twenty years later.

Dr. Lower, now back in Cleveland, wrote to Dr. Crile of the situation at home. "We are in the throes of a very serious epidemic of influenza. Hospitals are crowded to capacity and overflowing with Flu cases, and the mortality rate is very high. It has reduced surgical work very materially. In fact, we are asked to operate on only essential cases. Many nurses are sick."[114] In the coming weeks, some Unit members would receive word of the deaths of parents or siblings.

While Mobile Hospital No. 5 coped with the casualties of the Argonne offensive, back at Rouen, the first and only death occurred among the personnel at No. 9.

This afternoon we buried the first member of our Unit to die — a nurse who joined us a few weeks ago, and had never been on duty a day. She was from Wisconsin. It is against censorship rules for me to give her name. The <u>Flu</u> has been very virulent here, and the St. Louis Unit has lost two of its enlisted men in the past three days. In fact, it seems to hit the Yanks harder than the Tommies around here. There were two Yanks buried with this nurse.[115]

The 20 nurses who went forward with the mobile hospital all eventually returned unscathed to No. 9.

By the end of October, the earlier intensity of the offensive was over. Returning to No. 5 after a brief visit to Rouen, Dr. Crile remarked in his diary that "all was serene, but few patients were in the house. Peace rumors were rife. In the evening there was a masquerade party with dancing....Many officers from neighboring areas dropped in and with infinite eagerness danced with the nurses." Another medical officer explained the "infinite eagerness" of both officers and nurses for dancing and socializing: "There was no place or time for recreation until after the main part of the offensive had ended. The old adage 'Work when you work and play when you play' was very closely adhered to."[116]

Finally, after more than one false rumor of the war's end, the real armistice came at last, on November 11, 1918.

On the night before the Armistice was actually signed the word was received to the effect that it would be signed at 11 the following morning.

44

Daybreak came and the heavy artillery moved out and the doughboys went over the top as usual and there were more than 300 casualties before the cease-fire orders came through. The hospital unit was so busy caring for the wounded that it was many hours before they knew that the war was over.[117]

Back at General Hospital No. 9, Unit members likewise learned that the war had ended while they were in the midst of caring for its casualties. "I was working on the wards when the news of the Armistice came," recalled Constance Hanna. "I was treating the gassed patients — putting drops in eyes, spraying noses and throats."[118]

Armistice and Home

"The celebration of Armistice Day need not be described. Its outward features were like those everywhere else — informal parades and hysterical rejoicings. But work went on for though the streams of freshly wounded ceased they were replaced by streams of returning British prisoners from Germany." Unit members devoted little ink to describing the celebrations of Armistice Day. Once the war was over, thoughts turned elsewhere. "I think the realization that at last we could really go home made us all homesick, whether or not we were aware of it at the time," mused Ida Preston. "Just as the Tommy always speaks of 'Blighty,' so the Yank always calls home 'God's own Country.' I was amazed to find what a home-loving race we really are!"[119] By this time, most Unit members had been away from home for a year and a half, and since there was no transatlantic telephone service, they had neither seen nor spoken to their families since May 1917.

The mobile hospital nurses returned to Rouen in late December 1918, the officers and men in January 1919. While at Bois de Placys, they had cared for 994 patients, of whom 135 had died.

In January of 1919 orders were issued to close General Hospital No. 9. Colonel Frank E. Bunts, the commanding officer at the time the war ended, wrote a report on the Unit's activities. At peak levels, 103 nurses, 34 officers, and 292 enlisted men served with the Unit at one time. During the 20 months that Lakeside Unit personnel had staffed No. 9, they had treated more than 68,000 cases and performed nearly 9,000 operations, plus 14,000 ambulatory treatments. Dr. Bunts summed up his report by declaring that in a situation in which"officers, nurses and enlisted men worked devotedly and to the point of physical exhaustion, it would be manifestly unjust to select individuals for special acknowledgment, where everyone is worthy of the highest praise for their cheerful, self-sacrificing conception of execution of their duty."[120]

Finally, on March 24, 1919, Chief Nurse Elizabeth Folckemer cabled that the Unit's nurses were departing France and sailing for the United States. Two weeks later they were mustered out at the demobilization headquarters in New York City; on April 9, at about noon, 39 of the Unit's nurses who lived in the Cleveland area arrived at Cleveland's Union Station. Gertrude Schnaitter, Nettie Eisenhard and Inez McKee, who had preceded their colleagues by a few hours as an "advance guard," remained at the station to greet them.

"Violets and Lilies for War Heroines!" proclaimed the newspapers. "The girls in blue are back."[121]

The publicity surrounding the return of the 'girls in blue' made a striking contrast with their quiet departure, when the Unit had "slipped away" almost

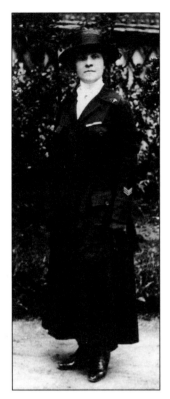

ARMY NURSE'S UNIFORM
At first, the dress uniform for Lakeside Unit nurses had been Red Cross capes over white dresses, and close-fitting white caps with the Red Cross insignia on the front. Duty uniforms, made for them in Europe, consisted of gray dresses (to save on laundering) with white aprons and stiff collars and cuffs. Eventually, as Reserve Nurses of the U. S. Army Nurse Corps, they acquired official dark blue military uniforms for outdoor wear. Army regulations specified that "white, tan, or black shoes, high or low, may be worn, but pumps, French heels and fancy shoes, will not be allowed; the U. S. pin and the insignia of the A.N.C. should be worn but not fancy pins or furs." Chevrons worn on the sleeve indicated length of overseas service; as members of the first American unit "over there," Lakeside Unit nurses could take pride in being the first to acquire them.

without notice. Now, as they prepared to slip back into the obscurity of the civilian nurse's life, Cleveland paid its tribute. Since the Lakeside nurses were "the first of [Cleveland's] war units home...and the longest of any from the city in service," their arrival marked the beginning of a two-day celebration the city put on to greet its daughters and sons returning from "over there."[122] An infantry unit and an engineering unit were scheduled to arrive at Union Station later on the same day.

"It was a pretty sight, as the long train drew past the hospital on the Lakeside avenue hill, to see scores of white-capped, blue-gowned nurses waving and cheering their returning sisters from the hospital windows. " At the train station, welcomes both public and private awaited them. "Mayor Davis had been scheduled to make a speech of welcome, but all idea of an orderly celebration went by the boards as the girls jumped from the train and rushed into the arms of friends and families." Asked by reporters to describe their experiences, nurses disclaimed the role of war heroines. "Why, we didn't do anything," nurse Isabel Bishop was quoted as saying.[123]

The Lakeside women also declined the honor of marching in the welcoming parade with the soldiers on the following day, being "anxious to spend the day in rest with their relatives and friends."[124] But they did turn out, in force and in uniform — by now the official U.S. Army Nurse Corps uniform, with four service chevrons on the sleeve — to greet their comrades, the Unit's officers, when the latter arrived home a few weeks later.

In May 1918, when the national nursing organizations had held their joint annual meeting in Cleveland, Grace Allison still had been in France. However, she had sent a report on the Lakeside Unit's work, which was read to the membership. In it, she had stated that "the true spirit of nursing prevails everywhere. Devotion to duty, with calm and steadfast courage amid indescribable scenes and conditions, has been a test of the contribution developed in each member thru their professional career. Every attribute of true character is given opportunity for expression, in which no member has been found lacking."[125]

The "true spirit of nursing" had been expressed in many ways by the Lakeside Unit nurses: by Marie Shields dressing the wounds of innumerable incoming patients and wishing she had more hands; by Minnie Strobel writing letters to the parents of the dead and dying men in her care; by Mary Roche giving anesthetics for 22 hours at a time, in her silk stockings.

Inez McKee matter-of-factly crawled under her bed, protected by a helmet and a washbasin, when the bombs began falling at the C.C.S. Arvilla Walkinshaw stated her forthright opinions on everything from the behavior of the enlisted men to Dr. Crile's weight ("he is — getting fat") in a letter to Mrs. Crile. Austa Engel hid a patient in the cupboard rather than send him back to the front. Caroline Smith stayed at the bedsides of wounded American soldiers at Mobile Hospital No. 5 during air raids, in the dark, even though she was frightened. They all, in their different ways, expressed "true character" — neither submissiveness, nor rebelliousness, but professionalism, and confidence, and compassion.

Four of the nurses still with the unit at the end of the war did not return with the others — Lillian Grundies, Katherine Devine, Margaret Tupper, and Lois Van Meter had requested and received additional tours of duty with the A.E.F. and remained overseas. So did Harriet Leete. Having returned to military nursing after her stint with the Red Cross child welfare project, she was stationed at a Red Cross military hospital when the war ended. An acquaintance wrote to Amy Rowland of her:

> A.R.C. Military Hospital #5, where Miss Leete is stationed, is being totally evacuated in about two weeks and the hospital itself is being made into a British rest camp. When I was there today, I saw Miss Leete and when I told her how glad I was to hear that the hospital was breaking up as I of course thought she would go home in view of her long service over here, she rather laughed and said - "No, indeed I am in the Army and I am here until the boys all go home and remember there are two million boys over here and I am glad to stay until they have all gone-".... I certainly admire her immensely. I guess I told you how the boys in the hospital adore her.[126]

Back to the Future

War makes strange bedfellows, the saying goes — and it makes for strange turnings in people's lives, too. Harriet Leete, who had devoted her career to reducing infant and childhood mortality, to working with babies and children and their mothers, took up a new duty born "amid the tumult of battle," among men. She became as beloved a figure at A.R.C. Military Hospital No. 5 as Florence Nightingale had been in the barracks at Üsküdar. Early in 1919 the Red Cross assigned her to service in Serbia. While there, she contracted typhus, which permanently weakened her health.

For most, the strangeness was no more than an interlude, although service in World War I was not an interlude that anyone could forget. Hundreds of memoirs, written by soldiers, nurses, and others who served on both sides of the front attest to this. Historians claim that the war shaped the experience, and subsequent attitude and behavior, of a generation. Nonetheless, life in the United States had continued to go on not so much differently than it had before. Members of the Lakeside Unit, like the rest of the American Expeditionary Force, took off their uniforms and returned to the lives they had left behind them, among their neighbors, co-workers, and families.

Several of the nurses were soon to have new families and would leave their careers upon marriage, as was customary. Joan Quinn, one of the "two brides" who married in France, had not had her destiny changed by wartime romance — she had been engaged to Captain David McClelland, a Lakeside Hospital physician, before going overseas with the Unit. Mary Roche, engaged to a naval commander, had also met her fiancé before the war. On the other hand, Mabel Horn did meet her future husband during service with the Unit — he was not one of the Tommies who drank the ale she saved for Christmas, but one of the Unit's enlisted men.

A number of the Unit's women remained in nursing. Elizabeth Folckemer, so successful as the Unit's second chief nurse, continued her career as a leader of nurses, becoming director of Cleveland's Visiting Nurse Association. Caroline Smith, who had tended wounded men near the front at Mobile Hospital No. 5, eventually left bedside nursing and became supervisor of the Crippled Children's Division of the Cuyahoga County Welfare Board.

Several of the nurses returned to Lakeside Hospital. Constance Hanna, the Unit's "baby," eventually headed the admitting office there, retiring in 1958, nearly 40 years after her return from Europe. Grace Allison, the Unit's first chief

A REMARKABLE CAREER

Harriet Leete's wartime service bore some remarkable parallels to the work of Florence Nightingale in the Crimea. Nationally known as a pioneer in child health nursing, Miss Leete, a Lakeside graduate (1902), went to Europe with the Lakeside Unit as assistant chief nurse. She was detached from the Unit to help organize the work of the American Red Cross Children's Bureau in France, but eventually returned to military nursing as chief nurse of A.R.C. Military Hospital No. 5. Like Miss Nightingale, she was "adored" by her soldier-patients. After the end of the war, she was assigned to the A.R.C.'s Commission to Serbia. The "deplorable" sanitary conditions she discovered, and remedied, were reminiscent of those Miss Nightingale had encountered during the Crimean War. Just as Miss Nightingale had contracted "Crimean fever," Miss Leete was stricken by typhus, which permanently affected her health. Despite this, she resumed her career in child and maternal health nursing after her return to the United States in 1919.

nurse, had already returned to her post as superintendent of nursing and principal of the hospital's training school. She remained at Lakeside until July 1923.

However, a new chapter in Cleveland's medical history was about to begin. In 1921 Drs. Crile, Bunts, and Lower, along with Dr. John Phillips, established The Cleveland Clinic Foundation.

Lillian Grundies, who had been in charge of the surgery at "the Office" of Drs. Crile, Bunts, and Lower before going to France, resumed her career in a new setting, as the Clinic's head surgical nurse. Eventually, Margaret Lane, trained as a nurse anesthetist while with the Unit, would briefly join her at the Cleveland Clinic, as an anesthetist at its hospital. Edith Morgan, too, came to the Clinic and there ended her career. These three women, veterans of the Lakeside Unit, had already had the experience of "acting as a unit" in an organization established by Dr. Crile. They not only represented, but lived, the connection between the Lakeside Unit and The Cleveland Clinic Foundation; between nursing and war; between Cleveland and the wider world; between doing their duty and going beyond it.

As the President of all the Nurses in the British Empire, I am most anxious to express to every individual Nurse my heartfelt and grateful appreciation of their unselfish devotion and patriotism in ministering to, and relieving the suffering of, our brave and gallant soldiers and sailors who are fighting for their King and Country.

With the whole Nation I wish to convey to our invaluable Nurses the undying debt of gratitude we owe them.

Alexandra

CITATION FROM QUEEN ALEXANDRA

British nurses caring for fallen soldiers and sailors received a certificate from the Queen Mother, expressing her gratitude on behalf of the nation. An identical certificate was also presented to each of the Lakeside Unit nurses, in token of their service in General Hospital No. 9 of the British Expeditionary Force. It depicted the Angel of Pity watching over a wounded soldier and his nurse, and also included the Queen's portrait and her message of thanks.

2

A New Era

[I do recognize] the splendid service that nurses have rendered in the past,
and the constant obligations under which I have been to them
for service to my patients, without whose aid I am sure such success
as I have had would not be possible....
— Dr. Frank Bunts, "A Discussion on
the Present Status of Nursing"

After the War

The First World War marked the shift from the traditions of the nineteenth century to the modern world of the twentieth. The Cleveland Clinic, founded in 1921, had its formative years during the postwar era known as the "Roaring Twenties," a period of economic prosperity and also of social change. Women's roles were in transition; so was the health care system. In Cleveland, new buildings were going up downtown, at the same time as the suburbs were expanding. This growing city, and this changing society, served as the backdrop to the Clinic's early history. The Clinic's first nurses lived and worked in the Cleveland of the 1920s. Their street dresses, and even their uniforms, had shorter hemlines. Many of these nurses lived in the Clinic neighborhood and walked to work; others rode the streetcar. During their leisure hours they could go shopping at nearby Doan's Corners, or listen to a brand-new form of entertainment, the radio broadcast. During their working hours, they cared for ever-growing numbers of patients at the new Clinic, which quickly established its reputation as a major referral center.

Less than two months after the Lakeside Unit nurses were mustered out of the U.S. Army, on June 4, 1919, the U.S. Congress passed the Nineteenth Amendment to the Constitution, guaranteeing American women the right to vote. By 1920, more than eight and a half million women worked for pay. Secretaries, sales clerks, and telephone operators were joining, in ever-increasing numbers, the teachers, nurses, factory workers, and domestic servants who had until then made up most of the female wage labor force.

But the American woman who came to symbolize the 1920s was not the suffragist or the secretary; she was the flapper, with her short skirt and bobbed hair, remembered for dancing the Charleston and drinking bootleg liquor, not for putting in a full day at the typewriter or the switchboard. The 1920s have been regarded as America's adolescence, a decade when, recoiling from the sacrifices of wartime and buoyed up by prosperity, the nation threw off old restraints and lived for pleasure; and of this, the flapper was certainly an apt representative.

Even before the war, hemlines had begun to rise and waistlines to loosen. Changes in women's fashions had a liberating effect, but brought with them constraints of their own. Short, tight skirts could be more confining than long, full ones (and trousers were still not a real option for women). Tiny waists and tight corsets were out, but thin was beautiful. Girdles, chest flatteners, and

49

even ankle bands — guaranteed not to show through stockings and meant to create the appearance of slender ankles — were worn by women in quest of a fashionable figure. As more of the body was exposed, women had to devote more time and effort to grooming. Bobbed and marcelled hair meant frequent visits to the hairdresser; cosmetics, formerly not worn by "respectable" women, grew in popularity.[1] Fashionable women powdered not only their faces, but also their necks, backs, shoulders, and even their knees. After gaining the right to vote in the postwar years, women also gained the right to compete for the title of Miss America; the first contest was held in Atlantic City in 1921.

In the economic sphere, the 1920s brought prosperity and expansion. Successful businessmen were admired, envied, and emulated. The average family had more consumer goods from which to choose, and more money with which to buy them, than ever before. With prosperity came easy credit; installment buying increased greatly, and was used for everything from cars to furniture to clothing to medical bills.

Along with consumer spending habits, advertising also changed. The "Somewhere West of Laramie" ad campaign for the Jordan "Playboy" — a high-priced car manufactured by the Jordan Motor Car Company of Cleveland — exemplified the new style. The advertisement provided virtually no information about the car itself. Instead, it used images of the Wyoming landscape, the wild horse, and the free-spirited cowgirl to suggest that excitement and romance could be bought for the price of a car. It was also one of the first automobile ads to appear in women's magazines.

Just as advertising helped to accelerate consumer spending, so the development of a new communications medium — radio — provided a new vehicle for advertising. The nation's first regularly scheduled radio broadcasts began in 1920, and Cleveland's first radio station, WHK, began broadcasting in 1922. Americans flocked to movie theaters; in 1920, films were still silent, but sound was added before the end of the decade. Grandiose "movie palaces," replete with red velvet, marble, and gilding, welcomed the audiences.

Another product of the media, particularly the print media of newspapers and magazines, was the celebrity. The popular press churned out reams of articles on film stars, athletes, gangsters, tycoons, and even scientists. The major accomplishments (good or bad) and also the trivial doings and random remarks of famous people were relayed to the public, on the radio, in mainstream newspapers, and also in the tabloid press alongside stories of sensational murders or bizarre stunts like dance marathons and flagpole sitting. Newspaper publisher William Randolph Hearst, who started the tabloid New York *Daily Mirror*, was a celebrity in his own right (and, eventually, a Cleveland Clinic patient).

Cleveland in the 1920s

Cleveland, too, was changing in the 1920s. Although the greatest proportion of the county's population lived in the city proper in 1920, suburban growth had begun in earnest. At the same time as the city's population grew from 560,000 in 1910 to 900,000 in 1930, the number of people living outside of Cleveland increased from 80,000 in 1910, to 150,000 in 1920, to 300,000 in 1930. The extension of streetcar lines to the suburbs and the popularity of the automobile made this possible.

In 1920, much of Cleveland's population was of immigrant stock — 75 percent of the people in the city were either themselves foreign-born, or had foreign-born parents. Increasingly restrictive laws slowed immigration to the United States, but migration from one part of the country to another contin- ued, helping to boost the number of African-Americans living in Cleveland from 4.3 percent of the city's population in 1920, to 8 percent, or 71,899 people, in 1930. Most lived in the area south of Euclid Avenue between East 9th Street and East 105th Street.[2]

New buildings on a monumental scale went up in the city center in the postwar years, including familiar landmarks like the Public Library, Public Auditorium, the Federal Reserve Bank Building, and Terminal Tower. However, a number of institutions moved eastward, following the residential population away from the center of the city and contributing to the growth of University Circle and the surrounding area.

Western Reserve University, Case Institute of Technology, the Cleveland Museum of Art, the Western Reserve Historical Society, and Mt. Sinai Hospital had all located in the University Circle area before 1920, along with some wealthy families who had built imposing residences nearby. In 1924, The Temple opened its new synagogue in the Circle, and the Western Reserve University schools of medicine, dentistry, and nursing were dedicated. In 1925 Babies and Children's and Maternity Hospitals opened adjacent to the med- ical school, and in 1931 they were joined by a new Lakeside Hospital building, completing the long-projected University Hospitals complex. In the same year, Severance Hall, just across Euclid Avenue from the hospitals, was dedicated as the Cleveland Orchestra's new home.

Lakeside Hospital and Western Reserve University School of Medicine had been located in the central part of the city, as was Huron Road Hospital (750 Huron Road). Mt. Sinai Hospital (East 37th Street) and St. Luke's Hospital (Carnegie Avenue near East 66th Street) had been located between downtown and University Circle. Huron Road Hospital moved in 1925 to a temporary site at East 89th Street and Euclid Avenue near University Circle; St. Luke's moved in 1927 to Shaker Boulevard near East 116th Street, parallel to the eastern edge of University Circle but farther south.

University Circle took its name from a streetcar stop and turnaround on the Euclid Avenue streetcar line which formed a huge circle around Euclid at East 107th Street. Just west of East 107th, the blocks along Euclid Avenue known as Doan's Corners were home to a lively commercial center, with hotels, banks, restaurants, businesses, and theaters. The Park, the Alhambra, the Circle, the University, and Keith's East 105th drew crowds to the area, especially on Saturday afternoons, for vaudeville, other live entertainment, and movies. Shoppers and moviegoers who did not yet have automobiles could ride the streetcar down Euclid to the University Circle stop for six cents.

Euclid Avenue itself, formerly a fashionable residential street, was left behind by Cleveland's wealthy as they, too, moved east, especially to the exclusive new suburb of Shaker Heights. Euclid Avenue became a commercial thoroughfare, although people continued to live in the more modest houses and apartment buildings on the side streets.

Manufacturing was of overwhelming importance in the city's economy. In 1920, Cleveland's 3,000 manufacturing companies employed 157,730 wage earners. Cleveland was the nation's fifth-largest industrial city. Even at the time of the 1930 census, after the Depression had begun, 41 percent of Cleveland's employed workers were in manufacturing and mechanical industries, compared to 20 percent in service industries. The number of Clevelanders employed as salaried clerical workers, however, had tripled between 1900 and 1930.[3]

Higher Standards

The importance of health care in Cleveland's economy was also growing. In the early 1870s, Cleveland had 7 hospitals; in 1920, the Cleveland Hospital Council had 20 member hospitals with a total capacity of 3,088 beds.[4] The 1920/21 Cleveland city directory listed 37 hospitals, although a number of them were actually nursing homes, sanitariums, or small private hospitals run by individual physicians or nurses. In Cleveland, as in the nation at large, health care had moved increasingly out of the home and into the hospital during the time between the Civil War and the First World War.

A variety of social and scientific reasons had contributed to the transformation of the hospital from a social welfare institution to a temple of healing, where an ordinary person could go with confidence, to be treated by expert physicians employing the latest medical techniques based on the most sophisticated scientific knowledge. Asepsis, antisepsis, and anesthesia had helped make possible advances in surgery, and advanced surgery could not be done on the kitchen table. Thus, surgery, in particular, came to be associated with an institutional setting. Also, city dwellers, with their smaller families, smaller houses, and higher standards of living, found it increasingly difficult and distasteful to care for sick family members in the home.[5] And, finally, the advent of formal hospital-based nurses' training in the United States provided staffing for hospitals, and gave the public increased confidence in the order, cleanliness, competence, and respectability of hospitals.

Beginning in the first decade of the twentieth century, a number of states enacted legal standards to regulate the practice of nursing. In Ohio, the governor signed the state's first Nurse Practice Act in 1915, after more than 10 years of effort on the part of nurses to have a satisfactory bill passed by the state legislature. Their task had been made more difficult by the fact that, as women, nurses were not able to vote. For the first time, graduate nurses in Ohio could attain the status of "registered nurse" (R.N.) by taking an examination administered by the state. An applicant for examination had to be over 21 years old, "of good moral character," and a graduate of a recognized nurse training school.[6] Registration was permissive, not mandatory; that is, even after the act went into effect, any person could practice as a nurse whether or not she met the qualifications for registration, so long as she did not call herself a "registered" nurse. Mandatory registration, and periodic license renewal, was still decades in the future for Ohio nurses. Nonetheless, the first Nurse Practice Act, by setting minimum standards for registered nurses and for nursing schools, represented a great step forward in transforming nursing in Ohio from an unregulated activity to a skilled profession. Some nurses, of course, had always met not only minimum, but high standards in their practice. However, the public had no way of judging a nurse's qualifications until the R.N. gained legal status in 1915.

By the time the Cleveland Clinic registered its first patients in 1921, institutional health care was an established fact of life for Americans, poor, wealthy, and middle-class alike. But the Cleveland Clinic took the concept a step farther, by moving not only hospital care, but "doctor's office" care as well, to an institutional setting. This combined the independence of the private practitioner with the technological and scientific resources of the large medical center.

The role of nursing at the new institution developed out of the ways nurses had worked in other settings with the Clinic's four founding physicians, Frank E. Bunts, George W. Crile, William Edgar Lower, and John Phillips. The three most important of these settings were: the Lakeside Unit; Cleveland hospitals, particularly Lakeside Hospital; and "the Office."

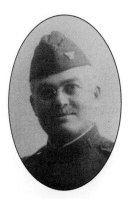

LILLIAN GRUNDIES

The Office

Three of the Clinic's founders, Dr. Bunts, Dr. Crile, and Dr. Lower, were surgeons. They had served as senior officers with the Lakeside Unit, and before that had worked in partnership for more than 20 years. They had a large private practice, and in the early days also did a considerable amount of accident and emergency work for several railroads and a number of large industrial firms. Charles Adams, the president of the Cleveland Hardware Company, in later years remembered how an accident call to the partnership eventually led to the hiring of an industrial nurse by his company.

DR. FRANK E. BUNTS   DR. GEORGE W. CRILE

> One time a young lad was terribly burned in the Mill. [Mr. Adams] said he laid the lad out on the stone floor, the only place available, and stayed with him until [Dr. Crile] came. As [Dr. Crile] left, he said, "Mr. Adams, you should never be without some first-aid in a case like this, and I am going to fix you up a little kit for emergencies," which he did. Mr. Adams said they still have that little kit, which not only proved to be the raison d'etre of the "hospital" at the Cleveland Hardware Company, with its nurse in attendance and every means for first aid, but it was the seed of all such hospitalization ideas in modern industry, for the Cleveland Hardware was the first industry to set up a first-aid plant, with a nurse, within their walls.[7]

In 1897 "the Office," as it came to be known by the three surgeons and their associates, moved to the Osborn Building in downtown Cleveland, at the corner of Huron Road and Prospect Avenue. Here the practice stayed for nearly a quarter of a century, until it was supplanted by the Clinic. The Office, initially housed in 3 rooms at the Osborn Building, grew to occupy 17 rooms. The doctors added to the staff more surgeons and a radiologist, along with nurses, secretaries, an artist, and laboratory researchers. In 1912, Lillian Grundies came to work at the Office as a surgical nurse. She was 25 years old at the time and would remain with the Office, and then the Clinic, until her retirement 40 years later.

Another nurse employed at the Office was Bertha Melcher, who had joined the staff in 1908. Miss Melcher was not a graduate nurse. She had worked at Lutheran Hospital as a probationer nurse before being hired at the Office and in 1911 went back to complete her training at Lutheran. Unfortunately, in her

The Cleveland Clinic was founded by four physicians. Three of them, surgeons Frank Bunts, George Crile, and William Edgar Lower, had been partners in a private practice, referred to as "the Office," before serving with the Lakeside Unit. They performed surgery in homes, in factories, in the Office, and as visiting staff members at several Cleveland hospitals. Lillian Grundies, surgical nurse at the Office, became the Clinic's first head nurse.

words, "after 1 years work I found that I was not strong enough to proceed" with the rigorous duty schedule that was the student nurse's lot at that time.[8] She returned to the Office for a few months in 1913 and 1914 and then, on a permanent basis, from 1915 through May 1920.

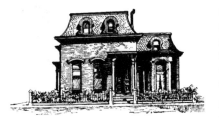

16 CHURCH STREET
1886-1889

> When I began my work with the doctors I was hired as office nurse. Later, under Dr. Lower's teaching I was able to do all the urinalysis work, both chemically and microscopically. At that time the doctors also took care of all accident work at the office for the Big Four, Nickel Plate and Erie Railroads that did not require hospitalization. There were many surgical dressings to be taken care of at all times. Goiter incisions to be dressed, also dressings where a breast had been removed etc.

> On first entering the employ of [Dr. Bunts], Dr. Crile and Dr. Lower, there were many dressings to be made and sterilized, for each doctor had his out of town bag which I always had to keep ready for any out of town operation, usually house operations, of which they performed quite a number for several years. These bags contained every dressing necessary as well as hypodermics and anesthetics and a few medicines. The only things necessary to add at the time of call were the instruments and these were put into a flat pan in which they could be boiled.[9]

Although Miss Melcher left before the Clinic building was completed, she witnessed a considerable growth in the practice during her time with the founders.

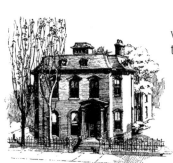

380 PEARL STREET
1890-1897

> They... were always enlarging the office space during the time I was employed there. That is no doubt why they conceived the idea of having a building of their own. Dr. Lower came to me at the time with the plans and asked my opinion as to where I thought would be the most convenient place to have the cystoscopic room, dressing room and sterilizing room.[10]

When Miss Melcher left in 1920, Dr. Bunts, Dr. Crile, and Dr. Lower presented her with a wristwatch, engraved with the words "In appreciation for faithful service" and their names. "I can gladly and proudly say that I was never reprimanded by them nor did they ever find fault with my work. They were very wonderful men to work for."[11]

The three surgeons also held academic appointments at the Western Reserve University School of Medicine, and were on the visiting staffs of several Cleveland hospitals. All three men served on the medical staff at St. Alexis Hospital. Dr. Crile and Dr. Lower were the chiefs of surgery at Lakeside Hospital and Mt. Sinai Hospital, respectively. Dr. Bunts had been affiliated with St. Vincent Charity Hospital since 1886. He became Charity's chief of staff in 1911, a position he held for the rest of his life.

Dr. Bunts and the Roman Catholic nuns who ran St. Vincent Charity had a strong mutual regard. In 1926, through what he called a "fool slip of the tongue," he let out that it was his 40th anniversary at Charity; when the sisters found out, they could not be stopped from throwing a party for him. A newspaper reporter asked Dr. Bunts what had impressed him most during his years at Charity.

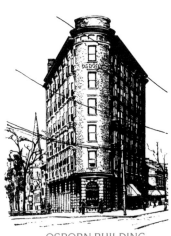

OSBORN BUILDING
1897-1920

> "The self-sacrifice of the sisters," he replied unhesitatingly. "When I first came to Charity they were compelled to scrub, paint the walls and do all the menial tasks. But I never heard a complaint despite the fact that many

times they were called to work twenty-four hours at a stretch. Now it is the same, although the sisters are all graduate nurses. They're forever finding work to do and — doing it."[12]

"Angel of Little Attentions"

Dr. Bunts had been affiliated with Charity Hospital for more than 10 years when the hospital opened its training school for nurses in 1898. From the beginning, he demonstrated his confidence in the school's graduates by calling on them to assist at his operations in patients' homes.

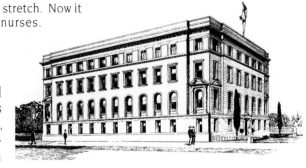

The graduate nurses were few. The school was in its infancy, yet there were many calls from the country and nearby towns for the surgeon and nurse. The surgeons from Charity Hospital, especially Dr. Frank E. Bunts, [were] called quite frequently to the country, and he summoned the nurse, gave her instructions and sent her on ahead to the farmhouse to make the necessary preparations.

The nurse would start off full of good cheer for the task she hoped to accomplish; her hand-bag filled to the brim, which included a box of tacks and a hammer. As soon as she arrived at the residence, she made a survey of the home and selected the room in which the operation was to be performed. Then she asked the farmer to drive out to the neighbor farmers to procure bed-sheets and towels, which she sterilized. The sheets were tacked to the ceiling and side walls of the room. Thus an operating room was improvised. She assisted the doctor in every way, and her efficiency and cheerfulness cajoled many a patient back from the border. She exemplified the school motto, "Charity Is Kind." Nor did her work go unrecognized. Doctor Bunts voiced his appreciation and was loud in his praise. He in turn was called by them "The angel of little attentions."[13]

When Dr. Bunts addressed the Lakeside Hospital graduating class in the first decade of the 20th century, he gave a list of the "ideal qualifications" of the nurse: "tact, human-ness, womanliness, appreciation of proportion, the attribute of sweet reasonableness, the rare sense of humor." Similarly, in 1913, speaking to another class of graduates, he stressed personal qualities as a nurse's greatest attributes. "The woman who will make the best nurse is one who is quick-witted, conscientious, resourceful and a good observer, and it is doubtful if any training will supplant these good traits." She should not be a "babbler" or a "gossip."[14]

Essentially, what Dr. Bunts said, over and over, to classes of newly graduated nurses, was that a nurse was not made, but born — and, importantly, born a woman. The innate feminine qualities and the skills in housewifely tasks a girl learned at her mother's elbow were the basis of the nurse's abilities; to them need be added only the discipline meted out by the hard school of hospital training, where the young woman learned by watching and then by doing. "Sleep, food, rest, recreation, health were often sacrificed that another's pains and suffering might be lessened, and now that those years are over you are going forth to do the same thing over in new fields and other surroundings."[15]

Dr. Bunts was voicing ideas common among physicians, with which the general public probably agreed. By the time he helped to found the Cleveland Clinic, he was 60 years old, and had been practicing medicine for 35 years.

THE CLINIC
AND BEFORE
Over the years, Drs. Bunts, Crile, and Lower moved their practice east, from houses on Church Street and Pearl Street (opposite page) on the city's west side, to an office building downtown (the Osborn Building, opposite page), and finally, in 1921, to the Cleveland Clinic (above) on Euclid Avenue at East 93rd Street. In the early years, the surgeons relied on their horses and buggies to take them to patients' homes. They also did a large amount of industrial work, much of it for railroads. Whenever the practice received a call to a serious accident, a team consisting of a surgeon, assistants, and a nurse immediately drove to the scene.

By the 1920s, automobiles had largely replaced horses, and patients came to the surgeons rather than the surgeons to them. Moving the practice from downtown to the less built-up east side had the advantage of providing more parking space.

During the 1920s, he grew increasingly troubled by changes in nursing that he felt were breaking down the traditional relationship between physicians and nurses.

In part, he blamed the spirit of the times. "Your problems are not peculiar to your profession. The medical profession, the world at large is meeting problems today which have been developed from the same crises, from the same universal spirit of unrest, from the same economic needs." Some changes he applauded, noting that women had "recently attained what has long been their due, equal suffrage." But he deplored the "spirit of self-promotion and self-aggrandizement" so prevalent in the postwar world, and saw the war itself as the great divide between the old, comfortable world, and the restless new one.[16]

> Many of the nurses, I think, who had served with wonderful effectiveness during the war returned to their homes dissatisfied with the idea of going back to private nursing and found positions in industrial pursuits and social service work and district nursing.... Hospitals found it difficult to secure sufficient nurses for training, and in many instances, found a spirit of intolerance of restraint and discipline that went far to destroy the proper running of a hospital and the care of the patient.[17]

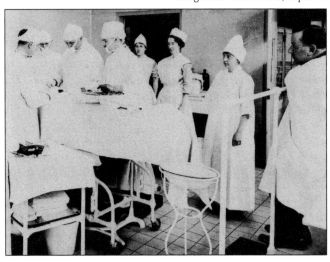

ST. VINCENT CHARITY HOSPITAL
Dr. Bunts was closely affiliated with St. Vincent Charity Hospital, serving as its chief of staff from 1911 to 1928. He held the hospital's nursing sisters in high regard. Here, he performs surgery in a Charity Hospital operating room, with three nurses in attendance. Lay graduates of Charity's nursing school assisted him with home surgeries. It was up to the nurse to transform a kitchen or bedroom into an operating room by sterilizing household linens and tacking them to walls and ceiling.

The commercial spirit of the age, plus the education nurses now received, created the attitude of the modern graduate nurse, he believed, who went out "with the idea firmly fixed in her mind that the first thing required of her is to fix her charges at 20 dollars a week and upwards," so that middle-class families not poor enough to receive district nursing services could not afford any nursing services at all.[18]

Many Cleveland physicians, like physicians across the nation, expressed worry during the 1920s and 1930s that private nursing care was growing too expensive for most people. They recognized the importance of the private duty nurse in both the home and the hospital; they saw that lack of nursing care could put their patients at risk, and spoke out of genuine concern for those patients. But they seemed not to recognize that the "twenty dollars and upwards" that a family was hard-pressed to spare from its weekly budget represented the entire weekly budget of the nurse, on which she might be equally hard-pressed to live.

The kind of education nurses received was determined at least in part by nursing leaders, and Dr. Bunts blamed them, also, for what he saw as problems. They were diverting nursing from its proper ends and souring nurse-physician relationships by promoting scientific education and even college degrees for nurses; by claiming that the "menial" services demanded of students by hospitals were keeping young women from entering nursing; and especially by emphasizing "the position of nursing as a profession and not as a calling. It has gone so far in some instances as to cause nurses to feel that they were really in a sense consultants in medical cases, and that they were better qualified to advise regarding the diet and hygienic care of the patient than the physician."[19]

Dr. Bunts was genuinely puzzled and hurt by the changes he observed. "In former days, it was a great pleasure, as well as a privilege to be allowed to speak to nurses," who, he felt, had been eager to be instructed by physicians. Now it sometimes seemed "that the nurse rather resents instruction or guidance from the physician and seeks by higher education to reach a position where any such advice will be entirely superfluous." He did not blame the rank-and-file nurse, for, in his words, "I have found her to be the same loyal earnest woman that we were proud to call our graduate nurse in the years gone by, the one ready...to devote herself, mind and body to the great object we all have in caring for our patient." He hoped that in the future nurses and physicians would continue "to work together in the same spirit of trust and confidence which they have...had in the past," for he recognized "the splendid service that nurses have rendered in the past, and...the constant obligations under which I have been to them for service to my patients, without whose aid I am sure such success as I have had would not be possible."[20]

Dr. Bunts may have had a tendency to see a rose-colored picture of the past, when the sisters got down on their hands and knees to scrub the floors at their hospital, and Charity's first graduates went with him, hammer in hand, to rig up makeshift operating rooms in farmhouse kitchens. But it was not a view he focused on nursing alone. Despite a dignified demeanor, he was, at heart, guided by sentiment. A desire to remain in practice with his long-time Office partners, as much as his enthusiasm for the practical advantages of the clinic system, led him to participate in founding the Cleveland Clinic. (He continued to perform surgery at St. Vincent Charity Hospital after the Clinic Hospital was built.) The old days with his partners at the Office, and with the sisters at Charity Hospital, always held their place in his affections.

Assistants and Collaborators

In some ways Dr. Crile had attitudes toward nurses similar to those of Dr. Bunts, believing that instinctive womanly qualities, especially intuition, made for a good nurse. He even went so far as to call the male nurse an "anomaly."[21] Sentiment, however, especially for the past, had little to do with his outlook in this regard, or indeed in any regard affecting his work. His physiologic view of life determined his view of women. During the war, there was some question of his college-aged daughter pursuing a career in science. Alarmed, he wrote to her:

> I have thought much about what course you should pursue and I am more and more convinced that you should not prepare for a personal career at all. What will be needed most in the world are splendid wives and mothers. There will be needed more than anything else splendid women to rebuild and restore good and humane standards of life and living. I want you to be the partner of some splendid husband and together make a career.[22]

Mrs. Crile in later years noted that her husband felt "that if work becomes too stimulating to a girl, it may easily become a menace to her health."[23] He did not hold these views out of respect to tradition, at least consciously, but rather because medico-scientific theories of the day, prominently including his own, linked mental exertion, emotional stress, and glandular activity.

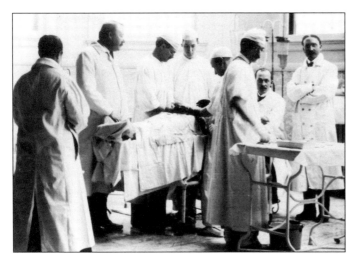

ST. ALEXIS HOSPITAL, 1903
Dr. Crile (third from left) and
Dr. Lower (across the table) also
worked with Roman Catholic
nursing sisters, as members of the
visiting staff at St. Alexis Hospital
on Cleveland's southeast side.
"I liked the philosophy that
motivated this hospital," wrote
Dr. Crile. "The achievement of
the Catholic Sisterhoods in giving
gracious care to the sick for so
little cost...was impressive."

DR. JOHN PHILLIPS
Dr. Phillips was the only one
of the Clinic's founders to
specialize in medicine rather
than surgery (and the only one
to marry a nurse). His skill as a
diagnostician complemented
the surgical expertise of his
colleagues, and was invaluable
to the young institution.

Dr. Crile in his own life depended heavily on women. Besides the operating room nurses and anesthetists so vital to his work, there was his devoted assistant Amy Rowland, who typed his publications, edited them, and even participated in the laboratory research they were based on. Another laboratory mainstay was Dr. Maria Telkes, a Hungarian-born biologist. His wife, Grace McBride Crile, daughter of a well-to-do Cleveland family, and by no means a meek or weak-willed woman, managed her husband's office and laboratory and kept tabs on his interests at Lakeside Hospital while he was overseas.

Unlike Dr. Bunts, Dr. Crile did not express much interest in how nurses were educated or what they felt toward physicians. He did not question the loyalty of his troops, and his outgoing, jovial personality attracted, rather than demanded, allegiance. Amy Rowland wrote that Dr. Crile

> not only took it for granted that everyone should be as interested in his investigations and the reasons for them as he was, but once a person was in his employ or was to be so, she must exhibit a like singleness of interest and of complete devotion to his problems. I know of only two instances in which he failed to secure such complete cooperation.
>
> Such was his own enthusiasm and appreciation that one could not work with him without being infected with a like enthusiasm. He never spoke of his assistants as working for him but always as working *with* him. He always referred to them not as *assistants* but as *collaborators*.[24]

Still, there was never the faintest glimmer of a question about who was "the Chief," as he was referred to by everyone from Agatha Hodgins to his own grandchildren.

Dr. Crile valued the nurses he worked with both at home and overseas, as he had expressed when he called the work of the Lakeside Unit nurses "beyond praise." He at one point used the metaphor of a "hive" to refer to Lakeside Hospital. At a time when it was rare for nurses to remain in the profession after marriage, this image equated nurses with worker bees — diligent, loyal, and unsexed, or, rather, barren, having given up woman's highest calling, motherhood, to care for the sick.

Judgment and Intelligent Care

John Phillips, the "quiet man" among the founders of the Cleveland Clinic — a highly respected medical man and diagnostician, rather than a surgeon, and the youngest of the four — had yet another view of nurses, as recorded in his writings on therapeutics. His detailed recommendations on the treatment of various diseases included his views on the significance of nursing care. Regarding acute lobar pneumonia, he stated: "There is no disease, which in its treatment demands from the physician and nurse, greater efforts or greater judgment." Although, in these pre-antibiotic days, treatment of the most virulent cases was "of no avail," there were also "the cases of mild infection where judicious nursing alone is required," as well as cases "of moderately severe infection, in patients with good resistance. In these careful nursing, watchfulness on the part of the physician for the indications as they arise, help to tide the patient through the disease."[25]

Nursing care for pneumonia patients included sponge baths every four hours to treat fever, since "as a rule it is not wise to give drugs for the reduction of temperature." If a patient's cough was due to pleurisy

> it can be best taken care of by strapping the chest, by the use of hot applications to the chest, or by giving codein sulphate 1/4 grain every two hours. If the cough is due to a bronchitis, inhalations of compound tincture of benzoin, two teaspoonfuls to a quart of water, often helps a great deal....If the patient is delirious, he should be watched carefully, he should be given plenty of fresh air, hydrotherapy such as mentioned above under fever should be tried, an ice bag should be kept on the head and certain drugs may be given.[26]

Local applications to the chest Dr. Phillips recommended were Priessnitz compresses or mustard plasters "made large enough to cover both the front and back of the chest and...left on only until the skin is reddened." For care of the bowels, calomel, petrolatum, and a variety of enemas could be used. The latter included plain water, olive oil, soap suds, peppermint, asafoetida, or milk and molasses ("warm the molasses and add warm milk, have the temperature a little above the body temperature, give with funnel and tube"). For local application to the abdomen, he recommended turpentine stupes. The mouth, teeth and eyes could be kept clean with boric acid solutions; bed linens, utensils, and the sputum itself had to be disinfected to prevent the spread of the disease.[27]

"Judgment"; "careful"; "judicious." These were the words Dr. Phillips used when speaking of the nurse, rather than "womanliness" or "intuition." The American nursing leader Isabel Hampton Robb, echoing Florence Nightingale's observation that "In no case is the physician or surgeon always there," had declared that although "doctors may be temporarily off duty, the nurse is always in charge. Her candle goeth not out by night, and it is to her watchfulness and intelligent care that the patients are in the main committed through the night."[28] It was precisely a nurse who could provide "intelligent care" that Dr. Phillips had in mind, a nurse skilled in carrying out all the therapeutic measures of the day and capable of exercising nursing judgment.

Lakeside Hospital

Dr. Crile had held the position of visiting surgeon (chief of surgery) at Lakeside Hospital since 1911. Dr. Lower and Dr. Phillips had also been members of the visiting staff there since before the war.

Lakeside Hospital fit the classic pattern of the 19th-century hospital. Tracing its origins to the "Home for Friendless Strangers" established in 1863 to aid Civil War refugees in Cleveland, the hospital opened in 1868 in a refitted

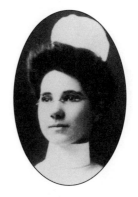

CORDELIA SUDDERTH PHILLIPS
Cordelia Sudderth was studying nursing at Lakeside Hospital when Dr. Phillips was a house officer there. A classmate, confined to the isolation ward during a bout of erysipelas, and being nursed by Miss Sudderth, noticed that Dr. Phillips's visits were very frequent. After graduation in 1904, Miss Sudderth worked briefly as a private duty nurse. She left nursing upon her marriage to Dr. Phillips, but enrolled as a Red Cross volunteer during both world wars, teaching classes in hygiene and first aid.

LAKESIDE HOSPITAL
Many of the Cleveland Clinic's first nurses were educated at the Lakeside Hospital Training School for Nurses. Lakeside's pavilion plan hospital, which opened in 1898, was located between East 12th and 14th Streets

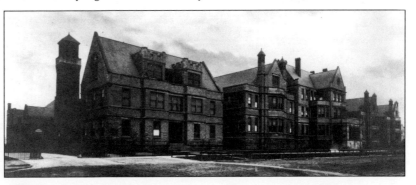

and overlooked Lake Erie. As the largest member institution of University Hospitals, Lakeside moved to University Circle in 1931.

frame house on Wilson Street.[29] In the 19th century, the metamorphosis from refugee home to hospital was not really an unnatural one. The voluntary hospital grew out of the same philanthropic roots from which institutions like poor relief societies, orphan asylums, and, later, social settlements also sprang; at this early date it was still an offshoot of the movement for social welfare rather than of advances in medical science.

Initially, as was common in voluntary or public hospitals, the Lakeside patients themselves did some of the nursing and other work. Many of them suffered from chronic, rather than acute illnesses, as well as low social status. Hospital workers were equated with domestic servants at best; many hospital patients were in fact domestic servants, or factory workers. Factory owners and mistresses of households alike were encouraged to endow beds so that their employees or household help would be sure of a place in the hospital

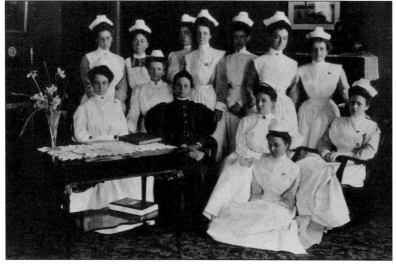

LAKESIDE NURSES, 1905
Elizabeth Maude Ellis (in black), Principal of the Lakeside Hospital Training School for Nurses, posed for this photograph with her nursing staff. Miss Ellis, along with an assistant, a night supervisor, a supervisor of probationers, a "diet instructress," and seven or eight graduate head nurses, directed the school's pupils (97 of them in 1905) in caring for the hospital's patients. Many other hospitals used senior pupils, rather than graduates, as head nurses.

when sick or injured. Even after Lakeside opened its "modern" pavilion-plan hospital and its nursing school in 1898, the rules for patients still stated: "Such free [non-paying] patients as are able shall perform such service as may be reasonably required of them."[30]

However, the hospital administration expected that the students of the new Lakeside Hospital Training School for Nurses would provide the gentle hands, willing hearts, and level heads to carry out doctors' orders and manage ward routine. In 1868, when Lakeside Hospital first opened, no hospital school for nurses existed in the United States; by 1900 there were 432.[31] By the time Lakeside opened its training school in 1898, a more skilled level of care than could be provided by one's fellow patients had become not only a reasonable expectation, but a necessity, due to advances in medical science and surgery. Social change accompanied medical innovation in the hospital.

Thorough Education and Practical Training

The development of the modern hospital and the development of modern nursing were interdependent. Trained nurses — or, at least, nurses in training — provided the technically skilled workers needed by the nation's hospitals, which were growing in numbers and medical sophistication. On the other hand, these hospitals created both a training ground where the skills could be learned and a new labor market where they had value. Without the aid of the hospital, the nurse could receive no training; without the aid of the nurse, the hospital could not function.

When Lakeside Hospital opened on January 17, 1898, it included an entire "private pavilion" to attract "pay" patients along with the traditional open wards and multiple-bedded rooms for "part pay" and "charity" patients. In another step away from the hospital's charitable origins, it was hoped that a greater share of its expenses could be covered by operating revenues. The hospital had a nursing staff of 17, including 8 graduate head nurses, 7 assistant nurses (also graduates), and its first student nurse. This number grew to about 40 (mostly through the addition of student nurses) during the course of the year, even though some graduates left for service in U.S. military camps after the outbreak of the Spanish-American War. The number of patients cared for by these 40 nurses fluctuated wildly. Relatively few other attendants, like orderlies or ward maids, were employed by the hospital. Nurses provided nearly all of the patient care.

By 1900, Lakeside had a nursing staff of 60, 35 of whom were students. M. Helena McMillan, the school's principal and the hospital's matron, reported that the 13 assistant graduate nurses

> with the exception of two, are employed in the private wards; of these two, one is on duty in the General Operating Rooms, and the second on night duty in ward 'G.' This ward has a mixed service and the character of the work is such that the pupils are not yet prepared to take the entire responsibility during the night. With these two exceptions, the pupil nurses, under the |10| head nurses' supervision, receive their training and do all the nursing in the operating rooms, dispensary, diet kitchen, and in the public wards on both day and night duty.[32]

In addition to working eight hours a day in the hospital, training school pupils had classroom work in subjects like principles and ethics of nursing, materia medica, bacteriology, hygiene and ventilation, household economy, and dietetics, as well as lectures by visiting staff physicians on various clinical subjects — medical diseases, surgical diseases, obstetrics and gynecology, and pediatric diseases.

Under this system, a large portion of the hospital's patient care was entrusted to nursing students, some of whom were not high school graduates. The educational background of physicians entering medical school at this time was not much different. A physician who had studied at the medical department of Wooster University when Dr. Crile taught there in the 1890s reminisced about his classmates: "We were a sad lot to teach. Only one or two of us had ever seen the inside of a college. Very few had full high-school education." Not until 1904 did the American Medical Association stipulate that physicians should have at minimum four years of high school before entering medical school, and in the early 1920s most state licensing boards still required only two years, at most, of premedical college education.[33]

The Lakeside nursing school must be judged by the standards of its own time. And by those standards, it had one of the most advanced programs in the United States.

Isabel Hampton Robb

The best schools are beginning to increase the time of training from two to three years, and ... have, at the same time, introduced the non-payment system, ... asking the nurse to forego a present remuneration, |guaranteeing| to her in return for her work a thorough education, as well as practical training. Under these circumstances, it was only just that more time for study, lectures and demonstrations should be given to the pupil nurse, and that her energies should not be exhausted in the routine work of the

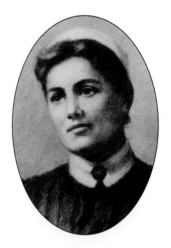

ISABEL HAMPTON ROBB
One of the country's foremost nursing leaders, Mrs. Robb had great influence on the Lakeside Hospital Training School. Born in Welland, Ontario, she graduated from the New York's Bellevue Hospital Training School for Nurses in 1883, and went on to head the Illinois Training School for Nurses and the Johns Hopkins Hospital Nursing School. She married Dr. Hunter Robb in 1894 and moved to Cleveland, remaining active in nursing through her role in professional organizations and her volunteer activities. The new Lakeside nursing school, which opened in 1898, was organized to meet the high standards of nursing education promoted by Mrs. Robb. She served on the Lakeside women's board and its training school committee until her tragic death in 1910 at the age of 50. (She was crushed between two streetcars while trying to help a companion avoid an oncoming automobile.)

wards, which should now occupy her only for eight hours out of the twen-ty-four....It is to be regretted that at present in only one or two hospitals have the hours of daily practical work been reduced to eight, the average time required still being usually from ten to eleven hours.[34]

Lakeside offered a three-year course and an eight-hour day largely at the recommendation of the woman who spoke the above words at the hospital's dedicatory exercises — Isabel Adams Hampton Robb, a national leader in nursing practice and education. Mrs. Robb had not been brought in for the day to add luster to the event. She lived in Cleveland, served on Lakeside's women's board and its training school committee, and, as one of her fellow board members put it, "so far as the training and care for nurses [at Lakeside Hospital] was concerned, she was...a dictator in that line."[35]

Formerly superintendent of nurses at Johns Hopkins University Hospital, Isabel Hampton had retired from nursing in 1894 at age 33 when she married Johns Hopkins gynecologist Hunter Robb. She accompanied him to Cleveland when he assumed posts at the Western Reserve University School of Medicine and Lakeside Hospital.

Isabel Robb continued to contribute to the development of the nursing profession, both locally and nationally. Her influence on the Lakeside Hospital nursing service and training school — and thus on the women who graduated from it, including many Cleveland Clinic nurses — cannot be overestimated. Her guidance ensured that the Lakeside school would spring, full-grown from the moment of its birth, into the first rank of the nation's nursing schools, serving as a model and an encouragement to weaker schools.

Fitted for the Work

The Lakeside trustees had given three reasons for resolving to open a nursing school: first, providing nursing "of the highest order" to the hospital's own patients; second, providing aspiring nurses with training to "successfully [fit] themselves for their chosen work"; and, third, filling the Cleveland area's need for "graduate nurses of high standing."[36] From the hospital's point of view, providing nursing care for its patients came first. In 1898, before the school was in full swing, Lakeside had tremendous difficulty in finding and keeping enough graduate nurses to staff its wards.

At this time most graduate nurses worked as private duty nurses, either in patients' homes, or as "specials" in hospitals, paid directly by the patients. A smaller number of graduates served as head nurses or sometimes as operating room nurses, mostly in larger hospitals; others worked in public health; and a few found positions as nursing educators and administrators, or as hospital superintendents, usually in smaller hospitals.[37]

LAKESIDE WARD, 1905
Supervised by head nurses, Lakeside nursing school students cared for patients in large, high-ceilinged wards. This photograph shows the children's ward.

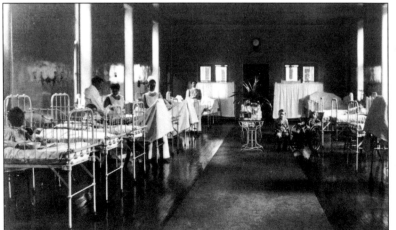

Graduates did not expect to make careers in general duty hospital nursing; this would have been something like a professional soldier spending his entire life in boot camp. The restrictions, the regimentation, the drudgery, the lowly status of the student were stigmas attached to hospital nursing. Nurses also believed they could earn higher incomes in private duty work, although this was less the case as time went on. For their part, many hospitals preferred student nurses, who were considered more docile, more trainable, and a less expensive labor source.

But if Lakeside, like other hospitals, saw its school first as a labor pool, it did make a serious effort to educate its students to the best standards of the day, thanks to Isabel Hampton Robb. In a number of hospitals, not only the general staff, but many, or even all, of the head nurses were students. Lakeside employed graduate nurses as head nurses whenever possible, ensuring that the students actually did receive training and supervision in their practical work from experienced nurses. At other Cleveland hospitals, as at most hospitals nationwide, such practical work was supplemented by little or no theoretical and scientific classroom training. At Lakeside, a complete and systematic course of lectures, classes, and demonstrations was offered, and ward duty assignments were made with the goal of giving each student experience in all areas of nursing — including special nursing, so that the young women would have a taste of the private duty work likely to be their bread and butter after graduation.

By early 1917, on the eve of the Lakeside Unit's departure for France with its 43 Lakeside nursing graduates, the school was well established. Grace Allison, who had graduated from Lakeside in 1908, was the school's principal. Minnie Strobel, a member of the class of 1907, served as her third assistant and supervisor of probationers. Twenty-one graduate nurses staffed the hospital and its operating room and supervised and instructed the school's 113 pupil nurses.

Not all of Lakeside's nurses worked on the combined training school-nursing staff. The hospital's housekeeper (a position derived from that of the hospital "matron"), who was in charge of not only cleaning, but also supplies, laundry, and the general running of the hospital "household," was a nurse, an English-born widow named Emma Oxley. Three of the hospital's four social service workers were nurses; one of them was Edith Morgan, who served as a special worker for children. She made home calls in the morning, with the Children's Department's new automobile; in the afternoon she registered children at the dispensary and made arrangements for hospital admissions and discharges. The anesthesia department, consisting of Agatha Hodgins and her two assistants, was a separate department and maintained its own training program, a postgraduate course in anesthesia.

Agatha Hodgins: The Intelligence and the Gift

Nurse anesthetist Agatha Hodgins was a key associate of Dr. Crile's during his years at Lakeside Hospital. A graduate of Boston City Hospital, she had come to Lakeside in 1906 as supervisor of the dispensary. At that time, most anesthetics were given by interns who had no intention of making a career in anesthesia, and who by definition did not give anesthetics long enough to gain expertise. Dr. Crile, following the lead of the Mayo brothers, decided to employ a nurse as his anesthetist.

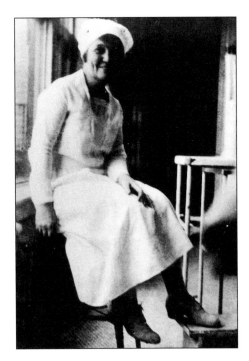

AGATHA C. HODGINS
Miss Hodgins was one of the
nurses most closely associated
with Dr. Crile, although she was
never employed by the Cleveland
Clinic. Born and raised in Canada,
Miss Hodgins remained in the
United States after graduation
from the Boston City Hospital
Training School for Nurses in 1900.
She became head nurse of the
Lakeside Hospital dispensary in
1906, and was chosen to be Dr.
Crile's first nurse anesthetist in
1908. In 1915, she organized the
Lakeside School of Anesthesia;
many of the Clinic's first nurse
anesthetists were educated there.
Miss Hodgins remained head of
the anesthesia service at Lakeside
Hospital until ill health forced her
to retire in 1933. The moving spirit
behind the founding of the
American Association of Nurse
Anesthetists in 1931, she served as
its first president.

In the entire domain of medicine no subject was at that time so neglected, so badly done and with such needless distress, not to mention direct and indirect disaster for its victims, as the administration of anesthetics.... I was convinced that a nurse of ability would, because of her natural intuition, make a better anesthetist than a man. So I looked over the nurses on our Lakeside staff and decided that Miss Agatha Hodgins... possessed the qualities necessary for such a responsibility.

One morning in 1908 while making rounds I drew Miss Hodgins aside and presented to her what amounted to an annunciation. She had received no warning whatever about the plan to make her my special anesthetist, but she told me promptly that she would undertake it if I would remember always that she was giving her best.... In order that she might become familiar with the symptoms of death, I started her to work administering anesthetics to rabbits and dogs. From anesthetizing rabbits she learned to anesthetize young babies. Her skill in amusing them with toys or my watch while she allowed the gas to play gently near the child's face until the sandman closed his eyes and he slipped back on the pillow was extraordinary....

The administering of an anesthetic is not only an art but a gift. In my mind it ranks close to the work of the operating surgeon.... Miss Hodgins made an outstanding anesthetist for she had to a marked degree both the intelligence and the gift.[38]

From being trained herself, Miss Hodgins quickly went on to teaching others. Although most of her pupils were nurses, doctors and dentists also came to Lakeside Hospital to receive instruction in the administration of anesthesia from her. One medical student sent for training "was admonished by his chief, 'George will talk a lot, but you watch Agatha.'"[39] In 1915 the educational requirements for the program and the course of study were standardized, and the Lakeside School of Anesthesia became the first formal postgraduate course in anesthesia in the country. The school accepted graduate nurses who had passed their state board examinations and physicians and dentists who had their degrees. It received far more applications than it had places for students.

But despite its success, the Lakeside anesthesia school had to close its doors in 1916. The Ohio State Medical Board questioned the right of nurses to administer anesthetics and declared that unless Lakeside stopped training nurse anesthetists, "all recognition of the Lakeside Hospital as an acceptable Training School for Nurses [would] be withheld." In November 1917, perhaps because of the pressing need for anesthetists at home and abroad, Lakeside was permitted to reopen its anesthesia school, but the nurse anesthetist did not gain legal status in Ohio until 1919. "The calm statement of this historical fact does not convey a picture of the fine fight waged to secure the law," remarked Miss Hodgins.[40]

When Dr. Crile chose Agatha Hodgins, he chose well. Although she was not the first nurse anesthetist in the United States, she was certainly an early leader in the field.[41] She was one of the founders and the first president of the American Association of Nurse Anesthetists. She trained hundreds of nurse anesthetists in this country, who in turn trained others, so that where there had been a few individuals working, there was now an entire profession. She took her technique overseas to the American Ambulance Hospital in Paris in

1915, as a member of Dr. Crile's surgical team, and stayed behind to teach after the rest of the team had returned home.

At Home and Abroad

Once the United States officially entered the war in 1917, Miss Hodgins' former pupil and assistant Mary Roche joined the Lakeside Unit as an anesthetist. Another, less experienced pupil, Margaret Lane, went as a general duty nurse. Miss Lane eventually worked as an anesthetist with the Unit after receiving additional training from Miss Roche. Although Dr. Crile wrote to Miss Hodgins from France, suggesting that she, too, return for a second stint overseas, she refused, evidently feeling her duties as chief anesthetist

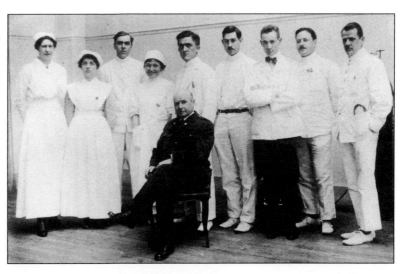

and head of the anesthesia school at Lakeside more vital. There, at times single-handedly, she kept the hospital's anesthesia service and school going, not without great difficulty.

During the First World War, the number of graduate nurses on the Lakeside staff fell to 17. However, the number of students in the school increased by a third, as both Lakeside Hospital and a large number of young women answered the nation's call for more trained nurses on the home front and abroad. An extra instructor had to be hired, and Lakeside's nurses' home did not have enough space to house the extra students. This problem was solved by using the second floor of the hospital's private pavilion for nurses' quarters, considered a far better option than allowing the young women to live off-premises.

The private pavilion had room to spare, because Lakeside visiting and resident staffs were also hard hit by the mobilization for war. Days of care and the number of operations dropped significantly — undoubtedly, the absence of Dr. Crile, a surgeon whose skill, speed, and efficiency were rivaled only by his popularity and reputation, was the major factor in this.

It was thus not surprising that the Lakeside trustees repeatedly wrote and cabled Dr. Crile to come home from Europe.

> I hear from Lakeside Hospital and Western Reserve Medical School how much you are missed and how greatly your services and skill as Surgeon and teacher are required at both places and I am venturing to ask you if you will undertake to see whether - in view of the early and whole hearted response of Lakeside to the Government call - by which we so largely denuded ourselves of the best men on our Staff and of our best nurses and aides - the United States Authorities under whom you are serving in France might not think it equitable and right to let us have you back for this coming year, and replace you with men from some Hospital and Medical School that has not yet done its comparable part.[42]

In fact, Dr. Crile later expressed the opinion that board president Samuel Mather, Cleveland's leading industrialist and philanthropist, never forgave

INDISPENSABLE
Dr. Crile's surgical team spent three months at the American Ambulance Hospital in Paris in early 1915. Dr. Crile himself left in February; Dr. Lower (in photograph, seated) took his place. The entire team departed for home in March — except for the indispensable Agatha Hodgins (4th from left), who stayed on into May to teach both physicians and nurses how to administer nitrous oxide anesthesia. A French surgeon wrote to Dr. Crile thanking him for the work of his team, especially Miss Hodgins: "I realize what a sacrifice it must have meant on your part to do without her...for this time."

him his refusal. He cited this rift as one reason for his own eventual decision to found the Cleveland Clinic.

The Clinic Is Founded

For this reason, and for several others, The Cleveland Clinic Foundation was, like nursing, a child of war. The founders, in retrospect, credited the idea for the Clinic to conversations that took place during walks in the "beautiful pine forest" just outside the base or evening "fireside chats" in the officers' quarters at No. 9. "The experience in a military hospital impressed these men with the efficiency of an organization that included every branch or specialty of medicine and surgery. They gained insight into the benefits that could be obtained when a group of specialists cooperated."[43]

Not only efficiency, but also an exhilarating sense of freedom characterized this interlude of military medicine. Dr. Crile, especially, had extraordinary liberty, as Director of the Division of Research in the American Expeditionary Force, to "move about and visit the stations wherever the action was." To him, wartime scarcities and the inevitable red tape spun out by the military bureaucracy were more than offset by the advantages of the situation: no medical school; no trustees; and no pressure to build a practice. "What a vast difference between this type of work and that at home! As a matter of fact, this to me is one splendid vacation," he wrote home to his wife, Grace, not long after arriving in Rouen. Small wonder that Drs. Crile, Bunts, and Lower — like many others among the Unit's members — despite the war's genuine horrors, hatreds, and deprivations, looked back to their service "over there" as a golden age in their lives.[44]

Our Own Masters

This emotional appeal may, in the end, have been the real motivating factor that led to the Clinic's founding. But there were many other reasons. On the positive side was the great success of the Mayo Clinic. Also, the three surgeons could look back to the long years of working together at the Office, as well as to the practical advantages of the base hospital model. On the negative side was the unsatisfactory condition of the status quo. Letters from home documented deteriorating conditions at Lakeside Hospital. "All of your skillful head nurses are gone....Sloan says work is so much easier at Mt. Sinai or White than at Lakeside. Nothing is so bled out as Lakeside....Phillips came up to the office the other day and sputtered to Miss Slattery over the difficulty in getting a patient to go to Lakeside and that when they did go, it was equally difficult to keep them contented there."[45] Ironically, the very existence of the Lakeside Unit, the embodiment of the base hospital concept credited to Dr. Crile, was a major factor in creating these problems.

Also, down the road, mandatory retirement loomed. Dr. Crile was due to retire as professor of surgery at Western Reserve, and therefore as chief surgeon at Lakeside Hospital, when he reached age 60 in 1924. Dr. Lower had agreed to retire from Mount Sinai Hospital when he had sufficiently trained junior men to take over the service there.

Diary entries and correspondence of Dr. Crile and Dr. Lower repeatedly refer to "great plans" they had in mind for the time when the war would be over. More definitely, in 1918, Dr. Lower, who had returned to Cleveland to keep the home fires burning, wrote, "I still think an 'association hospital' might be the best solution for the future. It could thus be run as we wish to run it." He later reminisced, "The general idea [of an association hospital] had quite taken possession of [me] and after the Armistice, when Dr. Crile was ordered home, [I] went on to meet him in New York City to present the idea anew. Crile was rather lukewarm about the proposition, having about decided to organize at Lakeside Hospital."[46]

However, Dr. Crile's differences with Samuel Mather and the Lakeside trustees, his general impatience with restrictions of any sort, and the flourishing state of his postwar practice, convinced him that his colleague was right. "In time I came to accept Ed's view about not building up our future in an institution governed by a Board of Trustees, but to be our own masters."[47]

In October of 1919, approximately six months after the Unit returned to Cleveland, Dr. Crile, Dr. Lower, Dr. Bunts, and Dr. Phillips (who was also a member of the Lakeside visiting staff and had served in the military, although not with the Lakeside Unit), signed a document creating the Association Building Company "for the purpose of financing, erecting, and equipping the Clinic building." The company leased land on the southwest corner of East 93d Street and Euclid Avenue on the streetcar line a few blocks west of busy Doan's Corners and the growing University Circle area. Dr. Lower had astutely observed that "the trend of activities for professional work was away from town and more toward the east," and so the Office left the Osborn Building and, like so many Cleveland hospitals, went east. A year and a half after the agreement was signed, the Clinic opened its doors in February 1921.[48]

From Home to Hospital

Initially, the Cleveland Clinic was something like a very grand version of the Office. Patients came there for examinations, consultations, and diagnostic work, just as they had gone to the Office. The physicians continued to admit patients and operate at Lakeside, Mt. Sinai, St. Vincent Charity, and the other hospitals where they were visiting staff members. However, the Clinic soon needed its own hospital facilities; two houses, also on East 93d Street, served this purpose for a time. Opened on April 1, their 53 beds were used for patients awaiting or convalescing from surgery or other treatment, as well as for patients who had to undergo extensive testing for diagnosis. Within a year, a brick addition was built behind one of the houses to accommodate the increasing number of operations Dr. Crile was performing on his own Clinic's premises. "The pressure of work, the lack of space at Lakeside, their continual complaint of my barrage of patients and insistent waiting list made us organize our own operating room and staff at Oxley Homes, and in the first year we performed over 1200 operations."[49] The concept was very similar to the small proprietary hospitals run by physicians for their own patients, except that it was part of the not-for-profit Cleveland Clinic.

OXLEY HOMES
Initially, the Cleveland Clinic had no hospital building of its own, only outpatient facilities. Two houses on East 93rd Street were purchased to serve as a nursing home for patients who needed to stay over one or more nights. They opened in April 1921 and became known as the Oxley Homes, since their superintendent, Emma Oxley, had title to the property. In 1923, two more buildings on the street were converted, into the Diabetic House and the Therapy House for the care of patients receiving insulin and radiation therapy, respectively. Another nearby building, the Bolton Square Hotel, could accommodate convalescent patients. Although there was no nursing staff there, private duty nurses were occasionally called in.

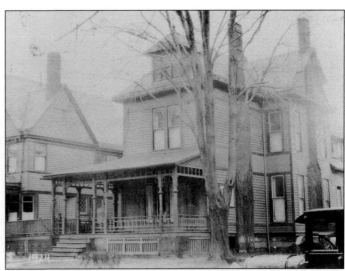

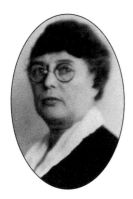

EMMA OXLEY
Under the direction of Mrs. Oxley,
nursing staff and other employees
cared for patients in the Oxley
Homes. An English-born nurse,
Mrs. Oxley was a widow when she
went to work for the Cleveland
Clinic in 1921. She had served as
Lakeside Hospital's housekeeper
for 15 years, responsible for
the day-to-day running of the
hospital "household." Her skills
had impressed the Clinic's
founding physicians, and they
brought her to the new institution
as superintendent of its first
inpatient facility. She left
Cleveland a few years later, moving to Montreal, Canada, and then
to Cambridge, Massachusetts.

Although all narratives state that these houses were located by Dr. Lower and purchased by the Foundation, there is some indication that title to the property, at least at first, was in the name of Emma Oxley — housekeeper at Lakeside Hospital for 15 years before she took on the task of administering this new nursing home/hospital. Described as a "competent English nurse," and now entrusted as the first superintendent of the Clinic's private hospital, Mrs. Oxley obviously enjoyed the confidence of the Clinic's founders, three of whom had observed firsthand her administrative skills during her tenure at Lakeside. The two houses, in fact, bore her name — they were known as the "Oxley Homes."[50]

The founders were well aware that once Dr. Crile, in particular, had to retire from his position at Lakeside Hospital, the Clinic would need far more beds than the 53 at the Oxley Homes. Dr. Phillips later stated that "the building of a hospital was part of our original plan of development."[51] A new hospital building would make life easier for the staff, too — since the Oxley Homes had no elevators, orderlies, nurses, and physicians had to carry patients up and down the stairs.

On June 14, 1924, the day on which Dr. Crile's tenure with Lakeside officially ended, the new seven-floor 184-bed Cleveland Clinic Hospital opened. In moving its inpatient facilities from two old houses to a new, modern hospital, the Clinic had in three years made the same transition the nation's entire health care system was in the process of making — the transition from home to hospital. The new institution, conceived less than seven years earlier, was growing rapidly.

Technique and Perfect Teamwork

The construction of a new hospital was a heavy financial burden, which had to be mortgaged and, through financing, met out of the incomes of the founders.

Once The Cleveland Clinic Foundation was set up in 1921, the founders (as well as all other Clinic physicians and employees) went on salary, although apparently some vestige of the original partnership agreement dating back to Office days remained in effect up through 1925. The salaries the Clinic founders received fell far short of the dollar amount their work collectively earned. The remainder of the money went to the Foundation. For instance, in 1922, the first full year of the Clinic's existence, "donations" from the incomes of the four founders amounted to $150,304.76. More than half of this came from Dr. Crile, about a quarter from Dr. Lower. Goiter was at this time still endemic in the Great Lakes region, and Dr. Crile had come to specialize in thyroid surgery. Since thyroidectomy had become "not only safe but almost fashionable" as a treatment for goiter, due to improvements in controlling hyperthyroidism and in operative technique, many, many people came to Dr. Crile for the procedure. He, and the Mayo Clinic, were leaders in the field. In 1926, the peak year of Dr. Crile's earnings, in which he saw 2,773 patients, Clinic receipts from his operations were $346,876.25. He received a salary of $80,000.00; his "donation" was therefore $266,076.25.[52]

These earnings — phenomenal in their day — were based partly on the Clinic's method of setting fees, which one visitor to the institution described thus: "The patients pay for the operation from $100 to $10,000. The fee for operation is fixed before admission, by a secretary in the clinic. It is regulated according to the patient's income, number of dependents, and so forth. Free work is done in some instances."[53] Fees for surgery generally ran between $50 and $1,500, with most being in the $150 to $300 range.

Also phenomenal was Dr. Crile's operative schedule. For example, on January 19, 1926, he had 25 operations scheduled from 8 a.m. to 2 p.m., all but two of which were thyroid operations. Six other operations by four other physicians constituted the Clinic Hospital's entire operative schedule for the day. It was not unusual for Dr. Crile to be scheduled for 30 or more operations on a single day. The visitor quoted above, Dr. John Hammond Bradshaw, recorded his reaction upon receiving a copy of the January 19 schedule. "As one takes up the paper, he involuntarily gasps to find under Dr. Crile's name a program of 25 operations slated at about 15 minutes headway each for the morning. But the impossible becomes possible as the technic and perfect teamwork develop."[54]

This "technic and perfect teamwork" had already been developed and put into place on Dr. Crile's service at Lakeside Hospital. It was based on several factors. First was the fact that thyroid surgery could be performed quickly, under light anesthesia, by a skilled surgeon with the help of well-trained assistants. Second was his trademark use of local anesthesia supplemented by "a whiff or so of [nitrous oxide] gas and oxygen...used off and on" so that there was "no time lost in getting the patient 'under.'" Third was his practice of operating in the patient's room. The original reason for this was to reduce the "shock of operation" for the patient, minimizing the risk of initiating thyroid crisis: a real danger to the lives of patients with severe hyperthyroidism, and one in which Dr. Crile felt emotional factors played an important role. But operating in the patient's room also had the effect of overcoming limits created by the number of operating rooms available, and soon thyroid operations on all sorts of patients, not just high-risk cases, were being performed with the patient remaining in her own bed.[55]

Several written descriptions of thyroid surgery as performed by Dr. Crile at both Lakeside Hospital and the Cleveland Clinic exist. All praise the coordinated work of Crile and his assistants in words similar to those of British surgeon W. H. Bowen, who saw him operate at Lakeside — "the finest demonstration of the perfection of a team system I have ever witnessed, or, I believe, am ever likely to witness."

Mr. Bowen continued:

> Surgical skill combined with an almost perfect team system is what enables Dr. Crile to complete a thyroidectomy in fifteen minutes, not in a special show case, but in a series of cases....[He] has...five assistants, and a highly trained set of theatre nurses....

"A THING TO SEE"
This is how one Cleveland newspaper described a surgery by Dr. Crile. "Into the operating room he marches, clad from head to foot in gleaming white, followed by a cortege of associates, assistants, anesthetists and nurses, while students and spectators watch him pop-eyed and awe-struck from the sidelines.

"To visitors he is beaming, at ease. He smiles at the patients; confidence oozes from him. He growls at the nurses, and they adore him for it." In this photograph, taken at Lakeside Hospital in 1914, Dr. Crile is partially visible in the center just behind the heads of the two nurse anesthetists.

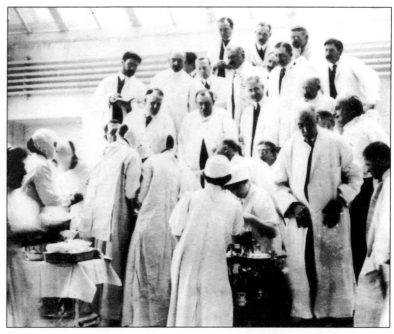

The nurse anaesthetist is ready at the patient's head with a gas oxygen apparatus; but this is only given at the surgeon's orders. Infiltration anaesthesia with 1/2 per cent. novocain is the usual anesthetic. If this local anaesthetic only is used the anaesthetist sits close to the patient's head and talks to her all the time very quietly and soothingly, or firmly, as may be necessary.[56]

Dr. Bradshaw described the rest of the operation from his observations at the Clinic Hospital:

Dr. Crile operates with 2 assistants and 2 nurses. One assistant is the artery clamp man and the other the 'retractor.' A marvelously efficient instrument nurse, using the sheet covered abdomen and legs of the patient as her chief table, slaps with decided audition and with great rapidity, each artery clamp into the extended hand of the first assistant. As Dr. Crile cuts more than he dissects...the snap, snap, snap of each successive clamp into the assistant's hand follows in succession almost like the tick of the clock, for in 5 minutes' time 5 dozen clamps are likely to be applied....It rarely took longer than 5 to 10 minutes for the removal of the gland. Sometimes Dr. Crile would begin and finish each case, but often he would leave the wound to be closed by his highly trained assistants and rapidly go to the intermediate room, change his gloves and gown and go to the next case that was ready (the skin and muscular incisions having been perhaps already made), for the removal of the growth itself. As half a dozen or so cases were kept in the preparatory stage at one time, there was great economy of time.[57]

There was one other component of the process which Dr. Bradshaw particularly noted:

I do not believe this unusual rapidity but safety of work could be possible if it were not for the "Crile Lamp." Now, this is an absurdly inexpensive article. It consists of an ordinary Mazda lamp on a stick! This stick is, say 30 inches long, a little larger than a curtain roller. It is made of a hollow broom stick painted with enamel. The lamp cord is passed through the hollow of the stick. The lamp painted on two-thirds of its surface, is coated first with quicksilver and then painted dark green and is held, wrapped in a sterile towel, by the only second operating room nurse in the room, who stands on a stool above the patient's head and by holding one end of the long stick is herself out of the way but is able to give mobile illumination and that with absolutely no interference nor glare to the operator, an intense and most satisfactory light projected into any and every part of the wound; thus at the expense of a few cents is furnished an operating lamp that not only is able to be taken anywhere at any time...but is by actual working demonstration better in many cases than the $500. or $1000 operating room illuminants it has been my experience to witness in use.[58]

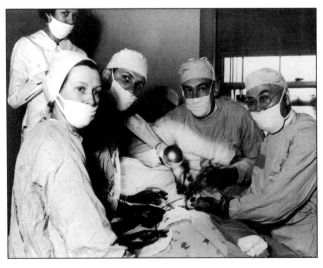

THYROID SURGERY
In 1936, Dr. Crile (far right) performed his 25,000th operation, in a Cleveland Clinic Hospital patient room. Eloise Fisher (left, foreground) was the scrub nurse; nurse anesthetist Elizabeth Thompson is barely visible here behind the two assisting surgeons. The round metallic object in the center is the "Crile lamp," attached to a broomstick wrapped in a sterile towel, which is being held by the nurse in the upper left corner. A staff or private duty nurse, she wears a mask but no gown while providing "mobile illumination" for the operation.

There was another reason, too, why the whole system of "shockless surgery" on the thyroid depended on its performance in the patient's room. One physician, writing in later years, called it a process of "stealing" the thyroid gland, "by which the patient was lightly anesthetized two or three times before the day of operation, and thus kept in ignorance of when it was to take place,...avoiding the emotional stress of worry."[59]

Margaret Boise, chief anesthetist at Johns Hopkins, gave a similar description of the technique in a newspaper interview.

> "This is really a process of delusion....For several days before an operation is to be performed the anaesthetist visits his [sic] patient and injects water with a hypodermic syringe. He also administers plain air or oxygen with a gas mask. This accustoms the patient to the process, and on the last day morphine is substituted for the water and nitrous-oxide oxygen gas for the plain air. Then the operation is performed, accompanied by local injections, and the patient awakes to find to his amazement an operation has been performed."[60]

Difficult as it would have been to schedule 30 procedures in a few operating rooms during a five or six hour period, it would have been impossible at the same time to wheel in and out 60 or 70 more people for dress rehearsals.

The pace of such a schedule could create stress, especially in an established institution like Lakeside, which already had its own routines and workload, onto which these additional tasks had to be grafted. When patient rooms had to be used as operating rooms, with the surgical team moving rapidly from one room to the next, the preparation for and aftermath of the operation had to be handled by the nurses on the ward. At Lakeside Hospital this meant the nursing students supervised by the head nurse. Grace Allison declared that she could not find a Lakeside graduate willing to serve as head nurse on one ward where many thyroid patients were admitted.

Even the use of the "Crile lamp" so praised by Dr. Bradshaw was a problem from the perspective of the nurse administrator: it was not such an "absurdly inexpensive article" when a nurse's time had to be added to the cost of the Mazda lamp and the broomstick. However, to Dr. Crile, the mobility and accuracy of the illumination that could be provided by a living holder was apparently worth the extra expense, since he continued with this system in the new Cleveland Clinic Hospital. There, patients' special nurses were often assigned to hold the light, minimizing use of hospital staff nursing time for the purpose. Florence Kempf, president of the Massachusetts League for Nursing Education in 1939, remembered doing this task as a nursing student at Lakeside Hospital and as a private duty nurse at the Clinic Hospital: "Many were the times when I was the tail end of the procession as you moved from room to room on the private pavilions doing thyroidectomies. I did private duty at the Cleveland Clinic for about eighteen months after graduation in 1923."[61]

For many years Dr. Crile relied on two individuals for the success of his thyroidectomies and other operations at the Cleveland Clinic: Emma Barr as Operating Room Supervisor and Lou Adams as Chief Anesthetist. Both had attended the Lakeside Training School for Nurses.

Miss Adams, a member of the Lakeside class of 1909, was one of the school's earliest graduates to work at the Clinic. Though not a pupil of Agatha Hodgins, she was a nurse anesthetist, having studied anesthesia in Philadelphia; though not a member of the Lakeside Unit, she did serve overseas during World War I as a Navy nurse at a base in Scotland. She came to the Cleveland Clinic Hospital in 1924 as head nurse in the Equipment Room, but a year or two later transferred to the Anesthesia Department.

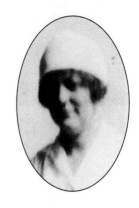

LOU E. ADAMS
Miss Adams was born in Columbia Station, Ohio, in 1886, and graduated from the Lakeside nursing school in 1909. Like most of her classmates, she did private duty nursing immediately after graduation. At the time the U.S. entered World War I, she was working as a surgical nurse at Stanford University Hospital in California. She entered military service and was stationed at a naval base in Scotland. Although she had studied anesthesia, she was first employed by the Cleveland Clinic as head nurse in the Equipment (central supply) Room. She transferred to the Department of Anesthesia in 1926, and served as Chief Anesthetist from 1928 until her retirement in 1952.

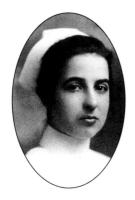

EMMA BARR

Miss Barr grew up in small towns
in Pennsylvania and Ohio, and
graduated from the Lakeside
Hospital nursing school in 1920,
at age 25. She was head nurse of
an operating room there before
coming to the Cleveland Clinic
Hospital in 1924, as head nurse
on the sixth floor. She soon
transferred to the position of
Operating Room Supervisor.
For twenty years, Miss Barr was
responsible for making sure that
the Hospital's operative schedule
ran smoothly. In the 1920s and
1930s, this included Dr. Crile's
thyroid operations in patient
rooms, scheduled at fifteen
minute intervals over five or six
hours. Miss Barr herself went from
room to room ahead of Dr. Crile,
making sure that table, gown, and
gloves were ready for him.

Emma Barr was a more recent graduate of Lakeside. Immediately after
finishing her nursing education in 1920, she took a position on her alma
mater's operating room staff, before coming to work as head nurse on the sixth
floor and then Operating Room Supervisor at the Clinic Hospital. Dr. Crile's
son, Dr. George ("Barney") Crile, Jr., remembered her as a "black-haired, handsome" woman in charge of the operating room and the "mobile units" used to
perform thyroidectomies in patients' rooms. He described how she and Miss
Adams worked together with the surgeons on these cases.

> The patient was sedated in the early morning and allowed to sleep until
> the nurse anesthetist came in and talked to her soothingly....[Miss
> Adams] was one of the world's greatest conversationalists. With her
> stream of fact, fancy, and query, the patients were distracted from their
> fears and intoxicated by analgesia provided by inhalation of a little
> nitrous oxide, sometimes called laughing gas. One of the residents would
> come in and prepare the neck with iodine and alcohol. Miss Barr would
> then open the table and the scrub nurse would arrange the instruments.
> The chief resident would bustle in and infiltrate the neck with novo-
> caine....Then the resident would make the incision and expose the thy-
> roid. At this time, or soon after, Dr. Crile would charge in, change into the
> new gown and gloves provided by Miss Barr, and spend five or ten min-
> utes removing the thyroid. Then off he would go to the next operation,
> leaving the resident to close the incision.

Dr. Crile, Jr., finished the story with an important observation: "This was the
organization that enabled my father to do so many operations....And it was
Miss Barr and Miss Adams coordinating their efforts with the other nurses and
the house staff that made it possible."[62]

Swarming to the Clinic

To Dr. Crile, it seemed that not only Miss Barr and Miss Adams, but
the whole Lakeside staff had left the old hospital to join him at the new
Clinic Hospital.

> As previously stated, I said good by to the tried and faithful nursing and
> professional staff of Lakeside on the day I left, and lo and behold, when I
> came back from abroad to the new hospital, here they all were down to
> the orderlies and porters, to greet me. Lakeside, like a hive of bees,
> swarmed and landed in the new clinic hospital.[63]

This was an exaggeration. Of the 71 visiting and resident staff physicians
on Lakeside's roster at the beginning of 1924, only 7 — including Drs. Crile,
Lower, and Phillips themselves — appeared among the 34 M.D.s (including
fellows) on the roster of the Cleveland Clinic a year later, although a few more
men from the 1924 Lakeside staff did join the Clinic in subsequent years.

More nurses than physicians "swarmed" to the Cleveland Clinic. Many of
the key nursing positions at the Clinic proper, the Oxley Homes, and the Clinic
Hospital during the early years were filled by nurses from the staff or training
school of Lakeside Hospital. By no means all, and probably not even half, of
the graduate nurses actually working at Lakeside as of 1924 left for the Cleveland Clinic. However, a substantial number of Clinic nurses had graduated
from the Lakeside school or had worked there at some point during their
careers. Of the 23 nurse administrator, head nurse, anesthetist, and operating

room nurse positions on the Cleveland Clinic staff at the beginning of 1925, at least 12 were held by women who had worked or been educated at Lakeside Hospital.[64]

Emma Barr had worked in Lakeside's operating room; Abbie Porter, the Clinic Hospital's Superintendent of Nurses, had supervised Lakeside's private pavilion. Blanche Snyder, the Clinic's Operating Room Superintendent in 1925, had been Lakeside's operating room supervisor. Preceding her co-workers in departing the Lakeside hive, she had moved to the Oxley Homes by 1922. As head nurse of the new operating room there, she held a position second only to that of Mrs. Oxley herself — another early arrival and former Lakeside employee. Clinic Hospital head nurses Frances Seitz and Anna Tulloss had been head nurses at Lakeside Hospital. Clinic anesthetist Margaret Lane, a veteran of the Lakeside Unit, had received anesthesia training both overseas and at Lakeside, and had worked as second, and then first assistant anesthetist at Lakeside Hospital from 1922 to 1923.

As she had in 1917, Agatha Hodgins remained at Lakeside after Dr. Crile's departure. However, mutual respect and admiration between her and Dr. Crile remained strong. "To me you will always be 'The Chief' held in constant, appreciative and affectionate regard," she assured him.[65] Likewise strong was the connection between Lakeside's anesthesia school and the Clinic anesthesia service. In her annual report for 1924, Miss Hodgins wrote:

> May we here express our feeling of deep gratitude and appreciation to Dr. Crile, our former chief, for the constant help and encouragement extended to the department of anesthesia, throughout his years of service to Lakeside Hospital. We like to think that in entrusting the work of anesthesia in his new hospital to our graduates, he is still showing to the world his always loyal belief in the nurse anesthetist.[66]

Not only did the Lakeside school furnish the Clinic's anesthetists; the new Clinic Hospital (along with several other area hospitals) furnished additional facilities for the clinical training of Lakeside anesthesia students, some of whom spent a month there during their course of study.

At this time the school was graduating more than 30 students a year. Agatha Hodgins remained at her post as Lakeside's chief anesthetist and head of its anesthesia school until her career was cut short by ill health in 1934. Even then she continued to support the cause of nurse anesthetists with intelligence and grace, determination and humor, remaining active as an advocate and a mentor to younger members of the field she had pioneered early in the century.

The All-Graduate Staff

Just as some Lakeside nurses had chosen to go overseas during World War I, each for her own reasons, so some had now chosen to become Cleveland Clinic nurses. Like the physicians who followed Dr. Crile to the new clinic and hospital, they felt respect and affection for him as a leader. There was also an element of excitement in being associated with his scientific and medical work, which frequently made both local and national headlines, and in being associated with a grand new venture like the Clinic. For some, the supervisory positions they obtained at the Clinic were in effect promotions. And, finally,

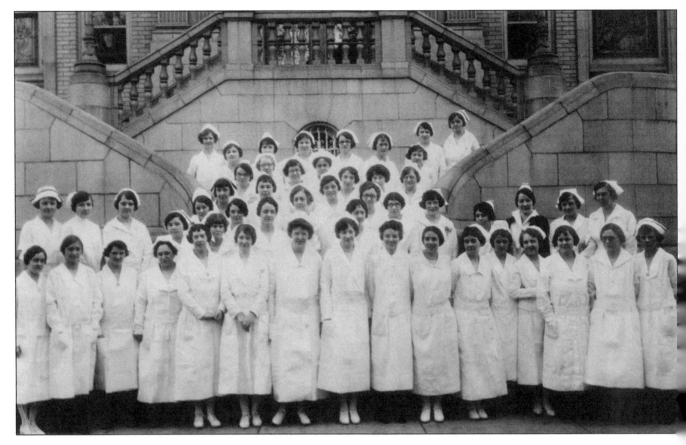

NURSING STAFF, 1925
This group photograph shows 52 members of the Cleveland Clinic Hospital nursing staff posed in front of the Hospital building. In March 1925 there were 42 general duty nurses, 7 head nurses, 4 operating room nurses, and 4 nursing administrators employed at the Hospital.

there was the joy of the craftsperson — the joy of the job well done, of performing as part of a precision team that excelled in what it did.

Fortunately, too, the Clinic and its Hospital were custom-built and staffed for the sort of work that Dr. Crile and his colleagues did. The Hospital was constructed "in such a manner that each and every room is an operating room....The rooms accommodate 1, 2, or in a few instances 4 beds, and have wide doorways (44 inches)."[67]

The nursing staff itself was part of the solution:

> Every effort is made to make the patient as comfortable as possible and to prevent the hospital routine from being so iron-clad that it is a burden and an irritation to him. There is no nurses' training school, but a post-graduate course is offered to the Nursing staff which consists entirely of registered nurses. In emergencies they act practically automatically, and furnish a very valuable cooperation to the doctors.[68]

Undoubtedly, the practice of operating in the patient's room was not such a fearsome burden to a head nurse when her staff consisted of fully-trained colleagues who acted "practically automatically," rather than inexperienced students whom she had to teach as well as supervise.

In 1924, 16 of the 44 hospitals listed in the Cleveland city directory had nursing schools listed as well: City, Euclid Avenue, Fairview Park, Glenville, Grace, Huron Road, Lakeside, Lakewood, Lutheran, Maternity, Mt. Sinai, St. Alexis, St. Ann's, St. John's, St. Luke's, and St. Vincent Charity. All six of the hospitals that the 1920 Cleveland Hospital and Health Survey had designated as major hospitals serving the entire population of the Cleveland area (as opposed to community or other more narrowly based institutions) — City, Huron Road, Lakeside, Mt. Sinai, St. Luke's, and St. Vincent Charity — had nursing schools in 1924.[69] The newly founded Cleveland Clinic Hospital, which also attracted patients from throughout the area and from greater distances as well in the 1920s, was at that point the only major hospital in Cleveland relying on an all-graduate staff.

Patient Satisfaction

In 1925, at the Clinic's annual meeting for staff and employees, Dr. Phillips spoke about his ideals for patient care:

> A great deal has been said in the last 3 or 4 years about the standardization and efficiency of hospitals. I read somewhere not long ago about the importance of these elements but also of retaining a genuine humanity. The patient coming into the hospitals should feel the touch of human kindness all through his treatment. It is not enough to take care of him medically and surgically but he should feel that he is among friends who are trying to ameliorate his ills; who are not only trying to cure his bodily complaints but also his mental fears.[70]

When the Cleveland Clinic Hospital opened in 1924, its directors characterized it as a "'hotel for the sick' to meet the needs of patients of moderate means." At the dedication of the Clinic in 1921, Dr. Crile had cited "the rapid advance of medicine," and the need to engage in the "active investigation of disease" as a "duty to the patient of tomorrow" as well as the patient of today, as among the reasons behind the Clinic's founding. The Cleveland Clinic Foundation was a thoroughly modern, scientific institution; for better or for worse, it was not burdened with the 19th-century philosophical baggage earlier voluntary hospitals had carried. Unlike Lakeside Hospital, the Clinic Hospital began not as a "Home for Friendless Strangers," but as a "hotel for the sick," to care for the increasing numbers of middle-class people for whom home care during serious illness was no longer an option.[71]

Patients and referring physicians were very happy with the treatment they received at the Clinic. A patient from Tennessee wrote a letter of thanks after his return home, praising the staff of the floor he had stayed on, as well as Nursing Superintendent Elizabeth Hinds:

> There was absolutely nothing during my twenty-three days stay on the sixth floor to disturb the equilibrium, not a jar, not a harsh word from any of the attendants, but all seemed eager and willing to go the full length of their ability to make everyone happy.
>
> ....Miss McCrea who presides over the sixth floor was a very fine example of efficiency and delightful in her attitude every way. So also were her attendants. She possesses the diplomatic qualities that are so essential in dealing with the intricacies of such a position. Miss Hinds with her fine spirit and friendliness was constantly on hand making everyone happy as a result of her presence.... The esprit de corp of the whole institution is so marvelous.[72]

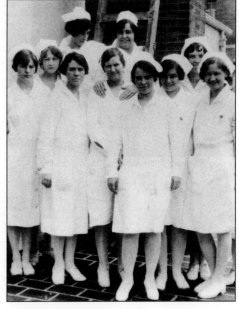

ON THE ROOF
Several Cleveland Clinic Hospital nurses, including 1922 Lakeside graduate Elizabeth Pratt Graber (front row, center), posed for this 1920s-vintage photograph on the hospital roof — a favorite spot for picture-taking. From the beginning, the Cleveland Clinic Hospital was staffed by graduate nurses. This was often not the case in early twentieth century hospitals. Those with nursing schools frequently got by without any general staff nurses. Nursing students, supervised by a few graduates, did nearly all of the patient care.

Word spread by mouth and by newspaper. Although most of the Clinic's patients came from northeastern Ohio and the surrounding states, others came from across the nation, and a few from across the world. Dr. Crile, and in a way the Cleveland Clinic itself, had become celebrities, and success bred success, as fame drew increasing numbers of patients while the growing numbers of patients added to the fame of the Clinic and Dr. Crile. Although the founders had specifically decided on an impersonal name for the new institution, many people called it the "Crile Clinic."

In August 1925, Dr. Crile performed 344 operations, a personal record. He had at this point performed a total of 10,214 goiter operations (also 1,020 stomach operations, 1,664 operations on the gall bladder, and 418 on the large intestine). "The endowment is now $400,000. We hope to raise this to $1,000,000 in four years. We also hope to build a laboratory building for research. My personal earnings are running at about the rate of $300,000 a year, and I am receiving $72,000."[73] The growing endowment, on which the

A Favorite Patient

In 1921, Dr. Frederick G. Banting of Canada isolated the hormone insulin for use in treating diabetes. Within a year, insulin was being distributed to a small number of physicians working with diabetic patients, including Dr. Henry John of the Cleveland Clinic. Patients had to be kept under observation, since very little was known about possible reactions to this new treatment. Dr. John's patients stayed in the Oxley Homes, and, as of 1923, the Diabetic House on East 93rd Street, cared for by the Homes' nursing staff.

One young patient stayed not for weeks, or months, but for years. Madeleine Bebout, the first child to receive insulin in Cleveland, was brought in to the Clinic, in a coma, at the end of 1922. She was 4 years old, and motherless since babyhood. There was no one able to pay for her treatment.

The Cleveland Clinic "adopted" the child, providing not only treatment —

four daily injections of insulin — but also a home, and a loving "family." Just before Christmas in 1926, when Madeleine was 8, the *Cleveland Press* featured her story.

"To all appearances, Madeline is a normal, healthy child. And she will continue as such so long as the insulin treatment is continued and there is no other disease to fight....

"Madeline says she has 'three mamas' — Miss Myra Cassell, head nurse in the diabetic hospital

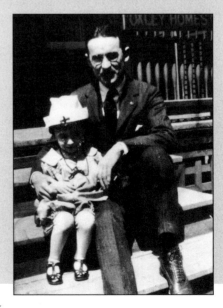

entire financial future of the institution rested, was thus based largely on the volume of operations performed by Dr. Crile — in turn made possible by the coordinated efforts of the entire operative team, including nurses and nurse anesthetists, as Dr. Barney Crile had observed.

Staffing and Salaries

The concept at the heart of The Cleveland Clinic Foundation was the concept of the Clinic itself — a group practice of specialists modeled on the base hospital and the Mayo Clinic. The Clinic Hospital began as a sort of appendage, as a private hospital to take care of those patients of Clinic physicians who could not be cared for on an ambulatory basis. The hospital developed out of the Oxley Homes, two ordinary houses originally purchased to be used as a nursing home for patients under observation. Soon they were equipped with an operating room and began to function more like a small hospital; from there, the next step was the construction of a full-scale, built-

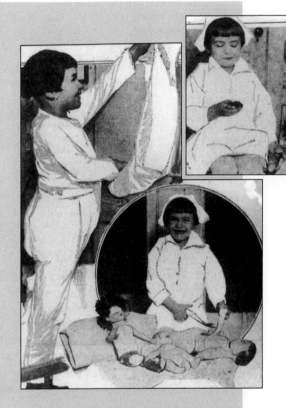

attached to the clinic, and her assistants, Miss Jane Swanson and Miss Elizabeth Berkey.

"The child is now enrolled in Laurel School all thru the good offices of the Cleveland Clinic.

"And Madeline's 'three mamas' make very real financial sacrifices to see that the child has a real home. They buy her clothes.... They buy her toys and all sorts of knick-knacks.

"Madeline is quite happy. She will tell you so. You can see it for yourself, too."

The newspaper photographs (this page) show Madeleine hanging up her "ether sack" Christmas stocking; and, dressed in a nurse's uniform just like the ones worn by her "three mamas," caring for her doll-patients.

Although a patient of Dr. John, Madeleine was everyone's favorite. In photographs taken circa 1923 (opposite page), the tiny girl sits on the steps of the Oxley Homes with Dr. Thomas Jones of the Department of Surgery, and with four of the nurses who made the hospital a real home for her. (This is the earliest known photograph of Cleveland Clinic nurses.)

Best of all, Madeleine's story had a happy ending. In those early days of insulin therapy, diabetic children did not have a long life expectancy. Madeleine, however, was a survivor. She grew up, moved to New York City, and lived well into middle age.

for-the-purpose hospital. However, despite the importance of the Clinic proper (that is, the ambulatory group practice), most of the institution's nursing staff, from the days of the Oxley Homes onward, worked on the hospital side. "We do not have a great number of nurses," remarked Lillian Grundies, the Clinic's head surgical nurse, in 1929.[74]

In April of 1921, two months after its opening, the outpatient Clinic had a nursing staff of 4. They had a collective monthly salary of $435, which meant an average of $110 each per month, or $1,320 per year. The clerical staff was much larger — 25 women, with an average salary of $1,620 per year.[75] (In both groups, particularly in the clerical group, a few employees had significantly higher salaries than the others, skewing the averages.) Six night cleaning women, a telephone operator, and possibly 2 of the 6 laboratory workers comprised the rest of the Clinic's female staff, for a total of 38 out of 60 employees (not including the 4 founding physicians). The 22 men included 10 physicians, 6 engineering and building maintenance workers, and art department and laboratory workers. Actual yearly salaries for individuals (again, excluding the founders) could be as high as the $15,000 paid Dr. Harry Sloan; most physicians received from $4,000 to $6,000, except for the fellow doctors, who received $1,200.

Nurses Bessie Thomas and Blanche Young received $1,200 each; nurse Bessie Hull is listed as receiving $1,020. Head surgical nurse Lillian Grundies, who had worked for the founders since first being employed at the Osborn Building Office in 1912, earned a salary of $1,800. Dr. Crile's secretary, editor, and research assistant Amy Rowland and artist William Brownlow — both, like Miss Grundies, veterans of the Office and the Lakeside Unit — were paid $3,600 and $4,000, respectively. "Building" workers Wilhemina Coffey, Lester Liebrock, and George Messner earned $936, $1,300, and $2,080. Secretaries Dorothy Daniels and Henrietta Scherwitz had salaries of $1,320 and $1,560. Reception room worker Charlotte DeHart earned $1,200, as did X-ray assistant Harry Clark Smith. In Cleveland in 1920, a skilled laborer working a 44-hour week in the manufacturing industry earned an average yearly wage of $1,571.86; an unskilled laborer, $1,210.35.

In 1922, four individuals — Lillian Grundies, Blanche Young, Harry Jones, and Lelah Parkhurst — were listed in the "Nursing" department of the outpatient Clinic. At this time, 11 women, at least 7 of whom were nurses, were working at the Oxley Homes, along with a male orderly and a custodian. In March 1925, during the first year of the Clinic Hospital's operation, the number of female employees in the outpatient Clinic who might possibly have been nurses (in fact, most of them were probably secretaries) was 28; the Oxley Homes employed 16 nurses and an orderly. The Hospital employed 61 nurses (including anesthetists), 4 postgraduate students, 6 female ward helpers, and 8 male orderlies.

The Nurse Administrator

The first Superintendent of the Clinic Hospital was a nurse, Charlotte Dunning, who remained in the position for three years. Abbie Porter, the Hospital's first Superintendent of Nurses, succeeded her in 1927, remaining in the post until 1949.

It was not unusual for a nurse to serve as a hospital superintendent at this time, especially in smaller hospitals. The female hospital superintendent, like

ALWAYS THERE
A lifelong Clevelander, Lillian Grundies was born in 1887, and grew up in the city's old Brooklyn neighborhood. In 1912, beginning an association that would last 40 years, she went to work as a surgical nurse for Drs. Bunts, Crile, and Lower. She served with the Lakeside Unit during WWI, and in 1921 became the Cleveland Clinic's first head nurse. She was most closely associated with Dr. Lower, working on his corridor in the Clinic building and often assisting him during cystoscopies and other procedures. In later years, she became head nurse of the Equipment Room, and then, in 1937, the Clinic's purchasing agent, a position she held until retiring in 1952.

the hospital housekeeper and the hospital superintendent of nursing, was an occupational descendant of the 19th-century hospital matron, who had often combined these three roles in one person. A list of superintendents of 15 Cleveland hospitals in 1927 shows only five male superintendents, of whom three were M.D.s. Of the 10 hospitals headed by women, 3 were run by Roman Catholic orders, and 3 more were hospitals specializing in work with women or children. That still left 4 non-Catholic general hospitals — the Clinic, Glenville, Lakewood, and Lutheran Hospitals — with female superintendents. At Lakewood Hospital and also at one of the Catholic hospitals, the hospital superintendent also served as the superintendent of nurses. However, Lakeside, Mt. Sinai, St. Luke's, and Huron Road, which were among the city's largest and best-established hospitals, had male superintendents.[76]

At the time Abbie Porter was called on to take Charlotte Dunning's place as the Superintendent of the Clinic Hospital, she had been employed as its Superintendent of Nurses for three years. During the First World War she had served as a nurse with the U.S. Army, although not in the Lakeside Unit. After the end of the war, in 1919, she was appointed supervisor of the private pavilion at Lakeside Hospital. The private pavilion had proportionately more graduate nurses on its staff than any other part of Lakeside Hospital, and Dr. Crile's patients filled many of its beds. For Abbie Porter to take on the job of Superintendent of Nurses at the new Clinic Hospital, with its all-graduate staff, was a natural transition.

During Miss Porter's tenure as Superintendent of Nurses, Helen McBride served as Assistant Superintendent of Nurses. Miss M. O. Sloan held the position of night supervisor, and Hilda Beam was assistant night supervisor. Besides Miss Adams and Miss Barr, Florence Barnett, Sara Cunningham, Ida Johnsten, Frances Seitz, and Anna Tulloss served as head nurses during the first year of the Hospital's existence. The Operating Room had a staff of four nurses headed by Blanche Snyder.

About 50 members of the Clinic Hospital nursing staff worked as head or general duty nurses. Since each of the Hospital's six floors had only one ward helper and one orderly, and since not more than about 30 of the nurses could have been on duty at any one time, six or seven people, at most, must have handled all patient care-related tasks for each floor (there was an average of 30 beds per floor). This included everything from passing trays and feeding patients to wound care to bed making to keeping records to passing medications to giving baths and back rubs. However, all nursing care did not fall to the Clinic-employed nursing staff.

Undivided Attention: The Special Nurse

Since the Cleveland Clinic Hospital did not rely on training school students to supplement or take the place of a full staff of graduate nurses, the "special nurse" — a private duty nurse engaged to care for an individual hospital patient, who was paid directly by that patient — had an especially important role there. The hiring of special nurses was such common practice that the Clinic Hospital's brochure for incoming patients in 1926 noted that the regular room rates included meals, attendance by the resident staff, and "the *divided* attention of a floor nurse [emphasis added]"; it also gave instructions regarding the hiring of specials.

IN THE 1920s
By 1923, the Clinic had 120 employees. On some days, more than 200 outpatients were seen. With the addition of the Hospital in 1924, the number of employees grew, to 470 by 1929.

In 1926, Hospital room rates ranged from $6 a day in a four-bed room, to $40 for a suite with two bedrooms, a sitting room and two baths. An ordinary single room cost from $10 to $20; a bed in a double room was $7.50. A 60-member nursing staff, plus an average of 90 special nurses, cared for Hospital patients. The usual postoperative stay was one to two weeks.

Operating room charges ranged from $10 to $50. Surgeons' fees varied widely depending on the operation, but most were in the $150 to $300 range. A typical day's operative schedule consisted of 20 to 25 thyroid operations and 2 laparotomies by Dr. Crile; 2 thyroidectomies by Dr. Dinsmore; 2 or 3 tonsillectomies by Dr. Waugh; 2 laparotomies by Dr. Jones; and a few orthopaedic procedures by Dr. Dickson.

> The Hospital will charge the patient for the board of each special nurse who may be employed on the case at the rate of $2.00 per day, and, on the order of the patient's physician, at the request of the patient or of the relatives of the patient, will secure such special nurses as promptly as possible. In rendering this service the Hospital acts as an agent only, and assumes no responsibility except that the nurses secured shall be competent in respect of their professional duties.
>
> The fees of special nurses are payable to the nurses only, not to the Hospital.[77]

After the world war, bearing out Dr. Bunts' observations, a substantial number of former Lakeside Unit nurses had turned to industrial nursing or to social service and public health nursing. However, several of the Unit women who preferred to work as private duty nurses did frequent stints as specials at the Clinic Hospital. Their competence "in respect of their professional duties" had been tried and tested at Rouen under the eyes of the Clinic's founders. Ara Agerter, Laura Miller, and Elizabeth Bidwell — who had demonstrated her devotion to her wartime patients by stealing potatoes from Dr. Lower's cherished vegetable gardens — were among those Lakeside Unit veterans who found ready employment for their skills as special nurses at the Clinic Hospital.

The usual rate for 12 hours of attendance by a private duty nurse in Cleveland at this time was $6, or $7 for some categories of cases, like obstetrical, contagious, or mental. During the first few months of its operation, when the Clinic Hospital's average daily census of patients numbered 75, the number of special nurses on duty at the Hospital averaged 31 per day. The number of the Hospital's own employees at work on a given day, including office workers and support department employees as well as nursing personnel, averaged 88. Private duty nurses could also be hired by the Hospital for general duty on a temporary basis, but this was a situation distinct from the private duty nurse's more usual role as a special, hired for and paid by an individual patient.

Traditionally, private duty nurses had cared for patients in their homes. For the nurse, the advantages of this were non-institutional working conditions, independence from the hospital nursing hierarchy, and the chance for a higher income than could be obtained as a hospital employee. Disadvantages included the tendency of some patients and their families to treat nurses as servants, the lack of hospital equipment, and the long hours and intermittent nature of the work. As the care of the sick moved increasingly out of the home and into the hospital, private duty nursing followed.

In 1926, according to the Cleveland Central Committee on Nursing, 87.6 percent of private duty nursing in Cleveland was done in hospitals, and only 12.4 percent in patients' homes. The city's Central Registry for Nurses reported that more than three hundred calls for nursing in private homes went unfilled that year, and that nurses were registering against home assignments.

Private Duty Nursing in Cleveland

The Cleveland-area affiliate of the American Nurses' Association (ANA) was District No. 4 of the Ohio State Nurses' Association (OSNA). Later known as the Greater Cleveland Nurses Association, District No. 4 served as the primary membership organization for the area's professional nurses, and operated a non-commercial nursing registry as "a service to the public, to the physician, to the hospital and to the nurse." It operated under several different names

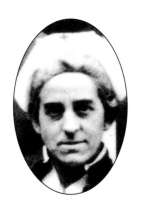

ARA AGERTER
During the 1920s, many graduate nurses preferred to work as private duty nurses, rather than as general staff nurses in hospitals. Called to the home or hospital on a case-by-case basis, a private duty nurse devoted her entire attention to one patient. Many Cleveland Clinic Hospital patients, probably more than half in the first decades, were "specialed" by private duty nurses. Some Cleveland nurses cared for so many cases there, they seemed almost like members of the staff. Among them were Lakeside Unit veterans Elizabeth Bidwell, Laura Miller, and Ara Agerter. Miss Agerter, a classmate of Lou Adams, graduated from the Lakeside Hospital Training School in 1909. With the exception of her wartime service, she spent her entire career in private duty nursing, retiring in 1940.

over time — the Central Registry for Nurses, the Official Registry of District No. 4, and the Bureau of Nursing Service — and was, for a number of years, Cleveland's main registry for private duty nurses. For a service fee of $12 a year, a qualified nurse could put her name on the Central Registry's roll of nurses as being available for private duty calls by physicians, patients, and hospitals. Unless a particular nurse, or a particular type of nurse (like a graduate of a specified school) was requested, nurses were assigned in order of call. Graduates of at least five years' standing could choose whether they wanted to work days or nights, in the hospital or in the home. The Central Registry set rates and recommended hours. The usual day was 12 hours, from 7 a.m. to 7 p.m., and the usual rate was $6 per day. This meant that a nurse was paid 50 cents an hour for an ordinary case, plus two meals, or $2 for board. When a nurse specialed in a hospital, the usual practice was for the patient to pay the board fee to the hospital, which would then furnish the nurse's meals.[78]

In this same period — the mid- to late 1920s — the possibility of making changes in the system of private duty nursing, particularly in hospitals, was being discussed. Under the auspices of the Cleveland Central Committee on Nursing, a subcommittee was set up, including several local nursing leaders, as well as representative hospital administrators and physicians, one of whom was Clinic founder Dr. John Phillips. The problem with the current system, from the viewpoint of the nurse, was that she was "unable to maintain the same professional standing as other groups, because her work is intermittent and her earnings as a rule average only about $1500 a year; her hours are very long and she can have no social life."[79]

Frank Chapman, the administrator of Mt. Sinai Hospital, ranged himself squarely on the side of the nurses, despite possible disadvantages to hospital economy. He noted that the state factory law mandated a 44-hour week, and asked why nurses should be expected to work 12-hour days when hospital engineers or maids worked for only 8 hours. Moreover, he pointed out, the system of patients paying nurses' board directly to hospitals was actually a windfall for the latter; it cost Mt. Sinai, for example, only 66 cents to provide the meals for which it was receiving $2.

In the end, the committee recommended that the nurse's compensation should be raised to $8 (the $6 rate plus the $2 board fee), and that, although 12 hours should remain the basic period of service, individual hospitals should try to reduce this to 10 hours. However, little was done to enforce these recommendations.

If she was physically and mentally able to endure the long hours and curtailed social life, a private duty nurse — especially one who had established a good reputation in the community, or a strong working relationship with a particular doctor or doctors — could earn an adequate, if not a "professional" income by the day's standards. Besides Lakeside Unit veterans like Elizabeth Bidwell, several other private duty nurses found regular employment at the Clinic Hospital; for some, so much that they listed it as their working address. Ella Chown, whose private duty career at the Clinic and other nearby hospitals spanned more than 30 years, was one such nurse; another was Flora Short.

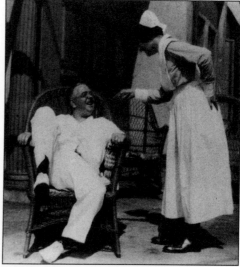

ELLA SCOTT CHOWN
In addition to the three Lakeside Unit veterans, a number of other private duty nurses had much of their practice at the Cleveland Clinic Hospital. One of them was Ella Chown, shown here with Clinic fellow Dr. Cecil Hodgkinson. Another native of Ontario, Mrs. Chown graduated from the Lakeside Hospital Training School in 1919. Known at the Clinic as "Ma" Chown, she may have received her nickname during her nursing school days, since she had already been married. Many nursing students did not come directly from high school. Some, like Isabel Hampton Robb, had obtained certificates and worked as teachers. However, it was very unusual for a woman to have been married before entering nursing school.

One Nurse's Story

Miss Short was a member of the first graduating class of the Kahler Hospital Training School (associated with the Mayo Clinic) in Rochester, Minnesota, in 1921. Many young women in her class had begun their training "in response to the world war cry for more nurses." The school's annual, or yearbook, remarked on Miss Short's "constancy" and her "sweet disposition" — qualities that served her well in her long career. During the first few months after graduation, she did private duty work in Rochester. One of her patients was Dr. Will Mayo's wife, whom she nursed at home through two days of bronchitis for a fee of $10. She was then named assistant superintendent at Kahler. After a year in that position, Miss Short moved to Saranac Lake, New York, where she did private duty for a year and a half. At the beginning of 1925, she moved to Cleveland, and, having registered with the Central Registry, began her first case, a six-year-old boy with a fractured pelvis and ruptured bladder, at St. Alexis Hospital on January 16. She was subsequently called to several home cases, as well as to Lutheran, Mt. Sinai, St. Luke's, and, in June, the Clinic Hospital. There, she served for two days as a special nurse for one of Dr. Crile's thyroidectomy patients, a man from Pittsburgh. On the following day she cared for two of Dr. Lower's appendectomy patients (the fee for nursing two patients at the same time was $4.50 apiece, rather than the usual $6).[80]

After that, more and more of Miss Short's calls came from the Clinic Hospital. Although she continued to take cases at other hospitals and in private homes, she had obviously become a favorite at the Clinic. In addition to her attractive personality, she must have had a steady hand, since she would have had the task of holding the "Crile lamp" when she specialed for Dr. Crile's patients. Many of her cases were thyroid operations, but Miss Short cared for people with medical and surgical complaints ranging from fractured skulls to cancer to tonsillitis to "nerves." She also at one time cared for E. C. Daoust — son-in-law of Dr. Bunts, Clinic trustee, and later President of the Cleveland Clinic Foundation; another of her patients was the mother of Clinic neurosurgeon Dr. Charles E. Locke. Certainly, the Clinic physicians had great confidence in her abilities, and it is certain that she could have obtained a permanent position on the Clinic Hospital nursing staff had she wished to do so.

During the 1920s, after her arrival in Cleveland, Miss Short worked from 225 to 252 days a year. In most years she earned from $1,400 to $1,500; in 1926, she earned $1,839. This was slightly higher than the incomes of most nurses working as Clinic employees at the time; however, Miss Short was working longer hours. In the wider world of Cleveland wage-earners, a skilled construction worker employed year-round, working 44 hours a week, would have made $2,402.40 per year in 1920. In 1930, his earnings would have been $3,157.44 per year. Work in the construction business, like private duty nursing, did not guarantee continuous employment; only those building tradesmen fortunate enough to be always on the job would have had such high yearly earnings. But even on a daily basis, the construction worker earned more: $8.40 per 8-hour day in 1920, and $11.04 per 8-hour day in 1930. Between 1925 and 1930, Flora Short's daily wage (averaged out on a yearly basis) ranged from $6.08 to $7.30 for a 12-hour day.[81]

Reversal of Fortune

On the whole, these first years were good years for Cleveland Clinic nurses, employees and specials alike, just as they were for the Cleveland Clinic itself. The Clinic employed a large number of graduate nurses; it also could provide a steady market for the free-lance labors of private duty nurses. The number of patients registered at the Clinic and admitted to the Hospital continued to grow steadily, along with the young institution's local and national reputation. A large addition to the Hospital opened in 1929, bringing the total number of beds to 275.

These happy days abruptly came to an end as the decade closed. Private and public disaster alike fell upon the Clinic, and its nurses suffered their own share of the consequences.

A foreshadowing of the dark times to come was the sudden death of founder Frank Bunts late in 1928. This was a sorrow rather than a disaster — Dr. Bunts had enjoyed a long, successful career, and earned the respect and affection of patients and co-workers alike. But with him, another remaining bit of the old world seemed to pass. His dignified and respectable presence, of which his old-fashioned, fatherly attitude toward nurses was a part, was beginning to fade into memory when the first bitter blow struck the Clinic.

The Disaster

What came to be called in Clinic annals, simply, "the disaster" took place just before noon on May 15, 1929. Slow combustion of nitrocellulose X-ray films stored in the basement of the Clinic building released carbon monoxide and nitrogen oxides, deadly fumes that noiselessly filtered up through air shafts and ducts. By the time the basement burst into flames and explosions blew off the skylight of the building, sending a huge cloud of brownish-yellow smoke into the sky, the human damage had already been done. One hundred and twenty-three people died in the tragedy, most on that same day, most from the effects of the toxic fumes. Forty-three Cleveland Clinic employees, including Dr. Phillips, lost their lives; most of the other victims were patients unfortunate enough to have made appointments to be seen at the Clinic that morning.

People had already started to evacuate the building before any flames or explosions alerted those outside that something was wrong. Clinic employees later told how they began noticing a brownish, dusty smoke coming out of vents, electric outlets, or small holes in the walls. Many at first assumed the problem was electrical. A financial clerk called a co-worker to see if the bookkeeping machine had shorted out. Dr. J. J. Faust and nurse/technician Mary Horning, in the X-ray department on the first floor, right above the deadly storage room, shut down their machines and told their patients to leave the building. Up on the fourth floor, one physician started in the direction of the stairs, but, embarrassed to appear in too much of a hurry, went back for his coat and hat.

Heroes and Victims

In the second floor reception area, described as the "heart" of the Clinic, Edith Morgan, a nurse veteran of the Lakeside Unit, marshaled the waiting patients and visitors toward the stairway at the front of the building. Miss Morgan had begun working at the Clinic only a few months before, not as a

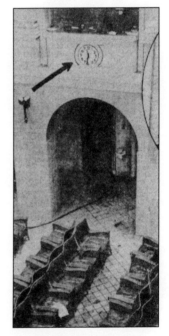

THE ELEVENTH HOUR
The Cleveland Clinic disaster, which occurred shortly before noon on May 15, 1929, claimed the lives of 123 people. The combustion of nitrocellulose X-ray films in the Clinic basement caused an explosion, which blew off the outpatient building's skylight, but most people died from breathing toxic fumes. In the Clinic's reception area on the second floor, a clock stopped at 11:32, the time the explosion took place.

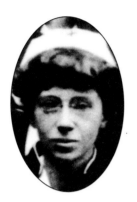

EDITH S. MORGAN
Miss Morgan was born in
Youngstown, Ohio, in 1886, and
graduated from the Lakeside
nursing school in 1905. She
worked as a private duty nurse for
several years, but then went into
public health, as one of Lakeside
Hospital's social service nurses.
While serving in France with the
Lakeside Unit, Miss Morgan
injured her back. She never made
a full recovery and eventually had
to find work less physically
demanding than nursing. She was
hired as a Clinic receptionist early
in 1929. She was one of five
nurses to die in the Clinic disaster,
temporarily trapped in the building by the crush of people on the
reception area stairway. Hearing
of her death, Grace Allison wrote:
"What a life of suffering she has
had since her accident in Rouen,
and now it is over."

nurse, but as a reception clerk. She had never fully healed from a serious back injury incurred while lifting a mattress during her wartime service, and after a "plucky fight" for recovery that had gone on for 10 years, she at least temporarily gave up on trying to return to nursing, and took a receptionist's job at the Cleveland Clinic.[82] Even if not a nursing position, the job did involve patient contact, and so put to good use the interpersonal skills Miss Morgan had developed in her nursing and social service work. It was not really so different from her afternoons in the Lakeside outpatient department before the war, when she had registered children at the dispensary and admitted and discharged them from the hospital.

Miss Morgan was talking to a patient when the fumes became noticeable. She started to take the woman down the hall for her examination, but, in the words of the latter: "At that moment the fumes became thicker. I asked her how to get to the stairway. She showed me and five or six others. I never saw her after that."[83]

Mary Slattery, financial secretary and a long-time Clinic and Office employee, was also in the reception room at the time of the disaster. She noticed "little streams of lava coming up through the center ventilator," and then an explosion.

> Then the patients who were waiting there...became panicky and left their chairs, and we had a hostess, Miss Edith Morgan...who tried to quiet them. I heard her say, "Don't get excited" and then patients started to go toward the stairs, and I went forward to help her re-assure them that nothing was wrong, and she said, "Go down quietly, one at a time, it is nothing but a little accident in the boiler room", and they were going down very orderly when someone on the ground floor called up and said, "Stay up there, it is worse here on the ground floor." Then they came back in a panic, but I am under the impression that a great portion that had started down had survived and left the building and had not been annihilated by the gas at that time."[84]

As it turned out, the people inside would have done better to brave the flames at the front door, because many were trapped and died on the stairway.

Lillian Grundies was on the second floor, where she worked as head nurse, usually on Dr. Lower's corridor. She was preparing a patient for physical examination and had just left her to get a gown, when

> I saw this puff of smoke and heard the explosion, not very loud and I assumed that it came from the basement. My first move was to see who was injured. I started for the back window...when a second explosion occurred, filling the back with a lot of fumes....Then I went down the corridor to warn some of the patients to get dressed. I met several doctors in the corridor but I did not take notice as to who they were as the fumes were coming in so rapidly. I then opened a couple of windows and started for the steps to see if I could get the patients down. I found the stairs blockaded....There were so many persons there, standing up, and coming from the second and third floor....I hesitated for a moment as to what to do, then a third explosion occurred, filling the reception room immediately....I went to the west corridor to see if we could get out there and found the corridor was filled with fumes and escape from the back of the building was utterly impossible.[85]

Mary Slattery remembered that "Our nurse, Miss Grundies, came running along the corridor and said 'Make for the windows' and with that we all made for the windows on the west side of the building. The ladders were put up by the billboard people and I went down the ladder."[86]

Miss Grundies also got out by means of the ladder. She said that several people preceded her, but she was becoming dazed and could not tell who they were. "Fumes were coming around us and we were gasping to get our breaths and I did not notice who was there." She and others had also seen Edith Morgan "at the turn of the stairs, trying to reassure the hysterical patients who crowded above and below her."[87]

Miss Morgan, too, eventually was helped down a ladder from the second floor. She then walked to the Clinic Hospital, where the victims were being taken,

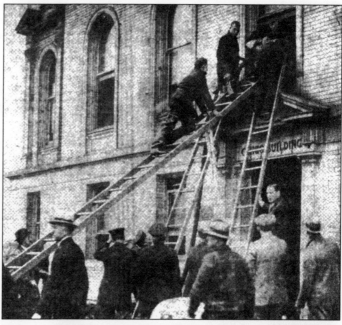

RESCUE ATTEMPTS
Rescuers used ladders to remove people from the Clinic.

> and started to care for those she said were worse off than herself, after she had telephoned her mother that she was all right. A little later she collapsed, was given a transfusion and every possible medical aid, but all in vain. Laura Miller and Elizabeth Bidwell [who had been working as specials at the Clinic Hospital that day] devoted themselves to her care until the end. Edith's mother and several friends were with her, and she was conscious until the last.[88]

The blood to transfuse Miss Morgan was donated by Elizabeth Folckemer, her comrade and commander from Lakeside Unit days. Miss Folckemer, now head of Cleveland's Visiting Nurse Association, had come to the scene like so many nurses, physicians, and ordinary citizens, to see if she could be of assistance. She and members of her staff "helped for several days and nights following the disaster."[89]

Lillian Grundies, too, began caring for others as soon as she left the building, first out on the lawn, and then in the Clinic Hospital. More fortunate than many, she suffered no ill effects other than a severe sore throat. She had covered her mouth and nose and breathed shallowly, by instinct, she said, not realizing the fumes were toxic, while making her way up and down the corridors through the smoke. She remarked, when asked, that she probably could have been confined to the hospital "if I had permitted myself to be, but I knew there was so much to be done. I worked in the hospital all that day until later into the night and also the following day...trying to help them out over there."[90] One of the patients she tended was William Brownlow, photographer and artist from the Office and the Lakeside Unit. She found him out on the lawn, sitting in a wheelchair, his arm bandaged. He had cut himself while breaking open a window on the third floor, after which he helped others out onto a fire department ladder before exiting himself. Despite his injuries

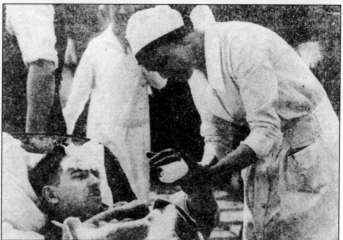

If Edith Morgan's Lakeside Unit service led, indirectly, to her death, Lillian Grundies (lower photo, right) possibly owed her life to military survival training. Able to exit the building by a ladder, she was well enough to care for others including the fatally injured William Brownlow, a long-time co-worker (left).

85

EMERGENCY CARE
While Clinic employees, firemen, policemen, and passers-by brought more people out from inside the building, physicians and nurses gave first aid on the lawn.

he was apparently his own dauntless self all afternoon, going about in a wheelchair, joking with the newspaper men, posing for a newspaper picture with Miss Grundies at his side. In the early evening he took a sudden turn for the worse, and in spite of everything Dr. Paryzek and others could do, passed out. Miss Grundies cared for him to the end. Brownlow leaves a wife and four sons, the oldest twelve years old.[91]

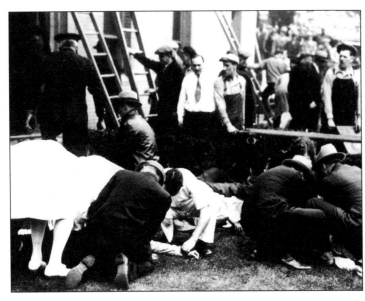

Nurse Louise Swant Morton left behind her husband. She was so newly married that many of the eyewitnesses who saw her that day referred to her as "Miss Swant." Mrs. Morton, aged 31, worked in the Dental Department on the third floor with oral surgeon Dr. W. J. Peart. Dr. Peart was seeing his last patient before noon, a woman from Washington, D.C., when the explosions took place. He got her out of the chair, and Mrs. Morton took the patient out of the room through a side door and into the corridor. Both nurse and patient died. Dr. Lawrence Weller, a Clinic fellow, saw Mrs. Morton run out of the back of the building, through the fumes choking the doorway. She immediately collapsed onto the ground, and Dr. Weller picked her up.

A Cleveland *Plain Dealer* reporter described the scene: "Nurses at the Cleveland Clinic Hospital went about their task of caring for the injured, stunned by the realization that...fellow nurses had been suddenly killed or terribly hurt. Many of them cried from the shock and the strain."

A private duty nurse, on a break from her case, "was downtown when she first heard the news. She went tearing out in a cab, could not get closer than four blocks because of the traffic jam.

"She ran all the way to the hospital, and, out of breath, found the electricity off and the elevators not running. At top speed she ran up four flights of stairs. Her private patient released her and she was assigned, with the other nurses, to the cases of emergency patients from the Clinic.

"At the hospital annex, on E. 93rd Street, nurses were kept busy answering queries. They had a list of known dead, which lengthened steadily during the afternoon."

I realized then that there was something wrong in regard to the aeration of the place, because she was breathing heavily and laborous [sic] and there was a froth to her mouth and she seemed very toxic.... I immediately picked her up and put her in the hands of some nurse standing by - well, there was more than one, and they took her on to the hospital.[92]

Besides Edith Morgan and Louise Morton, three other nurses perished in the disaster: Zanna Fahey of the X-ray Department, Blanche Young of the Surgery Department, and Susanne Matz of the Clinic Hospital, who was at the Clinic that day not as a nurse but as one of the ill-starred patients, being seen for a cold. The newspapers were full of stories of the heroic deeds of Clinic physicians, nurses, other employees, and even visitors and passers-by. One story described the discovery of the body of a nurse collapsed across a wheelchair, in which was still seated the patient she had tried in vain to wheel to safety. For the Clinic nurses, two powerful urges had to be reckoned with. One was the overwhelming instinct for self-preservation; the other was the duty enjoined on them through years of training and experience, that the life of the patient was their trust. A newspaper story about Blanche Young's funeral illustrated the point.

Miss Blanche Young,...a nurse at the Clinic, who is said to have forfeited her life because she refused to forsake a patient, was buried at Calvary cemetery yesterday morning....Father Kirby revealed last night that another nurse who had been with Miss Young at the time of the catastrophe fled from the building and thus saved her life. But Miss Young stayed with her patient and was found in the Clinic building some time later by Father Kirby when he was giving absolution to the dying victims. She received the last rites from him.[93]

Nurses, even in ordinary times, had always been expected to sacrifice "sleep, food, rest, recreation, health"; in times of crisis, it seemed, they were expected to risk their lives.

Other hospitals in the vicinity, including Lakeside, Mt. Sinai, and Women's, opened their doors to the victims of the disaster in order to assist the overtaxed Clinic Hospital. Agatha Hodgins sent nurse anesthetists to help. Laura Grant, Lakeside's nursing supervisor, sent nurses, as did Maternity Hospital, the Visiting Nurse Association, the Central Registry, and the St. Barnabas Guild House for Nurses, where Minnie Strobel was in charge. The nursing directors at City Hospital, St. Vincent Charity Hospital, and Women's Hospital also offered the assistance of nurses from their staffs. Red Cross nurses helped relatives and friends of the victims identify the dead at the county morgue. Clara Noyes, National Director of the American Red Cross Nursing Service; Janet Geister, Director of the American Nurses' Association; and Annie Goodrich were among the nursing leaders from across the country who wrote to Cleveland nurses to express their concern and sympathy.

Dr. John Phillips had been the only one of the Clinic's founding physicians to marry a nurse, Lakeside graduate Cordelia Sudderth. Despite losing her own husband in the disaster, Mrs. Phillips did not forget the family of Edith Morgan, a fellow Lakeside alumna; she sent yellow roses to Miss Morgan's mother. When the Lakeside Unit women met for their annual reunion luncheon two weeks after the disaster, Dr. Crile, Dr. Lower, and the Unit's enlisted men sent baskets of flowers to express their sympathy. A single rose marked Edith Morgan's empty place.

Another rose lay at the place of Margaret Lane — the nurse who had looked so stunning in Colonel Gilchrist's dress uniform at the masquerade party at Rouen, who had been trained in anesthesia by Agatha Hodgins and Mary Roche, and who, after the war, had worked as an anesthetist at Lakeside Hospital and then at the Clinic Hospital. Miss Lane did not die in the disaster; she had been critically injured in an automobile accident the previous spring and had died at the end of August. Fortune had not been kind to the Lakeside Unit nurses hired by the Cleveland Clinic. Ten years after the Unit's safe return home, only one among them, Lillian Grundies, was still alive.

"Worse Than Anything I Saw in France"

To anyone who had lived during the First World War — and in 1929, that was everyone above the age of childhood — poison gas meant the chemical weapons used for the first time during that war. "This is like phosgene!" Dr. Crile is quoted as having said as he stood out on the lawn of the Clinic, directing rescue and treatment operations in the wake of the disaster. (He had been in surgery at the Clinic Hospital at the time, and rushed over to the lawn of the Clinic Building as soon as a nurse caught him between operations to give him the terrible news.) Later, in a letter to Dr. Franklin Martin, he stated, "The poison gas and flame made this worse than anything I saw in France."[94]

Battalion Fire Chief Michael Graham, on duty at the scene, "an overseas war veteran who [had] served in the front line trenches in France and encountered

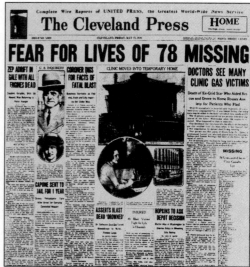

A HEADLINE STORY
Local and national newspapers gave the Clinic disaster front page headlines and extensive coverage. Some out-of-town papers erroneously reported that Dr. Crile, Dr. Charles Higgins, and Hospital Superintendent Abbie Porter were among the dead, resulting in a flood of telegrams and phone calls.

a number of gas attacks, declared that the fumes…were apparently as deadly and even more penetrating than the poison gas used in the war." A few days later, in Washington, D.C., Representative Hamilton Fish, another World War I veteran, made an appeal in the House of Representatives for the United States to sign the Geneva Protocol banning the use of poison gas in warfare. Declaring the United States the only civilized nation not to have signed the protocol, he cited the Cleveland Clinic disaster as an example "of the horrors of gas poisoning."[95]

To Lillian Grundies, the parallel was at first unconsciously recognized, but she later credited her war experience with saving her life. When she covered her mouth and nose and tried to take as few and shallow breaths as possible, she was remembering the lessons she had learned more than 10 years before, as one of the first women to attend the British Army's "Gas School" while preparing for duty in a casualty clearing station at the battlefront.

But the survivors of the disaster could not feel safe for some days after May 15. Not all of the eventual victims died, or even seemed to be affected, immediately after being exposed to the gas. Dr. Henry John remembered that in "the next two days there were so many of our colleagues who were OK at first, suddenly took ill and died in a brief time, that I began to think: 'Are all of us who were within the Clinic at the time, going to succumb?'"[96]

In 1929, the Cleveland Clinic disaster was the second-deadliest accident in the city's history (after the 1908 Collinwood School fire, in which 174 people had lost their lives). A commission appointed by City Manager William R. Hopkins to look into the cause of the tragedy presented its findings in August. The commission determined that an unshielded light bulb placed too close to X-ray films stored on top of open shelves in a room in the Clinic's basement (formerly a coal bin) had started the slow combustion of the nitrate films. This combustion was potentially more lethal, in its insidious release of toxic gases, than an out-and-out fire (which would have resulted from higher temperatures). But the commission did not fix responsibility for the disaster.

The hazardous nature of nitrate film was not well-known. The Kodak Company produced the film, and hospitals used it, in great quantity. The more advanced opinion of the time was turning to favor safety film, but most health care institutions, including the Clinic, still used nitrate. The Clinic disaster itself was perhaps the single most important factor in spurring users of X-ray film to change over more quickly from nitrate to acetate.

Meanwhile, the two surviving Clinic founders had to worry about lawsuits. "You can readily realize we are sitting on a volcano right now and will be for the next two years," Dr. Crile wrote as early as May 31, in his letter to Franklin Martin.[97] But long before the two years were up — in fact, less than six months after the disaster, on October 29, 1929 — the public disaster followed the private one. The collapse of the United States stock market on Black Tuesday signaled the beginning of the Great Depression.

Depression

Just as the 1929 event was always referred to as "the disaster" in the annals of the Cleveland Clinic, so the national and international economic disaster that began in the same year became known to future generations as "the" Depression, with no qualifier needed. During that period of economic decline, businesses collapsed, banks failed, and the unemployment rate soared to one-quarter of the working population, or about 13 million people nationwide, in 1932. The average wage went down by as much as 60 percent. According to various measures, economic activity dropped to less than half the level of the boom year of 1929.

In Cleveland, with its high concentration of manufacturing industries (only Detroit had a larger percentage of people employed in manufacturing), one-third of the work force was out of work by 1931.   Only four of Cleveland's seven largest banks survived long enough to reopen their doors after the bank holiday in March of 1933. And the effect of the Depression on the Cleveland Clinic was just as great as that of the disaster, if not greater.

When the Clinic reopened after the disaster, for the time being in a private school building across the street from its campus, patients returned, in as large numbers as before, to be treated at the famous Cleveland Clinic. (In fact, the Clinic was now more famous than ever before, since every newspaper from the *New York Times* on down had headlined the story of fire, explosion, poison, and death.) A group of prominent citizens got together and pledged contributions to make up for any financial losses caused to the Clinic by the disaster.

Within two years, these same citizens lost some of their own fortunes and were unable to make good on their pledges. And for the first time, the number of patients seen at the Clinic began to show a pattern of decline. People stayed away not because they were afraid of poison gas, but simply because they could not afford to come. However, the number of patients did not decline so fast as the Foundation's income; patients who came and were treated, paid less, and paid more slowly, or not at all.

This did not happen overnight. But during the course of the three or four years following the stock market crash, the economy of the Clinic, along with that of the nation, steadily declined. Things then began to improve slowly, but it would take another world war to end the Depression.

Disaster's Aftermath

Meanwhile, in purely financial terms, the disaster and the Depression worked together at the Clinic in strange and ironic ways. At first sight, the conjunction of the two seemed to be a double blow of fate. Because of the disaster, the Clinic lost operating income; it suffered damage to its structure and equipment, and ultimately had to construct a new Clinic building; lawsuits amounting to $3,000,000 were filed against it. And then, on top of that, came the financial woes of the Depression years.

But the alchemy of lawsuit and Depression had some unexpected results. Since the founders of the Clinic were salaried employees, no claims could be made against their personal fortunes and estates, diminished now in any case. The Foundation had $30,000 worth of liability coverage. The rest would have to come out of the income and assets of the medical facilities. The statute of limitations ran out on May 15, 1931, a time when the economy was still in free fall. At this point the lawyers began their negotiations on the 69 cases — 63 for deaths and 6 for injuries — that had been filed.

Nearly all of these suits had been filed by families of patients. Families of employees had received compensation from the Ohio State Industrial Commission and could not sue. The amount of compensation was determined by whether or not the deceased had dependents. The state referee had recommended that $6,500 be paid in compensation for Edith Morgan's death, the same amount recommended for Dr. Phillips and William Brownlow; $3,238 for Blanche Young; $150 for funeral expenses and possibly medical expenses for Zanna Fahey; disallowed any claim on the part of Louise Morton's husband, since he was not a dependent; and also disallowed compensation for Clinic Hospital nurse Susanne Matz, who had not been killed in the course of her employment.

More than a year later, in July of 1932, an out-of-court settlement was reached, for a total of $167,000 — the largest settlement in the history of Cleveland's common pleas court to that date. The settlement assigned no fault in the accident. Outside lawyers consulted by Dr. Crile and Dr. Lower had "strongly advised settlement." One of them, Cleveland mayor John Marshall, voiced the collective opinion when he said he believed the Clinic was "fortunate in the moderate amount involved."[98]

Paul Lamb, the lawyer who actually arranged for the settlement on behalf of the Clinic, modestly made light of his own efforts, remarking in a newspaper interview, "Of course, everyone was primarily interested in maintaining the services of that institution in this city and country." In fact, he had successfully made the case, in the words of a *Time* magazine correspondent, that "claimants for damages might easily wreck the institution, but claimants could squeeze no money from empty corridors."[99] With the decreased cash flow at the Clinic, it would not take much to "wreck the institution"; moreover, since the settlement was figured on the basis of Depression-level salaries and costs of living, the individual amounts were set at correspondingly low levels. The standard value set on a husband and father was $5,000; $2,500 was the amount for a wife and mother. Some claimants received only $750, if no dependents were involved. Since the state industrial commission had disallowed workers' compensation in her case, the family of young, single Susanne Matz joined in the lawsuits with the survivors of the other victims; it received $1,000 in the settlement.

It was calculated that, in the end, the disaster cost the Clinic nearly $840,000, after adjustment for insurance claim payments received. However, $440,000 of this was spent on the new Clinic building, and was therefore more a capital investment than a disaster loss.[100]

The Third Blow

The proverbial third misfortune was also beginning to darken the Clinic's skies at this time — or perhaps it was not so much a misfortune, as a decline of the good fortune that had prevailed in the Clinic's early years. If having a thyroid operation had been "almost fashionable" earlier in the decade, that fashion had finally run its course. It was, again, *Time* that pointed out the fact to the general public, in 1933.

> Not enough patients are going to the Mayos, the Criles, the Laheys to keep the plants running at efficient capacity....

> The Mayos, expert medical economists, do not agree with the run of the profession that Depression alone explains the lessened incidence of goiter. Like Dr. George Washington Crile in Cleveland and Dr. Frank Howard Lahey in Boston, the Mayos built a large portion of their clinic activities on goiter operations.

The Mayos commissioned a survey in their own state of Minnesota, which showed that there

> were actually fewer goiters in that goitrous State than any prior survey had shown. To the astonished surveyors it did not seem possible that Minnesota goiters had been operated or medicated out of existence. Unless depressed and worried existence prevented goiters, it seemed probable that five, ten years ago the State and the nation were in a goiter epidemic. If so, the epidemic now seems past....
>
> Theorists suggest that the present low incidence of goiters in the U.S. which the Mayos and other clinicians note, may be the result of the goiter scare last decade and the resulting exploitation of iodized salt.[101]

Fortunately, major institutions like the Mayo Clinic and the Cleveland Clinic had already established reputations as medical meccas and had never concentrated on thyroid operations to the exclusion of all other practice. Whatever their illnesses, people wanted to be treated at the hospitals and clinics they had come to regard as the best. In 1932, at the depth of the Depression, William Randolph Hearst, publisher of sensationalist newspapers, came to the Clinic to be operated on for a diverticulum of the esophagus. (Ironically, but not surprisingly, he desired that there should be as little publicity as possible about the matter.) Dr. Crile, in accordance with the Clinic's sliding fee scale, charged him $10,000, since Mr. Hearst reputedly had one of the highest incomes in the nation. He was accompanied by his mistress, actress Marion Davies (and her poodle), who presented Dr. Crile with a token of the publisher's esteem upon their departure — a Cartier watch. Income from wealthy patients like Mr. Hearst helped the Clinic maintain its solvency, but overall, receipts inevitably declined.

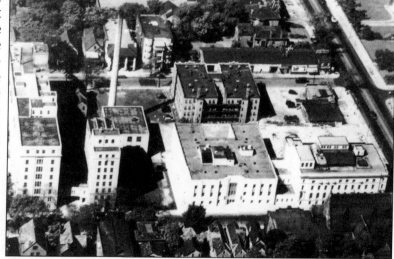

THE CLEVELAND CLINIC
This aerial photograph was taken in about 1931. At the center is the three-story Clinic Building, just completed to replace the damaged original building (right) as the outpatient area. To the left is the Research Building, and on the far left, the Hospital.

Hard Times

Yet, despite everything, throughout the entire Depression, the Cleveland Clinic never laid off a single employee. It did have to reduce salaries across the board. A letter that went out on January 19, 1933, to all employees on behalf of the Foundation's Board of Trustees read as follows:

> During the past year the Clinic has suffered a progressive loss of income. Rigid economies in all departments have been put into effect during the year.
>
> These economies have been carried as far as efficient service will allow but have not offset the great decrease in income due to the continued progressive decrease in the ability of the patients to meet their bills.
>
> It is with deep regret that the Board of Trustees finds it necessary to reduce the salaries in the amount of 10%, to take effect with the January 31, 1933, payroll.[102]

A 10 percent cut had been made before this, in September of 1932; later in 1933 an additional 25 percent cut was made. A senior level Clinic nursing employee who was making $150 a month in 1931 received $91.12 in early 1935. A general duty Clinic Hospital nurse, who might have received $125 monthly in 1931, now earned $67.50 to $75.98 a month. But having a steady job, with a dependable, if reduced, income, numbered them among the fortunate ones during these years of unemployment and despair.

In Cleveland, and all over the country, private duty nurses also were suffering a reversal of fortune. Considering that a private duty nurse's good fortune consisted of being healthy and popular enough to work 12 hours a day, six or seven days a week, to earn a living that was no more than decent, perhaps reversal is too strong a word. The line between that decent, precarious standard of living, and underemployed poverty, was not very great.

Even before the Depression, middle class people had been finding it difficult to afford hiring private duty nurses. The number of graduate nurses churned out by training schools in hospitals, which depended on students for their staffs, could not be absorbed by the private duty market. But until more hospitals began hiring more graduates, nurses had nowhere else to turn. Once the Depression hit, hospitals were less able to hire additional nurses. Instances where nurses worked at hospitals for room and board, or gave free service to hospitals and were promised patient-paid employment as specials in return, became more and more common. This issue came to a head in Ohio after March 1932, when an article in the *Bulletin* of the Cleveland Academy of Medicine suggested that more nurses should donate their time, "making it possible to give much needed service to the community at a lower price." State and local officers of the Ohio State Nurses' Association were dismayed by the article, and the OSNA eventually developed the following policy: voluntary private duty service was appropriate only in the case of the patient who was "a free patient in the hospital ward or under the doctor's care in the home. If the hospital or the doctor receives pay, the nurse should not be expected to give free service."[103]

But if some nurses found it necessary to donate their time in return for minimal employment, some people were desperate enough to donate, literally, themselves. Dr. Crile's celebrity brought with it the usual, and usually unwanted, correspondence that celebrities receive. In 1931, Grace Crile wrote to one of her children that "amusing letters still come in. One man was so interested [in the Clinic's medical research] that he wanted to arrange to sell himself for experimental purposes. He said he was a 'Failure' anyway."[104] The letter she was referring to went like this:

Here is a letter from a FAILURE in this thing we call life.

I have tried to make a success out of myself but I have found out I just could not get out of the rut. Now I dont give a care for myself but when one is married and you have to sit by and see your wife and child taken from you why then you wake up and realize just what a failure you are. Now doctor here is what I would like to do. I have about $1000.00 worth of insurance on myself and I would like to sell myself to you or your Clinic. By that I mean for you to use for experiment purposes with your different serums etc. Dont you think that you could accomplish more when you had a human body to work on than a guinea pig.

A LOW POINT
In 1933, statistics for the Cleveland Clinic and its Hospital hit their lowest levels: 8,321 new patients registered at the Clinic, compared to a pre-Depression high of 15,898 in 1926; the Hospital recorded 36,948 days of care, slightly over half the 63,191 total for 1930. Cleveland Clinic nurses, like other employees and staff, had their salaries cut twice during the year, but considered themselves fortunate in being able to keep their jobs.

Cleveland-area private duty nurses were also struggling, in some cases earning as little as $30 a month. Nurses enrolled on District No. 4's Central Registry, fearing there was not enough work to go around, repeatedly asked that the number of new registrants be limited. Some District members proposed setting higher standards for entry, both to reduce the number of nurses and to ensure quality care.

92

Now please do not misunderstand me I am not offering to do this for the sake of Humanity but for the sake of making money....I could find no work so as a last resort (except one) that is the reason I am making this proposition to you.[105]

The man added that he was 35 years old and in good health.

Throughout the Depression, private duty nurse Flora Short continued her career, and as before, she received many calls to serve as a special nurse for Cleveland Clinic Hospital patients. Although her income decreased somewhat, it decreased no more than that of Clinic-employed nurses. Other nurses who specialed at the Clinic on a regular basis also probably had better incomes than might have been expected.

Undoubtedly, for some, less work was available. In the single year between 1930 and 1931, the number of hospital care days at the Clinic Hospital dropped from 63,191 to 56,498; the average number of special nurses on duty per day dropped likewise, from 54 to 44. But it was not until 1933 that Miss Short worked fewer than 200 days a year. That year, and the two following, were the most difficult for her. In 1933 she worked only 150 days, and earned $980 — an income similar to that of the Clinic Hospital's general duty nurses.

By 1935 her income had dropped to $827, its lowest level. This was partly because in 1934, the working day for Cleveland's private duty nurses was finally shortened, not to 10 hours, but to 8 hours. At the same time, the rate was lowered to $4.60 a day. This, it was felt, would make nursing more affordable to patients who did not really need around-the-clock specialing, and it would also spread the available work around to a greater number of nurses. For a nurse like Miss Short, who had a large practice, this move probably hurt more than it helped, as far as income went, but at least she finally had a working day more like everyone else's. And in 1936, as the economy in general picked up, so did Miss Short's work. She spent 269 days on duty — the highest number ever — and earned $1,343, at the rate of $5 per 8-hour day.

Change for the Better...

As economic conditions improved, Cleveland nurses, perhaps feeling that they had sacrificed enough, began to make their voices heard, asking, demanding even, that their own fortunes should change for the better. In 1936, Cleveland's 105 city public health nurses delegated a committee to meet with city officials and demand "financial recognition of the value of their department." Their salaries, like those of other city workers, had been cut 25 percent in 1931. However, policemen and firemen were now receiving their full base pay, and the nurses wanted to know why the city could not do something for them, too, since, as a newspaper story noted, "all councilmen in their public statements profess to love the health department, which deals with the indigent sick."[106]

At University Hospitals, the whole system of payment for nurses was revamped in 1937. In 1936 nurses there had received $50 a month plus room, board, and laundry. In 1937 the hospital began, on a trial basis, to pay nurses completely in cash. Protests from nurses about the inadequacy of the new salaries (which covered the cost of the in-kind benefits but did not include an actual raise) resulted in hospital director Dr. Robert Bishop addressing a mass meeting of nurses and personally guaranteeing them a raise of $6.50 per month, whether or not the hospital board of trustees approved it. Subsequently, the board did approve the raise, and the nurses voted overwhelmingly to remain on the all-cash plan. A new graduate thus earned a salary of $91.35 per month, which went up to $101.71 after a year. The hospital charged those who wished to live in its nurses' residence $15 a month, and $3 for laundry.[107]

The Clinic's nurses and other employees had seen their salaries begin to go back up in 1935. The numbers of patient registrations and admissions, which had reached their lowest levels in 1933, were growing again. By the late 1930s, the post-Depression pattern of life at the Clinic was establishing itself.

During the early 1930s, the superintendent of nurses had also served as the assistant superintendent of the hospital, second in command to Miss Porter. Elizabeth Hinds, who had been praised by a patient for being "constantly on hand making everyone happy," was the Superintendent of Nurses and Assistant Hospital Superintendent until 1934, when she resigned and was succeeded by Maude Peters. Miss Peters was a Clinic Hospital veteran, having begun her career there as a general duty nurse in the first year of the hospital's operation.

One of the hospital's nursing floor supervisors, Sara C. Jones, took over as Director of Nursing at the Clinic Hospital after Miss Peters resigned in 1936. In her annual report for 1937, she thanked the administration for bonuses given to the staff during the year. She noted that due to the high turnover rate, and the fact that new nurses had widely varying backgrounds, it was important for the Hospital to provide instruction in various routine procedures: blood transfusions, diabetic treatment, starting and properly operating oxygen tents, "accurate recording of blood pressures and its importance in hypertension patients," setting up for thyroidectomy, preoperative and postoperative thyroid routine, and the admission and discharge of patients.[108]

A very important change for the nursing staff, which took place in 1937, was the institution of the straight eight-hour day — "a progressive step over the previous divided 9-hour day," according to Miss Jones. "I feel that this change has benefited both patients and nurses, as we have had fewer complaints of service and lights being left unanswered. It has also created more contentment and happiness among the nurses." The split shift schedule was standard for hospital nurses at the time — in 1940, three years after the Clinic Hospital had gone to a straight day, about 70 percent of American hospitals still used the split shift. This type of schedule, which gave a nurse a three or four hour break in the middle of her work day, was obviously inconvenient to her, but advantageous to the hospital, since service could be covered by two shifts per day. When the Clinic Hospital went to a straight-day schedule, it had to hire 25 more nurses to cover the additional shift, bringing the total number of nurses on the Clinic Hospital staff to 101.[109]

By this time, the Clinic Hospital was using private duty nurses, called from the Central Registry, on a regular basis as temporary relief general duty nurses. They received the regular private nurse's fee, now $6 for an eight-hour day, which was paid to them by the Hospital. However, in 1937, only 40 days of relief work were necessary, compared to more than 1,000 days in 1936. The number of calls made for special duty nurses for Hospital patients in 1937 was 3,610. At this time, the Hospital employed 10 ward maids and 10 orderlies, an average of 2 of each per floor.

IN THE 1930s:

In 1931, the total budget for nurses' salaries at the Cleveland Clinic Hospital was $119,860.75. Orderlies' and ward helpers' salaries came to $16,079.04. Medical and surgical supplies, including drugs, cost $34,979.46. A patient's care brought in $9.55 a day while costing the Hospital $8.27, including $2.42 for nursing. In 1936, Clinic nurses could have their uniforms cleaned at the Eagle Laundry for 20 cents, and caps for 5 cents. In 1937, 5 of the 63 nurses who resigned during the year "married and left to keep house." Thirteen left for private duty nursing, and 39 went to other hospitals. Equipment purchased by the Nursing Department in 1939 consisted of "12 electric heating pads; bakelite nourishment trays; 12 more beaver boards; one more inhalator."

District No. 4, investigating Cleveland hospital policies on private duty nurses, found that 7 of 16 hospitals required severely ill patients to have special nurses in some or all circumstances; 9 hospitals required special nurses for patients in isolation.

Also in the late 1930s, two important administrative changes occurred at the Clinic. In 1938, the third-party payor entered the scene when The Cleveland Clinic Foundation became a member of the Cleveland Hospital Service Association (CHSA), the forerunner of Blue Cross of Northeast Ohio. In that year, 117 patients insured by CHSA were cared for in the Hospital. The business office noted that "the remittances on these accounts were very prompt."[110]

At the beginning of 1940 the Foundation hired a general superintendent, George W. Grill, to take charge of both the Hospital and the Clinic. He was to have responsibility for all properties and affairs of the Foundation, except for finances and professional activities. Abbie Porter, as Hospital Superintendent, now reported to Mr. Grill, rather than to the Administrative Board of physicians. An additional organizational layer had been interpolated into the Clinic's structure; the traditional role of the nurse superintendent had lost some of its autonomy.

...And New Trials

However, one of Miss Porter's chief responsibilities remained ensuring that the Hospital had a sufficient number of nurses to provide the best patient care possible within the confines of the Foundation's finances. As the economy improved, and the patient load at the Hospital increased, financial constraints became somewhat less important (although, of course, they always necessarily set the upper limit) in determining the size of the nursing staff.

Another factor — the number of nurses available and willing to fill the positions needed — now came into play. In 1940, Miss Porter was concerned about the large number of nurses, 77, who had left the employ of the Hospital during the preceding year. "I believe that raising the salary might help to keep the most desirable nurses on our General Duty Staff. At the present time we are paying $80.00 for the first three months, if their work is satisfactory $85.00 is paid. The nurses live out and take care of their laundry. Their meals are provided."[111] The salaries still had not returned to levels anywhere near those in effect before the Depression. There were ominous signs of a nursing shortage in the offing.

In 1939, the Hospital had to use private duty nurses for 459 days of relief work, "due to the busy summer months and the inability to secure nurses for general staff duty." It had also taken the unprecedented step of hiring an undergraduate nurse, "to assist the night nurses in some of the routine work which did not include actual nursing care."[112] At the beginning of 1941, as the entry of the United States into the Second World War looked more and more likely, Abbie Porter made her prediction for the future, and also proposed a partial solution to the staffing problems with which she was already dealing.

> During the past year it has been increasingly difficult to obtain graduate nurses. I believe this is the beginning of a trying time. There is a decided shortage of nurses thru the country. The Government is calling 4000 for service. It was possible to obtain a group of young girls, which we will call nurses' aids. We hope to train them to do routine work and relieve our nurses, so that their time can be devoted to the bedside care of the patient. We may not be able to maintain our full quota of graduate nurses but I believe we can maintain our standard of care for the patients. I trust that we can keep the nurses that have been with us for some time.[113]

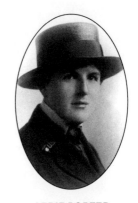

ABBIE PORTER
Born in Ravenna, Ohio, in 1889, Miss Porter is shown here wearing her WWI U.S. Army Nurse Corps uniform. After the war, Miss Porter was appointed supervisor of Lakeside Hospital's private pavilion, where many of Dr. Crile's patients were admitted. When the Cleveland Clinic Hospital opened in 1924, she became its first Superintendent of Nurses. In 1927, she succeeded nurse Charlotte Dunning as Hospital Superintendent. Elizabeth Ione Hinds, a Lakeside graduate (1910), became the new Superintendent of Nurses. Miss Porter remained as the Hospital's head through the disaster, the Depression, and the Second World War.

Less than a quarter century after the Lakeside Unit had gone overseas to care for the casualties of "the war to end all wars," another war loomed. The Cleveland Clinic, barely 20 years old, was again called into service.

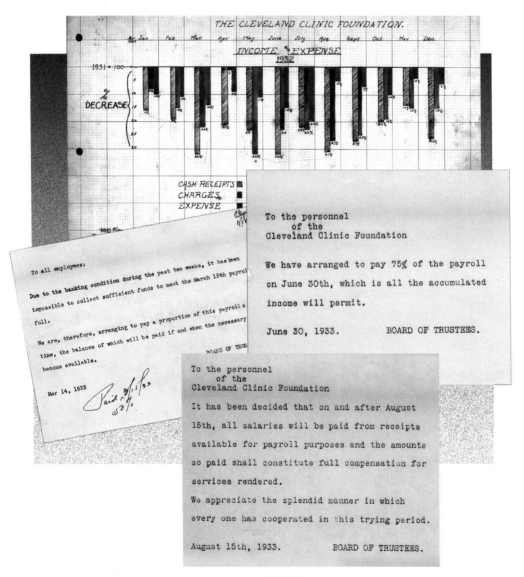

RED INK

A bar graph showed decreases in the Cleveland Clinic's receipts, charges, and expenses throughout 1932. Bank closings and low receipts caused difficulties in meeting 1933 payroll expenses, even though salaries had been cut equally for all personnel and medical staff. The cuts made it possible for the Clinic to get through the Depression without laying off a single employee.

3

They Also Serve

*Many nurses are in a state of confusion as to
what the real needs are and whether or not
they should give up their essential work in Civilian Service.*

— Sue Z. McCracken, General Secretary's Report,
OSNA District No. 4, January 12, 1945

Better Days

The ominous rumblings presaging another world conflict could be felt by the people of Europe even before Germany's Blitzkrieg conquest of Poland in September of 1939. Germany's continuing buildup of armaments, its absorption of Czechoslovakia, and its reoccupation of the Rhineland threatened the peace of other nations in the region. At first, the unsettling events in Europe and in Asia, where Japan had invaded China, seemed far away to Americans. At home, the nation had just climbed painfully out of the depths of the Depression and looked to the future for better times, not another catastrophe.

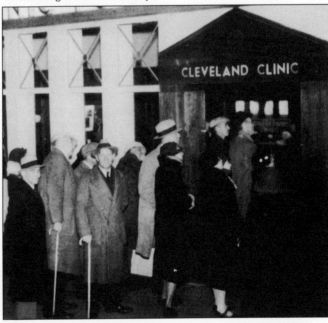

For Clevelanders, the hopes of the later 1930s were embodied in the Great Lakes Exposition of 1936-1937, a combination of civic celebration, trade fair and entertainment extravaganza that was touted as a stimulus to employment and business. Built on 135 acres along the downtown lakefront, the exposition was intended to celebrate the centennial of Cleveland's incorporation by showcasing the economic, scientific, and cultural achievements of the states and provinces bordering the Great Lakes. It featured exhibits like the "Streets of the World," the "Hall of Progress," and the "Aquacade" — the fair's biggest crowd-pleaser, where swimmers including Olympic champion Johnny Weissmuller (even more famous as the star of the Tarzan movies) performed in water ballet shows patterned after the dance spectacles so popular at the time. The exposition may not have brought any permanent benefit to the city's economic structure, but it did attract visitors from across the nation, as well as area residents.

CLINIC EXHIBIT
During the 1930s,
one way the Cleveland Clinic
communicated its work to
the public was through exhibits.
Here, people stand in line
to see a Clinic display
in 1933. The Clinic also
had an exhibit at the 1936-1937
Great Lakes Exposition.

Many Clevelanders, especially those who were children at the time, later remembered the two happy summers they spent riding the streetcars downtown for a day at the exposition. The Cleveland Clinic had its own exhibit there, and its employees were encouraged to join in the fun. The June 8, 1936 issue of the Clinic's *Bulletin* announced that "Miss Porter in the Hospital has a number of Ticket Books for the Great Lakes Exposition. These Books sell for $2.50, and they may be secured at the front office of the Hospital."[1]

Nurse anesthetists from across the country also had the opportunity to attend the exposition when the American Association of Nurse Anesthetists held its fourth annual meeting in Cleveland in 1936, in conjunction with the American Hospital Association convention. Agatha Hodgins, by this time the organization's honorary president, gave a welcoming address. Dr. Crile also spoke at the meeting, reiterating his belief in the nurse anesthetist's unexcelled skill, and singling out the Clinic's Chief Anesthetist, Lou Adams, for special praise.

Besides being able to buy exposition tickets at work, nurses and other Cleveland Clinic employees received another new benefit in 1936 — hospitalization insurance. Before this, the Clinic had furnished free medical and surgical services to employees, as well as hospitalization and drugs approximately at cost. The new plan, "The Cleveland Clinic Foundation's Mutual Benefit Fund," was based on the self-insurance model, and as before, provided service by Foundation physicians, at Foundation facilities only. For a small monthly contribution, staff, fellows, and employees would receive physicians' services, plus a maximum of 21 days a year of "general duty nursing, board and room." Services not covered included psychoses, tuberculosis, maternity care, and injuries covered by workmen's compensation. Dependents were not covered, but would continue to receive care under the old system. Employees who chose not to participate would now pay regular Clinic and Hospital rates for all services received, "without discounts and payable in cash."[2]

The proposed plan, which needed a high level of participation to be workable, was submitted to employees for their reaction. Only two "Clinic girls," one "boy in the research building," eight Hospital nurses, and two Hospital maids did not favor the new system.[3] In practice, it did not mean a great change for employees, since the premium was not high and its most noticeable effect, the elimination of hospital room charges, would be a positive one for those employees actually needing hospitalization. The Mutual Benefit Fund's greatest significance was more as a sign pointing to the future, when insurance would cover health care expenses for more and more people.

Assurance of Care

The Depression had given pause to the increasing use of hospitals by the average American. Although up-to-date care for serious illness or injury could be received only in a hospital, the costs of that care were often too great for an individual's or family's Depression-era budget. Spreading the risk by setting up hospital insurance plans, with large numbers of subscribers paying small premiums, appeared to be the answer. Although various commercial insurance schemes already existed, the future giants in the field — the "Blues" plans for hospital and medical coverage — proliferated during the 1930s.

In Cleveland, University Hospitals administrator John Mannix developed a plan featuring prepaid group hospitalization based on inclusive rates for hospital services. "Inclusive" meant that daily room charges covered not only nursing care, room, and board, but also items such as lab work, surgical dressings, and routinely prescribed drugs.

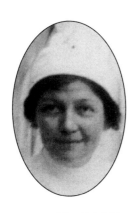

A NEW GENERATION
By the 1930s, nurses who had worked with the Clinic's founders before the Clinic itself had opened were retiring. Nurse anesthetist Agatha Hodgins (above) had retired from her position at University Hospitals in 1933. Young women like Elizabeth Meszaros Hartman (below), a 1932 graduate of New Castle Hospital in western Pennsylvania, were joining the Cleveland Clinic nursing staff, bringing a fresh outlook. Mrs. Hartman would go on to work as a head nurse and a supervisor during her long career at the Cleveland Clinic Hospital.

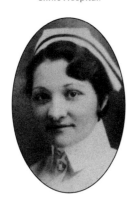

With the support of the Cleveland Hospital Council (the local hospital association), the Cleveland Academy of Medicine, and the Cleveland Welfare Federation, the non-profit Cleveland Hospital Service Association (CHSA) — a precursor of Blue Cross of Northeast Ohio — incorporated and began enrolling subscribers in 1934. The affiliated Medical Mutual of Cleveland, later Blue Shield, was established to cover physicians' services in 1945.[4] The hospitalization portion of the Clinic's Mutual Benefit Fund was very similar to the CHSA plan and may well have been modeled after it; its coverage of physician services predated Medical Mutual by almost ten years.

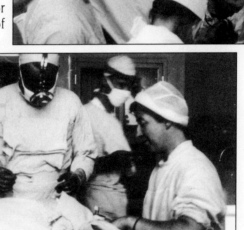

The Cleveland Clinic Hospital, not at this time a member of the Cleveland Hospital Council, did not join the Cleveland Hospital Service Association until June 1938, the year in which CHSA became the first plan in the country to reimburse hospitals on a cost basis. Until then, the many Clevelanders enrolled in CHSA did not have insurance coverage for hospitalization at the Clinic Hospital. Within a few years, a significant portion of the patients admitted to the Clinic Hospital had their stays covered by CHSA insurance. In 1941, for example, 1,323 CHSA patients made up 17 percent of the year's admissions.

Prepaid group hospital insurance had a substantial impact on Cleveland-area hospitals. During the early 1930s, admissions had decreased and hospitals had struggled to meet costs as patients struggled to pay hospital bills. The Cleveland Hospital Service Association offered subscribers assurance of care, and hospitals assurance of payment. Ironically, as hospital insurance came into its own, the Depression-era scarcity of money that had stimulated its development was becoming a thing of the past. As families'

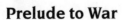

incomes grew, and as more employers signed on with CHSA, more people could afford hospital care. Empty hospital beds began to fill.

But nurses did not rush to join hospital staffs, in part because there were fewer new graduates. Nationwide, 60 percent more nurses had graduated in the 1920s than in the 1930s. In Ohio, high unemployment among nurses (a 1933 survey gave a figure of six thousand unemployed R.N.s in the state) was one reason that OSNA policy favored limiting the number of student nurses. The organization reversed its policy to one of encouraging prospective nurses in 1939, but as the war drew nearer, demand for nurses outstripped the available supply. [5]

Prelude to War

"Nurses Shortage Here Hampers All Hospitals," declared a headline as early as July 1941, five months before the bombing of Pearl Harbor precipitated America's entry into the war.[6] Members of the Cleveland Hospital Council prepared to eliminate morning visiting hours in response. By the end of the war in 1945, hospitals could only dream about having staffing levels as high as those that "hampered" them in 1941. They would be using measures much more radical than curtailing visiting hours to conserve nursing resources, and some of these measures would have a lasting effect on the way hospitals worked. Personnel in all categories would be siphoned off from their jobs in health care and drawn into the war effort, to fill ranks on the assembly line as well as on the parade ground and the battlefield.

The process of converting the American economy to wartime status had in fact been well underway before Pearl Harbor. In 1940, Nazi Germany, having begun the war with the invasion of Poland in 1939, defeated France and launched the Battle of Britain, an all-out bombing assault meant to prepare for the invasion of the country. Although officially neutral, the United States was, as in World War I, producing huge quantities of war materiel, mostly for use against Germany and its allies.

In September 1940 Congress passed the Selective Service Act, America's first peacetime draft. As early as December 1939, the Army and Navy had extended the upper age limit for nurses from 28 to 30, and reduced the minimum height requirement to 60 inches. As war drew nearer, the American Red Cross, still handling nurse recruitment for the armed services, put out a first call for 10,000 young women to join a reserve nurse corps.

In Cleveland, preparations for the mobilization of the Fourth General Hospital of the United States Army, successor to the First World War's Lakeside Unit, began in 1940. Olga Benderoff, Assistant Director of University Hospitals' nursing service, had the responsibility of recruiting and organizing 120 nurses for the Fourth General. Although the Unit was again informally known as "the Lakeside Unit," physicians and nurses from a number of area hospitals signed up with it. In March 1941 Miss Benderoff requested and received help from District No. 4 of the OSNA in contacting private duty nurses as well. The District office provided stamps and addressed 243 envelopes to the younger of its members engaged in private duty, and several private duty nurses did join the Unit.

FOURTH GENERAL HOSPITAL NURSES
The U.S. Army's Fourth General Hospital, with its core personnel drawn from the medical and nursing staffs of University Hospitals of Cleveland, was the World War II successor to the World War I Lakeside Unit. Elizabeth McCoy (at far left in the photo) was one of two Cleveland Clinic nurses to join the unit.

The Cleveland Clinic and World War II

Cleveland Clinic nurses who wished to join the military were on their own this time. Dr. Crile, Dr. Lower, and Dr. Phillips had severed their Lakeside and Western Reserve University ties long ago. Although the Fourth General Hospital was the original Lakeside Unit's military descendant, and the Cleveland Clinic was, in a sense, its civilian descendant, the two had no official connection. However, individual Clinic employees were of course free to join the Fourth General if they liked. When the Surgeon General's office summoned the Fourth General Hospital to active duty on December 24, 1941, this new Lakeside Unit was again the first U.S. armed forces general hospital called to overseas service. Two Cleveland Clinic nurses, Mary Gruber and Elizabeth McCoy, went with the Fourth General as second lieutenants.[7]

Meanwhile, the Cleveland Clinic was organizing its own unit for military service. On May 27, 1941, the old soldiers, Dr. Crile and Dr. Lower, went to Washington, D.C., to find out "at first hand what the Cleveland Clinic would be required to contribute."[8] It was determined that the Clinic would furnish a Naval Unit of medical specialists.

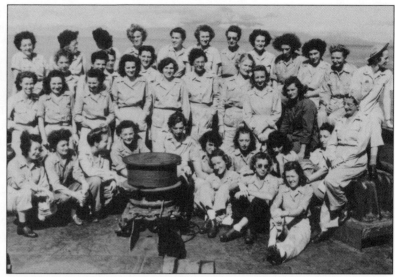

SOUTH PACIFIC
The Fourth General Hospital unit served in Australia and New Guinea. The photo above was taken near the end of the nurses' service, aboard ship after their departure from New Guinea. Cleveland Clinic nurse Mary Gruber is in the front row, third from the right. The fatigues the nurses wore on duty in New Guinea contrasted with the winter dress uniforms (opposite page) they had used as street wear in Australia. The contrast with the long gray dresses and white aprons of the World War I Lakeside Unit nurses was even greater.

Dr. Crile made a second trip to Washington in late December to meet with the Navy's Surgeon General, to impress upon him the importance of keeping a sufficient number of surgeons and physicians at the Cleveland Clinic. This was necessary to provide alternates for the Clinic's Naval Unit, as well as to maintain the Clinic as a working institution where the civilian population's needs could be met and young physicians who might be needed for service could receive training.

He explained the situation at the Clinic in a letter to the Surgeon General: "Many of the best men both of the permanent staff and of the fellowship group are very anxious to enter military service of some sort without delay. If they could now be assured of assignment as teachers, as research workers or as members of the active services, their patriotic impulses would be satisfied, and in future they would feel that they had done their part."[9]

Ironically, Dr. Crile now faced the same problem that had plagued the trustees and administrators of Lakeside Hospital and the Western Reserve University School of Medicine during the last war. He had to convince Clinic personnel that duty lay at home, as well as on the battlefield, and suppress their desire to be in the midst of the action, the same desire he and other members of the Lakeside Unit had found so irresistible 24 years back.

Eventually Dr. Russell L. Haden and Dr. W. James Gardner visited Washington to work out more definite plans for the Clinic's Naval Unit. They reported to a meeting of the Clinic's Administrative Board on January 13, 1942, that the Unit would be a neurosurgical one, headed by Dr. Gardner, and would leave March 1. It would include six nurses from the Reserve Corps, two neurosurgical scrub nurses and one or two anesthetists, as well as a hospital corps of enlisted orderlies.

In the end, the Unit included no nurses at all when it shipped out for duty in New Zealand that spring. Apparently, no one had ever seriously considered sending Cleveland Clinic nurses. The only tangible, recorded contribution of the Clinic's nurses to the Unit was a St. Christopher key ring, which anesthetist and Navy veteran Lou Adams gave to Barney Crile before he left Cleveland

ᅟ‌‌‌‌

ﾠ

ﾠok

with the Unit. Miss Adams (who adored the young Dr. Crile "like a son," and was very close to his family) said that she had carried a St. Christopher medal throughout her World War I service, and it had brought her luck.[10]

Fewer Nurses, More Patients

The Unit's organizers gave no reason for not including Clinic nurses in their plan in the way that Lakeside Hospital nurses had been included in the World War I Unit and University Hospitals nurses were part of the Fourth General Hospital. However, had nurses been required, the Clinic would have been even more hard-pressed to supply them than it was to supply physicians. The "trying time" envisioned by Abbie Porter at the end of 1940 had arrived by 1942. By the end of that year the Cleveland Clinic Hospital's nursing staff consisted of 62 general duty nurses and supervisors, down from 108 in 1940. At the same time (1940 to 1942), admissions had increased from 6,620 to 7,785, and bed occupancy from 73 to 94 percent. No one at the Cleveland Clinic or its Hospital needed newspaper stories to tell them that a nursing shortage existed.

The city-wide (and indeed nationwide) scarcity of nurses hit the Cleveland Clinic Foundation particularly hard, staffed as it was by graduates rather than by students. The military only accepted graduate nurses, as, in general, did industry, another war-era recruiter of nurses. Hospitals had to compete in the labor market with the glamour of military service and the better pay and greater independence of industrial nursing. But at least those numerous hospitals that still depended on students to do a significant portion of their nursing could continue to count on schools to supply them with staffing. In Cleveland, by 1945, the nursing staff at St. Alexis Hospital consisted of 29 graduate and 120 student nurses. At St. Luke's Hospital, there were 21 general duty nurses and 244 students.[11] The Cleveland Clinic Foundation had the difficult task of attracting and then keeping graduate nurses to do virtually all of the nursing at its increasingly busy Hospital and Clinic. The Hospital Nursing Department had to continue the practice it had begun in 1940, of hiring a few undergraduate nurses to supplement its staff.

Another factor unique to the Clinic among Cleveland-area health care institutions made the war years particularly trying. As area medical men departed for military service, more and more patients were left without their family physicians. The Cleveland Clinic, as a large group practice, was a logical place for these "war orphans" to turn, knowing physicians would always be available to care for them. In 1939, 12,748 new patients consulted Clinic physicians; five years later that number had more than doubled, to 27,950. The total number of patient visits rose from 148,574 to 246,413. This was at a time when the Clinic's physician staff was reduced by 25 percent; in 1943, 11 of the 40 active members of the Clinic's staff were commissioned in the armed services. The remaining Clinic physicians and nurses had to deal with this greatly expanded practice.

Since the Cleveland Clinic Hospital existed to provide hospitalization for the patients of Cleveland Clinic physicians, the increased number of Clinic patients was a major factor in the increased Hospital census. Harassed and

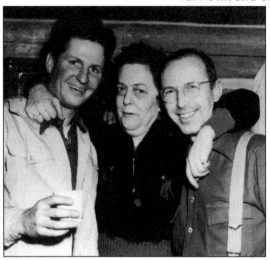

A FOND FAREWELL
The Cleveland Clinic sent a unit to serve with the U.S. Navy in the South Pacific during World War II. No nurses went with the 10-surgeon unit. The Clinic's Chief Anesthetist, Lou Adams (center), shown saying good-bye to unit members Dr. Barney Crile (left) and Dr. Gardner (right) at a family gathering, sent her best wishes for a safe return in the form of a St. Christopher medal that she gave to Dr. Crile. She said that a similar medal had brought her luck during her own Navy service in World War I.

overworked, Cleveland Clinic nurses, physicians, and other employees held the home front with honor during those war years. Dr. Barney Crile, with the Naval Unit in New Zealand, acknowledged their dedication in a letter to the Clinic's Chief of Surgery, Dr. Thomas Jones. "Don't think for a minute that we don't appreciate all that you people at home are doing for us or that we don't know what a load you are carrying. It must be hell to be at home these days with so much to do and with the restlessness that these days breed."[12]

Division of Labor

At the beginning of 1944, the Cleveland Clinic Hospital's nursing staff reached its numerically lowest level — a total of 50 graduate nurses, less than half the number on roll in 1940.[13] There were also 5 undergraduate nurses; 19 full-time and 2 part-time aides; 6 orderlies; and 4 nurse anesthetists. These 85 people, divided into three shifts, constituted the Hospital's entire roster of paid employees responsible for all direct patient care services, including operating room work, in a hospital with an average daily patient census of 223, and with seven thousand operations performed in a year. The average total number of employees on duty in the Hospital per day, including office workers, was 207, meaning that there was actually less than one employee per patient. "During the war, we never wrote a note," recalled a Hospital nurse. "We were too busy."[14]

Hospital workers in all categories were in short supply, but the shortage of nurses was by far the most critical staffing problem: first, because the nurse's high level of skill and training made it impossible to replace her by simply hiring someone off the street; and second, because registered nurses gave most of the direct patient care. Relatively few auxiliary nursing employees worked alongside them at the time.

A floor-by-floor list of staff positions from 1940, the last "normal" year before the war, illustrated this. The third and fourth floors, with approximately 75 beds per floor, were staffed identically, with 15 nurses, including a supervisor, a head nurse, 2 senior nurses, and 11 general duty nurses listed for the 7 a.m. to 3:30 p.m. day shift. Eight nurses covered the 3 p.m. to 11:30 p.m. shift, and 2 covered the 11 p.m. to 7 a.m. shift on each floor. Both of these two floors also had 2 ward maids and 2 orderlies assigned to them, with no shift specified. The fifth and sixth floors, with approximately 50 beds apiece, each had 10 day shift nurses, 6 or 7 evening nurses, and 2 night shift nurses, as well as 2 ward maids and an orderly. The small (17-bed) second floor had a total of 7 nurses spread over three shifts, and a maid.

The Hospital had an additional night staff of 13 nurses and 3 orderlies, who floated to the floors as needed. The Operating Room staff consisted of 13 nurses, 3 maids, and 2 orderlies; 4 nurses and 2 maids worked in the Equipment (or central supply) Room. Four nurse administrators rounded out the staff of the Nursing Department. Counting all of the floor personnel on all shifts, the Hospital had 107 nurses, 9 maids, and 9 orderlies working on the nursing floors, a ratio of almost 12 registered nurses to each maid and orderly.

Nurses were responsible for doing virtually anything and everything directly related to patient care, as well as many clerical and other tasks. Ward maids were responsible for seeing to the cleanliness of the patients' surroundings.

ON THE HOME FRONT
With many of their colleagues leaving for military service or industrial nursing in the defense industry, nurses who stayed at the Cleveland Clinic had a difficult and vital role. The number of Clinic outpatient visits doubled within the space of five years.

The number of Hospital admissions and operations also increased, while the Hospital staff of registered nurses shrunk to 50, less than half the prewar level, by 1944. The skill and dedication of Hospital nurses, including Elizabeth Graber (right, with nurse Rina Ritter and an unidentified colleague), made it possible to keep the Hospital open and running at an occupancy rate of 94 percent.

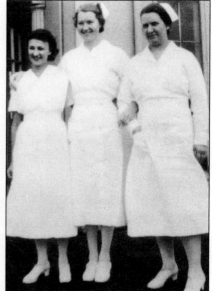

They, and not housekeeping employees, dusted the patients' rooms. Nursing Department personnel cleaned and made up vacated rooms, served trays and fed patients, transported patients to and from the Clinic, greeted and discharged patients, did all paperwork, and answered the telephone and delivered flowers and mail on the floors.

This division of labor could not continue as more and more staff nurses left, with no replacements to be found. By the end of 1941 the Housekeeping Department had created a team consisting of a housekeeper, a porter, and two maids. They worked from 1:00 p.m. to 9:00 p.m. and took care of all vacated rooms and beds, preparing them for immediate occupancy to meet the pressing demand for beds. At the same time, the Dietary Department hired extra maids and began taking all trays to patients.

"Real Assistance to the Nursing Staff"

In addition to reassigning tasks among existing departments, the Hospital found it necessary to create new job categories. Seven full-time and nine part-time "floor hostesses" — the precursors of ward or unit secretaries — were hired in 1942 and stationed on each floor at desks near the west end elevators. "Their duties are to receive all telephone messages for patients and personnel, deliver mail, flowers and packages, greet and establish new patients, list clothes and valuables. They are responsible for discharge of patients, checking clothes, valuables and notification to office, in preparation for patients' bills. We expect to train them to do graphic charts."[15]

By 1944, floor hostesses were also helping to pass trays, feed patients, and assist visitors. Asking the hostesses to transport patients to the Clinic on carts and in wheelchairs was less successful, since many of the older women employed for the job found themselves taxed beyond their limits. But on the whole, the innovation was very successful. "They have been of real assistance to the nursing staff and I have had many favorable comments from patients," reported Hospital Superintendent Abbie Porter, adding that although officially part of the Hospital's Office Department, the hostesses were really an auxiliary nursing service.[16]

The Nursing Department also created an important new category of employee: the nurses' aide. As early as January 1941, the Hospital began training "young girls" to "do routine work and relieve our nurses, so that their time can be devoted to the bedside care of the patient." Unfortunately, as production was stepped up in defense industries, and women were at first grudgingly admitted, and then warmly welcomed onto the assembly line berths vacated by servicemen, the young aides left for higher-paying factory jobs. The Hospital had to hire older women, and they, like the hostesses, found transporting patients difficult.[17]

NURSES' AIDES
Auxiliary nursing personnel, like the young women shown here with patients enjoying fresh air and sunshine on the Hospital roof, became an important presence at the Cleveland Clinic during World War II. Until this time, registered nurses, with the assistance of a small number of ward maids and orderlies, had handled all patient care, as well as paperwork, on the nursing floors. The wartime nursing shortage changed things. For the first time, nurses' aides were hired and trained to assist nurses. A "floor hostess" position was created to assume clerical and reception duties, and a volunteer director was hired to coordinate the large number of volunteer workers.

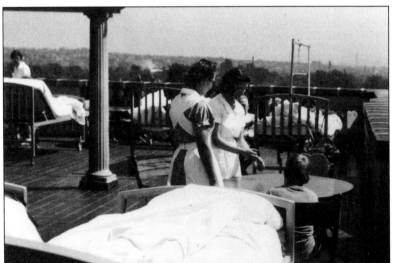

The lack of qualified male workers was a serious problem for hospitals. At the Cleveland Clinic, orderlies were even more scarce than nurses. During 1943, 11 orderlies came and went. "There were times when there was not a one on duty," reported Director of Nursing Sara C. Jones. Those men who did not go into the armed services went, like the nurses' aides, into the defense industry. The Housekeeping Department had to replace some male employees with female porters, when possible: "One painter and a wall washer left and it has been impossible to replace them." Turnover among both men and women was high in all departments. The Dietary Department complained of "a constantly changing group of unreliable workers."[18]

Although the turnover was also high among aides — for instance, in 1942 three aides left for every one that stayed — there were generally from 20 to 30 on the staff at any one time throughout the war. The "nurses' aide" was an upgrade of the "ward maid" position, which was phased out as the aides became an integral part of the patient care team on the floors. The number of ward maids decreased from 14 to 7 in 1941, the year in which aides were first hired; by the end of 1942, there were no maids. In 1943, the task of dusting the patients' rooms, which the aides had inherited from the maids, was turned over to the Housekeeping Department so that the

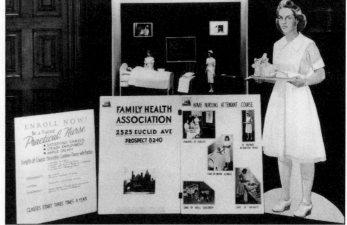

aides could concentrate on services to patients. In addition to the full-time aides, the Hospital hired high school girls to help out after school, on weekends, and during the summer, but they were rated as "generally unsatisfactory" and "a transient lot."[19]

Not all aides were paid employees. In the wake of Pearl Harbor, the Foundation's Administrative Board, and particularly its Hospital Committee, of which Abbie Porter was a member, had begun planning for a "Women's Emergency Unit." A questionnaire was drawn up to be signed by Miss Porter and sent out to prospective members, including "wives and sweethearts" of Clinic staff physicians and fellows. The key question was "Are you a registered nurse?...Practical nurse?" Office skills were also considered desirable, as were car ownership and the ability to drive. "Is your car available, with yourself as driver, for emergency service in case of air raid, sabotage, explosion or other disaster?"[20]

Although this emergency unit was apparently never organized, the Cleveland Clinic Hospital did make extensive use of volunteer aides during the Second World War, "to meet the situation involved due to the extreme shortage of nurses." Some of the volunteer workers came through the American Red Cross, and were trained at the Clinic in cooperation with the Red Cross. "The patients seemed to enjoy the attention and service rendered by this group."[21]

The Clinic Hospital also started its own course for volunteer workers. Taught by the Hospital's Assistant Director of Nursing, Josephine Hruby, the class met for three hours on three successive Sunday mornings and received instruction in practical work. A third group of volunteers was made up of doctors' wives, who met each Tuesday and Thursday afternoon to make dressings.

HOME CARE
The wartime nursing shortage affected the entire Cleveland community. Organizations like the Family Health Association and its Central School of Practical Nursing offered courses for practical nurses and "home nursing attendants," publicizing the programs in displays like the one depicted here. While graduates of these courses could not independently practice nursing, they were able to assist with patient care tasks like bathing, feeding, and bed-making, and often cared for convalescent patients or mothers and newborn babies in the home. Homemakers and other women were encouraged to take first aid and home nursing courses offered by organizations like the Red Cross, enabling them to care for the minor illnesses and injuries of family members, as well as to volunteer in hospitals.

The Hospital also obtained sponges and dressings made by volunteers at the Red Cross dressing center, with volunteer drivers picking up materials at the Hospital and returning finished dressings each day. In 1943 the Hospital hired Lila Kappan to coordinate and direct volunteer service. In 1944, 907 volunteers gave 17,521 hours of service, and the Clinic's Administrative Board approved the use of 10 Red Cross volunteers as Clinic Building ushers.

Aides, hostesses, and volunteers helped make it possible for the Cleveland Clinic and its Hospital to carry on through the war years with an increased patient load and a decreased nursing staff. However, simply managing this inexperienced, ever-changing group of auxiliary workers was a task in itself, as Abbie Porter recognized. "Our staff of supervisors numbering seventeen have made it possible to care for the patients with any degree of safety. The Fellow-Doctors, Staff Duty Nurses, Aides and Volunteers are changing constantly. I believe we should do every thing possible to keep this group, so long as they can stand the pressure physically and mentally."[22]

Private Duty Nurses — An Adjunct Staff

The one remaining source of reinforcement for the Foundation's embattled nursing staff was the legion of private duty nurses headquartered at OSNA District No. 4's registry, by this time known as the Bureau of Nursing Service. First of all, there were the private duty nurses called in as special nurses for individual patients. In addition, by the late 1930s, the Cleveland Clinic Hospital was paying private duty nurses by the day, or occasionally by the month, to supplement its general duty nursing staff during periods of high census or low staff levels. In 1943, the number of temporary nurses working at the Hospital ranged from 15 to 38 per month over the course of the year.

The special duty nurses had always served as an adjunct nursing staff, not only at the Clinic Hospital, but at many hospitals both locally and nationally. They provided "undivided" attention to individual patients, giving constant care that hospitals were not sufficiently staffed to offer. Along with Lakeside/University Hospitals, St. Luke's Hospital, and Mt. Sinai Hospital, the Cleveland Clinic Hospital had continually been among the top users of private duty nurses from District No. 4's Bureau of Nursing Service.[23] By the 1940s the Clinic Hospital and University Hospitals each often had three hundred or more calls for nurses filled by the Bureau per month, significantly more than other area hospitals.

Since the Clinic Hospital's own statistics showed over five thousand calls per year at this point, it was obviously getting some of its nurses from outside the Bureau. Some of these nurses may have come from commercial registries, or they may have been Bureau nurses contacted directly (rather than through the Bureau) by the Cleveland Clinic. These were common practices at area hospitals, which District No. 4 tried to discourage, without lasting success partly because the District's registry could not always furnish enough nurses.

The Bureau of Nursing Service also lost nurses during the war. During the years 1934 to 1942, from nine hundred to more than one thousand private duty nurses were registered with the Bureau during any given year. By 1945, there were only 561. Some of the "missing" nurses had joined the military. As of 1943, 382 District nurses, or more than 10 percent of its membership, had done so. Other former private duty nurses went into the expanding field of industrial nursing.

District members included not just the private duty nurses at the Bureau, but all qualified nurses in Cleveland and the surrounding area who had joined the organization and through it, the Ohio State Nurses' Association and the American Nurses' Association. The District had three internal sections to which nurses could belong according to their employment and interests: Institutional/Education, Public Health, and Private Duty. In 1942 the District created an Industrial Division within the Public Health Section for the increasing number of nurses working in industry. A partial survey of Cleveland industries in that year indicated that 192 nurses were so employed, 114 of whom were District members.

Group Nursing in Cleveland

In 1942 the District's Board of Trustees approved what it hoped would be a solution to the wartime shortage of private duty nurses: group nursing. Under this system, two (or occasionally more) hospital patients (preferably in the same or adjoining rooms) needing special nursing were "grouped" under the care of a single private duty nurse. The concept of group nursing was not new. The District had set a fee for nurses tending two patients at least as early as 1920, and group nursing had been instituted at the Clinic Hospital during the 1920s. Flora Short's second call there, in 1925, was for two patients at $4.50 each. However, grouping had been so little used in recent years that some members of the District's Board were uncertain about the policy regarding it.

Group nursing had always been controversial. During the Board's 1942 discussion of the subject, the District's long-time General Secretary, Lota Lorimer, stated that it had actually first been proposed in Cleveland for trial in home cases during the influenza epidemic of 1918-1919, but that only one physician had actually had patients nursed on a group basis. Some nurses believed it encouraged the provision of substandard care. Others believed that it would create friction between hospital staff nurses and nurses doing group nursing, because the daily rate for the care of two patients would be higher than the per diem salary of most staff nurses.

However, by 1942 it was clear that group nursing was better than no nursing. The Private Duty Section proposed that the District offer group nursing, at the rate of $8 for two patients per eight-hour day, "for the duration." (The daily rate at this time for nursing one patient was $6.) Margaret Lundberg, a private duty nurse and a District trustee, related to her fellow Board members the substance of a discussion that had taken place at a meeting of the Private Duty Section.

> The girls realize there are calls not filled, and the Section is very anxious to see that the sick of Cleveland are taken care of efficiently. The girls were very much concerned at the last meeting; quite a few girls turned out, showing an interest in it.

> There are patients who really need private duty care. I know one girl cited at the clinic [the Cleveland Clinic Hospital] that there were five combines that were done in one day, and there wasn't a nurse available at all to take care of them, and they are very, very difficult cases. There was one nurse on the floor to take care of five fresh 'ops' plus forty other patients, she said. At that time the girls felt if there had been one girl who could have come in and done group nursing to relieve the patients that were so very ill, it would have been a lot better than the care that they did receive, because they didn't receive any, and they could have gotten some care

107

that night until more relief could have been given to the patients by more nurses being placed. If there are ten patients on one floor, in group nursing the idea would be to have five nurses taking care of the ten patients, relieving the pressure on the hospital nurse, because more patients would be taken care of, it would be more reasonable for the patient, and most of the patients would be getting care where they are not now.[24]

Another trustee said that she believed all general duty and institutional nurses would "welcome such a plan wholeheartedly." However, it would have to be publicized carefully, so that nurses, physicians, and, above all, patients would know what to expect. One private duty nurse related an instance in which a patient said to his nurse, who had charge of two patients, "'You are giving him' (the other patient) 'too much attention. Come over here and take care of me a little bit.'"[25] It was suggested that nurses appeal to patients' patriotic feelings when explaining the new system:

> A patient just can't be told, "Well, now, you will have to share your nurse with another patient." He will have to be told that this is war time, that this is a time of sacrifice, and this is a time when sick people must realize a little care is better than none, and that if they will help the nurse in the hospital by being cooperative and not expecting too much care, and so forth, the plan will work better.[26]

The District Board of Trustees approved the group nursing plan. In February 1943, the Board also approved the Private Duty Section's wartime "Suggested Plan for Temporary Staff Nursing in Cleveland Hospitals." The plan basically took group, hourly, and temporary staff services already being offered by the Bureau of Nursing Service and promoted their increased use as a solution to the wartime shortage. Rates for nursing services were raised, from $6 to $7 for the care of a single patient. Group nursing rates would be $9 for two patients per 8-hour day, or $11 per 12-hour day, with $1 added to the total for each additional patient beyond two. Temporary staff nurses obtained through the Bureau would be paid the prevailing private duty daily rate, now $7 per 8-hour day.

To make sure that the distinction between temporary nurses and employee staff nurses was maintained, the plan reminded hospital administrators that they could not deduct laundry, meals, housing, or Victory Tax (the withholding of income tax was itself a wartime innovation on the part of the federal government) from private duty wages. Private duty nurses, whether specials or temporary staffers, were independent contractors. The plan included a proposal for the Bureau to contact inactive nurses through alumnae associations and "interest and encourage them to help in this emergency" as hourly or temporary general duty nurses, since the Bureau's existing private duty registrants would be fully occupied in filling regular private duty calls.[27]

The District called a meeting of hospital representatives, including directors of nursing, to discuss the plan. The hospital representatives were asked about their institutions' experience of group nursing. Only the Cleveland Clinic Hospital reported much success in using it. Other hospitals reported lack of cooperation by patients or nurses, as well as problems with the physical layout of patient rooms, in implementing group nursing.

"Not So Young Anymore"

Private duty nurse Flora Short, now well into middle age, shared in the trials, and the rewards, of work on the home front during these years. Her income finally rose back to pre-Depression levels. She recorded receiving payments amounting to $1,852 in 1942, when the base rate was still $6 a day. But to earn that money, she had to work an incredible 307 and 1/2 days, equivalent to six days a week year-round, with no vacation. She had worked 285 and 1/2 days the year before. In 1943, when the private duty rate went up to $7 a day, and Miss Short began doing group nursing at $9 a day, her daily income averaged $7.41; she was able to make nearly $1,900 while working a more reasonable 256 days.

Most of her cases were patients of Clinic surgeons — transurethral resections by Dr. Charles C. Higgins, cataract removals by Dr. A. D. Ruedemann, thyroidectomies by Dr. Robert Dinsmore, combined abdominoperineal resections by Dr. Thomas Jones — but she also cared for the occasional cardiac or diabetic patient.

Her time was evenly divided between group nursing and caring for individual patients, and often she would care for the same person on both bases. First, for a day to several days following surgery, she would devote her entire time to a single patient, and then, as that patient's condition improved, she would take on an additional patient, caring for both on a group nursing basis. In 1944 Miss Short did a brief stint of military nursing, working at the Army Infirmary at Western Reserve University for three-and-a-half months, for which she received $146 a month, less than she was earning in her regular practice at this point. She then returned to the Cleveland Clinic Hospital, where she continued to do by far the greatest part of her work.

Like Miss Short, many private duty nurses and also many staff nurses working at the Cleveland Clinic were middle-aged or older. Sara Jones, lamenting the difficulty of obtaining relief nurses, turned to staff nurses able to work extra time. "This, however, has dwindled to a minimum, the staff nurses finding it too hard with the exception of one or two. Most of the private duty nurses are tired and not so young any more and while they are willing and want to do their share, they feel that one and two patients are all that they can care for properly."[28]

But these "willing" women, however tired, served The Cleveland Clinic Foundation, its patients, and the community well, caring for the civilian population while their colleagues served in the Army or Navy. Civilian nurses did not always receive thanks for their service. While military nurses were admired and made into heroines of stage and screen, the public sometimes took for granted the nurses who stayed home, or even abused them as selfish and unpatriotic.

Nurse Recruitment

Younger nurses were subjected to tremendous pressure to join the military. "Patients in some of our hospitals are very disagreeable to the nurses caring for them, especially to those who appear to be of military service age. Much of this attitude upon the part of the patients is no doubt due to the radio appeal from one of our National Red Cross Nurses asking the public to boycott and not employ any nurses who are of military age."[29]

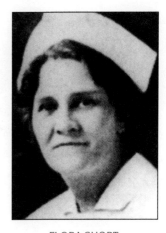

FLORA SHORT
Miss Short, a 1921 graduate of the Kahler Hospital Training School in Rochester, Minnesota, was a favorite private duty nurse at the Cleveland Clinic Hospital. She began caring for patients of Clinic staff physicians almost immediately after her arrival in Cleveland in 1925, and continued to do so until her retirement in 1956. Miss Short nursed both medical and surgical cases, but more of the latter. Her practice reflected changing trends in surgical treatment. During the 1920s, Miss Short cared for many of Dr. Crile's thyroid surgery patients; by the 1950s, she was nursing cardiothoracic and vascular cases.

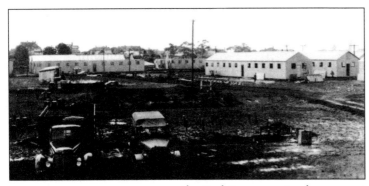

WORLD WAR II
MILITARY HOSPITAL
The Cleveland Clinic's
Navy unit was stationed
in New Zealand during the
war, where it established
Mobile Hospital No. 4, shown
here under construction in 1942.
Dr. Crile noted that the
routine operations the unit's
surgeons were performing —
appendectomies, hernia repairs,
and skin grafting, on young men
in good condition —
differed considerably from
the more unusual surgical
practice at the Clinic.

As it had in the First World War, the Red Cross took an active part in recruiting nurses for military service. Locally, there was some friction between the Red Cross and District No. 4. The District prided itself on being a purely professional organization, run by and for graduate nurses. Private duty nurses had a strong voice in District matters. The Red Cross's Board and committees had both professional and lay members. In 1943 the Cleveland chapter of the Red Cross received an urgent request from the Army's Fifth Corps Service Command for two hundred additional nurses. The Red Cross Nurse Recruitment Committee requested a list of names and addresses of all private duty nurses eligible for service from the District's Bureau of Nursing Service. The District offered to mail any notice the Red Cross wished to send, but would not furnish names and addresses. The Red Cross refused this offer, "as they want the names and addresses of the nurses for follow-up work."[30]

The two organizations also clashed over the refusal of the District Board to name a representative to the Red Cross Nurse Recruitment Committee. Some District trustees believed that supplying nurses for the armed forces was too important a goal to let past differences between the two organizations interfere. However, most felt that the District was already doing its share in the war effort through its participation in Office of Civilian Defense activities, and the entry of many member nurses into military service. This included the president of the District's Board, Margaret F. King, a private duty nurse who resigned from office in 1943 when she joined the armed services.

The national Bolton-Laird Act, sponsored by Cleveland-area congressional representative and nursing advocate Frances Payne Bolton, was envisaged as a way to provide the increased number of nurses needed for civilian and military duty alike. Under the program, known as the Cadet Nurse Corps, young women entering nursing schools agreed to work after graduation in military or essential civilian nursing for as long as the war lasted. In exchange, the U.S. Public Health Service would cover the cost of their nursing education and also pay them a stipend. In this way, the program had both patriotic and financial appeal. It also compressed the usual 36 months of nursing education into 30, so that the new nurses were available for military or other service as soon as possible. During their training, and until they were registered, the cadets served as much-needed additions to civilian hospital staffs.

In practice, the cadet nurses were unable to give much help to institutions without nursing schools, like the Cleveland Clinic, until the war ended. The Clinic Hospital hired some newly graduated cadets in 1944, but they stayed only until the completion of their state board examinations; "then pressure from the Red Cross to join the Army Nurse Corp. made it imperative for them to leave for service. This same pressure is being used on all graduate nurses. Twelve left in January [of 1945] and four in February."[31]

In all, 17 Clinic Hospital nurses joined the military in 1945, compared to 8, 7, and 6 in 1942, 1943, and 1944 respectively. During the early years of the war, the decrease in the Hospital's nursing staff had been attributed primarily to nurses leaving for new positions in industry and improving opportunities in the private duty field. Already, however, the number of younger nurses in military service contributed to the difficulty of obtaining replacements.

The Cadet Nurse Corps was very successful in recruiting young women into nursing.[32] But even the entry of the cadets into the military during the last year of the war could not satisfy the insatiable demand for nurses, as the United States occupied more and more territory in Europe, and a full-scale invasion of Japan seemed a distinct possibility. A nurse draft had been discussed in 1943, but since an act of Congress would have been required to draft women, the idea was dropped. By the beginning of 1945 it had resurfaced, and the President of the United States and the president of the ANA both supported the idea.

But at the grass-roots level of the profession, a "deluge of telephone calls" to District No. 4 headquarters revealed a great deal of bitterness among nurses. Some felt that they were being singled out for criticism by the media and at the same time betrayed by their own leaders. District headquarters received reports that Red Cross recruitment committees, desperate to fill their quotas, were hounding nurses with daily calls and letters, and even contacting nurses in other states.[33]

Nurses were genuinely uncertain where their duty lay. "Many nurses are in a state of confusion as to what the real needs are and whether or not they should give up their essential work in Civilian Service," commented Sue Z. McCracken, District No. 4's General Secretary. Miss McCracken also noted that she was receiving reports that the skills of military nurses were being "dissipated" and wasted on non-nursing or non-essential tasks.[34] And despite their stated need for nurses, the armed forces admitted African-American women to their nursing corps with great reluctance.

When the District contacted Ohio congressional representatives to urge them to oppose the drafting of nurses, the replies were not encouraging. Senator Harold Burton declared that he "was watching the situation carefully." Representative Frances Payne Bolton did not hesitate to blame the nurses themselves for their predicament. "A very sure and definite method to stop the passage of any measure to draft nurses would be for nurses who are qualified for work in the Armed Services to volunteer. Their failure to do so has created an exceedingly difficult situation which must be met." Under public pressure and the threat of a draft, so many nurses volunteered that the Army ended up with more than were needed. This, and the end of the war, ended the demand for a draft of nurses.[35]

First Line of Defense

From a certain perspective, the nation's insistent call for nurses was a compliment. Alone among women, they were singled out as vital to the national interest in a way that teachers, secretaries, and even mothers were not. But their choice of career also made them subject to pressures and criticisms that other women did not have to face. Society had always asked service of nurses;

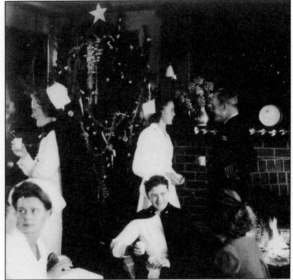

CHRISTMAS OVERSEAS, 1942
Military nurses, including the women attending this Christmas party, were in charge of patient care in hospitals like the one where the Clinic Navy unit was stationed. A Navy nurse known as "Smitty" served as "the excellent head nurse" of Dr. Crile's general surgery ward. Smitty and other head nurses directed the work of medical corpsmen, who gave much of the patient care on the wards and also worked in the operating rooms.

when that meant military service, white uniforms had to be changed for khaki or navy blue. During the Second World War, as in the First, nurses in some ways seemed to have more in common with men and soldiers than with other women, to the point of being considered for military draft. But at the same time, the U.S. armed forces refused to allow male nurses to serve in the nurse corps.

Cleveland Clinic physicians, especially the fellows (postgraduate physicians-in-training), felt pressures of their own during and even after the war. Young physicians, although subject to the draft, were also expected, like all

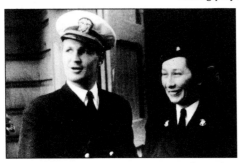

IN UNIFORM
Many physicians and nurses, like Barney Crile and Smitty (above), served in military hospitals overseas or in the United States. Younger nurses, especially, came under considerable pressure to join the armed services; there was even talk of drafting nurses. Those who stayed at home, however, also served their country, through serving the needs of their fellow citizens. Insofar as overwork and scarcity went, conditions were often more difficult at home than in the military.

young men, to volunteer rather than wait to be called. The Clinic granted salary increases to keep and attract fellows and interns during the war, even to the extent of giving extra pay to married men. After the war, the Foundation's Fellowship Committee reflected the general attitude of postwar America when it proposed "that it be the policy of the Clinic only to employ returning war veterans" as fellows.[36]

These contradictory demands placed many people, not only the District No. 4 nurses, "in a state of confusion." Did an 18-year-old son of a widowed mother do his duty by going overseas and risking death, or by taking a factory job at home and braving accusations that he was a coward? Would a young physician better serve his country by joining the Army right away, or by completing his education first? Who needed nurses more, the sick and injured in civilian hospitals, or the soldiers and sailors wounded in battle? Should hospitals encourage enlistment, or use all means necessary to hold onto their dwindling numbers of employees?

Some people declared health care and hospitals to be the country's first line of defense. Dean Marion Howell of the Western Reserve University School of Nursing said so as early as 1941, before America entered the war. Dr. Herbert B. Wright of the Cleveland Civilian Defense Committee said so in 1942, when memories of Pearl Harbor were still fresh. "'We must consider the Hospitals as our first line of Defense and furnish them with an adequate staff of nurses.'"[37] But as the war went on, and the threat of invasion grew more distant, nurses for home service came to be seen as something of a luxury, to be rationed like sugar or gasoline or nylon, with the biggest share going to the Army. If young nurses were under pressure to enlist, older nurses were under pressure to rejoin the work force. "More and more of the nurses who have retired will feel it necessary to return to active duty, in order to let younger nurses join the military services," stated an editorial in a Cleveland newspaper.[38]

It seemed logical for older nurses and physicians to take over responsibility for civilian medical care, whether or not hospitals were the first line of defense. But for nurses, this required a break with tradition. Because of the dynamics of a woman's life, many nurses left their careers after a few years, whereas physicians did not. Therefore, although there was a larger pool of "retired" nurses to draw from, there were relatively fewer older nurses in the active labor force. The necessities of wartime brought about changes, for example, the great increase in female workers in heavy industry. Just as some married women had returned to work during the Depression when their husbands were unemployed, married women (especially those whose husbands had gone off to military service) returned to work to help the war effort. At the Cleveland Clinic Hospital, they proved a welcome and necessary addition to the nursing staff.

The Home Front

Even for ordinary citizens who stayed quietly at home, for those who were too old or too young to think of joining the armed services, World War II was an everyday fact of life. The country mobilized its resources on a massive scale, and immediately after Pearl Harbor, in particular, people genuinely feared attack and invasion. Not since the Civil War had Americans felt war to be so near them. Compared with the hardships and dangers experienced by people who lived in countries closer to the lines of battle, air raid drills and gasoline rationing were no more than inconveniences. However, the intervention of the U.S. government in almost every sphere of private economic life did have a great impact on civilians.

Before the United States actually entered the war, a large number of federal boards, bureaus, and agencies had been set up to control war production and all that was associated with it. In part, this was a continuation of the activist stance adopted by the Roosevelt administration during the Depression, but it was equally a response to the crisis at hand. The War Labor Board, the War Production Board, the Office of Procurement and Assignment, the Office of Civilian Defense — all these, and others, became very well known to American producers and consumers, employers and employees alike.

Citizens not able to volunteer for military service could volunteer for service in their own towns and neighborhoods. Older men became air raid wardens or served on local draft boards. Teen-aged boys and girls could be Civilian Defense messengers. Women joined the Red Cross as drivers or nurses' aides. Everyone could participate in bond drives and scrap drives. Even gardening was patriotic, since growing the family's own vegetables in a victory garden meant that more of the nation's farm production could go to the armed forces.

The Cleveland Clinic Foundation and its employees, patients, and private duty nurses were swept along in the war effort with everyone else. Early in 1942 Dr. Higgins was put in charge of the institution's Civilian Defense program, to be responsible, together with Hospital Superintendent Abbie Porter and Administrative Board Chairman Dr. Ruedemann, for making plans "for the participation of the Foundation in problems relating to war at the time of emergency." Dr. U. V. Portmann looked into the possibility of converting the Research Building into a 100-bed hospital "if the emergency arose." Clinic space was set aside for conducting draft physicals. "An exhibition of the technic of extinguishing a Thermite bomb" took place one Saturday morning in the Hospital parking lot. In January of 1943 Superintendent and Secretary of the Foundation George W. Grill resigned to enter the armed forces; in December came word that his son, Lt. George Grill, Jr., had been killed in action in the Pacific.[39]

The U.S. Office of Procurement and Assignment limited the number of fellows the Clinic could employ. The 1943 quota was 25. Permanent staff members of military age had to be approved by the government as "essential" to remain at the Clinic.

During 1942 the government enacted wage and price freezes to control wartime inflation. Hospital nurses' salaries were frozen at rates "all the way from $184.50 per month for Miss Barr down to $119.50 per month for a few of

EASING THE SHORTAGE
Cleveland newspapers ran frequent stories about the measures that the local health care community was using to cope with the nursing shortage. Although some hospitals employed practical nurses, the Cleveland Clinic Hospital did not. In addition to the new nurses' aides, floor hostesses, and volunteers, the Hospital depended on private duty nurses to supplement the work of its own registered nurse staff. "Group nursing," which allowed a special nurse to care for more than one patient, became common in Cleveland hospitals.

Practical Nurses Praised for Easing Help Shortage Here

BY SEVERINO P. SEVERINO

Medical chores are being re-shuffled today to ease pressure on nurses.

Biggest assist comes from the practical nurse who proves herself capable of performing tasks once assigned only to registered nurses.

Practical nurses today work in hospitals, doctors' offices, in patients' homes. They release registered nurses to do tasks that call for highest training.

Doctors endorse the role of the practical nurses.

"They do an excellent job," a doctor said. "I call upon them often for home care of patients."

A practical nurse, for example, sets up a sterile tray of medical instruments today, a time-consuming chore which once was performed only by a registered nurse. A registered nurse could administer medicine to a full ward in the time saved by relief of sterilization duty.

In doctors' offices practical nurses administer simple medications. They give injections and aid with routine checkups of babies and children.

Practical nurses also play a role in the care of tuberculosis patients. There are a number at Sunny Acres Hospital where they receive a special short in-service training course.

Training of practical nurses takes 54 weeks. Sixteen weeks are spent at Central School of Practical Nursing, 3300 Chester Ave. Twenty-four weeks training is followed at University Hospitals, and 14 more weeks are used in preparing the practical nurse in various types of home care.

The Central School of Practical Nursing is an agency of the Family Health Association. Miss Etta A. Creech is director.

the more recently employed nurses."[40] Most nurses received $134.50 or $139.50. These figures included $19.50 for two meals a day, so that the typical base pay was actually $115 or $120. The nurses also received "adjusted compensation," or a bonus, a holdover from the old Office days, when a "distribution" was made at the end of the year from the money earned over and above the separate practices of the individual physicians.

The War Production Board (WPB) set priorities for all civilian and military production and determined what equipment could be purchased. When in 1943 the Clinic's Dermatology Department wanted to replace a 22-year-old X-ray therapy machine with a new unit, the WPB's priority restrictions had to be consulted. In 1944 Dr. James A. Dickson requested a new fracture table for the orthopaedic service, which the Administrative Board agreed to purchase if "a priority can be obtained."[41] Again, when the Administrative Board decided to purchase air conditioning units for the operating rooms, Mr. Daoust had to apply to the WPB for priority. Nothing escaped the WPB's attention. It even requested the Foundation to sell a quarter of its new typewriters to the government, and rent used ones instead. (The Foundation decided it could afford to surrender only 5 of its 95 machines.) And, like every American family, the Clinic had to cope with food rationing.

Essential Activity

Workers themselves, as well as their salaries, were "frozen." In 1943 the War Manpower Commission (WMC) prohibited approximately 27,000,000 "essential" American workers from leaving their jobs without official permission. When District No. 4 inquired into how this would affect nurses, the answer came back that all Cleveland area nurses were frozen into their current jobs, and each "must secure an availability slip when going from one essential nursing position to another." However, student nurses were not frozen into their training hospitals upon graduation, and a nurse who wished to leave an essential position to enter private duty nursing would be treated like a physician establishing a private practice; she did not need to secure a release. The local director of the WMC said that he "consider[ed] institutions giving care to the sick and injured more essential than industrial institutions."[42]

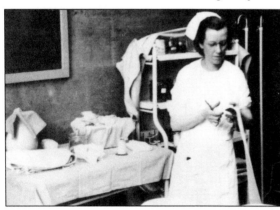

PREPARING SUPPLIES
Nurse Eloise Fisher is shown here preparing a bandage, with a supply cart visible behind her. Frequent dressing changes were part of the nursing care of Dr. Thomas Jones's colostomy patients, since there were no colostomy bags at the time. When Dr. Jones made rounds to examine his patients, he required that all dressings be opened up.

The need for military nurses was a consideration that overrode all others. Dr. Jones, Chairman of the Cleveland Clinic's Hospital Committee, reported at a meeting of the Administrative Board in February 1945 that

> the number of staff nurses has been reduced from 70 at the first of the year to 52 through resignations to join the Army, notwithstanding that the Nurses Procurement & Assignment Office has classified the Clinic Hospital nurses as 3-A and therefore employed in an essential activity; that with the present nursing force it will be impossible to continue operating the Hospital to capacity and that unless immediate relief can be found it may be necessary to close a floor or at least half a floor.[43]

At the Clinic Hospital, one general staff nurse cared for 12 patients on the day shift, 18 on the evening shift, and 40 on the night shift. Board members

	DAYS	HOURS	MEMO	EARNINGS			MEMO.	TAXABLE EARNINGS	WITHHOLD-ING TAX	DEDUCTIONS					TOTAL DEDUCTIONS	NET PAY	PERIOD ENDING 194_	N
				REGULAR	OVERTIME	GROSS PAY	FOOD			GR. A.	C.H.S.A.	OHIO SALES TAX	MISC.	BONDS				
1	½ mo.			80.00			9.75	89.75	7.60	1.50	.26				9.36	70.64	1-15	4
2	½ mo.			67.50			9.75	77.25	8.90		.75	.26			7.81	57.67	1-15	47
3	½ mo.		3 da. ill	77.50			7.50	85.00	18.00		.75	.20			18.95	53.55	1-15	47
4	½ mo.			67.50	.50		9.75	77.25	14.00	1.50	.26				15.76	51.74	1-15	47
5	½ mo.		2 da vac 1da L.A.	67.50			8.25	75.75	8.80		.75	.22			9.77	57.13	1-15	47
6	½ mo.		9 da. vac	67.50			3.75	71.25	8.90		.75	.10			9.65	51.85	1-15	47
7	½ mo.			87.50			9.75	97.25	7.60		.75	.26			8.61	78.89	1-15	47
8	½ mo.			70.00			9.75	79.75	8.90		.75	.26			9.81	60.19	1-15	47
9	½ mo.			70.00			9.75	79.75	8.90		.75	.26			9.81	60.19	1-15	47
10	½ mo.			70.00			9.75	79.75	8.90	1.90	.26				10.96	57.04	1-15	47

PAY ROLL SUMMARY — No. 5 — OR PERIOD ENDING Jan 15th 1944

suggested solutions ranging from pleading the Clinic's case with the government, to advertising for married nurses to work part-time, to hiring undergraduate cadet nurses. The Board approved all of these recommendations. The suggestion of providing nurse housing appeared for the first time in the record, but no action was taken. Physician staff members were again reminded to "more carefully scrutinize" their cases to admit "only those patients clearly requiring hospitalization."[44]

The 17 beds of the Hospital's second floor had been closed in 1943. Closing an additional, larger floor would be a last resort. The significance of nurses in the operation and financing of the entire Cleveland Clinic Foundation was never so clear as in a crisis like this.

> In connection with the consideration of the effects of closing a floor in the Hospital, Mr. Daoust stated that apart from the irreparable damage to the Clinic's good will and the disruption of both the In-Patient and Out-Patient Departments of the Hospital, he had estimated that the closing of 60 beds would probably result in a loss of about $425,000. per year in Hospital and Clinic cash income, and that such a loss would undoubtedly greatly interfere with the Foundation's research and educational programs.[45]

In May there were still only 55 nurses on roll, of whom only 30 were general staff nurses. Abbie Porter suggested that admissions be curtailed sharply during the vacation months, but the Board continued to resist any notion of closing beds: "It will be impossible for the medical staff to meet their obligations to provide necessary medical service if additional beds are closed."[46]

A shortage of surgical nurses was also affecting the functioning of the entire institution. In 1940, 13 was considered an appropriate number of Operating Room nurses. By June 1943, there were already too few surgical nurses to "serv[e] patients properly." Mr. Daoust requested Abbie Porter to employ "immediately...additional supervisors and head nurses for that service, paying, if necessary, the maximum allowable pay."[47]

When the situation had not improved by September, additional measures had to be considered, including using volunteer aides, doctors' wives with

NURSES' SALARIES
This handwritten payroll ledger from the beginning of 1944 shows that Cleveland Clinic Hospital R.N.s were earning semimonthly salaries in the range of $67.50 to $87.50. Employees received two meals a day, which were valued at $.75 per day and considered part of taxable earnings. The official working week for nurses was 48 hours — eight hours a day, six days a week.

surgical nursing training, or part-time general duty nurses as assistants. It was also suggested that outpatient Clinic nurses be trained in surgical nursing, so that they could assist in the Hospital operating rooms, or at procedures moved to the Clinic itself. One important innovation was the hiring of an additional anesthetist to accompany patients back to their rooms after surgery, which had been the responsibility of the surgical nurse up to this time. This might be considered the beginning of specialized post-anesthesia care nursing at the Hospital.

The Clinic's administration also decided to pay surgical nurses for overtime in order to lessen "the unusual pressure on the surgical nursing service." This was a delicate matter, since surgical nurses were in the same Hospital department as general duty nurses. Transferring Operating Room nurses to the Clinic side of the organization, where nurses worked as employees of the various clinical departments rather than in a unified nursing department, "in an endeavor to obtain more surgical nurses without so much disturbing the relationship with the general nursing service," was considered but not done.[48]

Between 1940 and 1945, the number of operations performed at the Cleveland Clinic Hospital rose from 4,720 to 8,180. In early 1945, the number of Operating Room nurses was at times as low as eight.

Chief Anesthetist Lou Adams disapproved of overtime pay, but requested salary increases for her staff members, who were also working long hours in the operating room for $150 to $175 a month. From 1940 to 1945 the number of nurse anesthetists remained fairly constant, generally at four, including Miss Adams. However, there was continual turnover in the other three positions. At least two nurse anesthetists left for military service, and at least three more married. Of these three, Elizabeth Thompson Fisher, a five-year Clinic employee, eventually returned to work, since her physician husband was serving overseas. Although there were continual efforts made to find and hire anesthetists to increase the staff, the new recruits generally ended up replacing someone else who left. A memo written by Abbie Porter to Edward Daoust in December 1944, relaying the recommendation of the Surgical Committee that the anesthesia staff be increased to six, explained how hard it was to obtain anesthetists.

> There are three anesthetists on duty at the present time....We had an anesthetist from Illinois, who was anxious to work here. A telegram was sent to her. The hospital where she is working refused to release her. An anesthetist from Buffalo was to report Dec. 15th. We received a message from her. She has a sick aunt and is unable to come until after the 1st of the year....[An anesthetist] who used to be with us, was to report the 26th of December and stay until our staff was complete. Her father and mother refused to let her come. We are now communicating with an anesthetist in Penn. It is doubtful that we can get some one before the first of the year.[49]

"On a Wartime Production Schedule"

From very early in the war years, as it became clear that a decreased number of physicians, nurses, and other employees would continue to face an increasing number of Clinic appointments and Hospital admissions, the issue of limiting the number of new patients who could register at the Clinic (which would also have the effect of limiting Hospital use) came up again and again. When

Clinic nurses were assigned to the various medical specialty "desks" in the outpatient area. During WWII, there were five Clinic desks: Desk 20, Surgery and Gastrointestinal; Desk 21, Diagnostic; Desk 30, Orthopaedics and ENT; Desk 31, Eye, Neurosurgery, Endocrinology, and Dental; and Desk 35, Dermatology and Genitourinary. There were also separate areas for Allergy and X-ray. Of a total of 107 examination rooms in use, the Diagnostic Desk had 26 examination rooms, and General Surgery, 11. The number of patient visits per year went above 200,000 in 1942. Clinic consultation fees were $10. In 1946, the charge for a physical examination was raised — to $25.

the Administrative Board discussed the matter in March 1942, the members decided unanimously not to close registration in the various departments, and declared that special effort should be made to give good, prompt care to the increasing number of Clevelanders seeking medical services. But a year later, with every department in the Clinic and Hospital "worked to capacity," Dr. Haden, the Chief of Medicine, proposed that new patient registration should be restricted to two thousand per month.[50] The Board set aside the proposal for further study.

At the same time, new regulations regarding Hospital admissions stated that as long as the Hospital census remained at capacity levels, admissions would be limited to 25 on Mondays, and 17 on all other days. Two beds, one each for male and female patients, would be held open at all times for emergencies. By the end of the year the Hospital found itself turning away as many as eight or nine patients a day.

Clinic registration continued under discussion during the spring of 1943, and minor changes were made, including requesting physicians to take fewer history notes, requesting local non-emergency patients to make appointments during the later part of the week, and adding a note to the patient information brochure stating that the reduced staff made delays inevitable. Dr. Haden still urged limiting registration and finally, effective April 30, the Board set a weekly limit of 450 new patients. Unfortunately, the plan did not seem to work as well as had been hoped, since 542 new patients registered the following week, with 24 patients deferred.

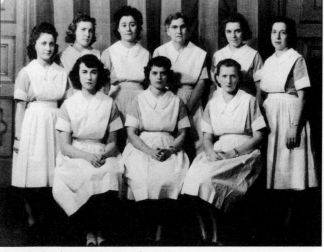

PRACTICAL NURSING STUDENTS, 1943
The hairstyles and uniforms of these practical nursing students show the influence of wartime fashions. After the longer hemlines of the 1930s, the knee-length skirts of the period helped conserve fabric, so that more production from the nation's textile mills could go to making military uniforms. Government regulations prohibited the manufacture of skirts with hems more than 72 inches wide or 2 inches deep, and discouraged the design of garments with excessive ruffles, pleats, pockets, or wide sleeves.

The Board concluded that the Clinic's entire registration and appointment system needed substantial changes. Certainly the system as it stood was haphazard and lacked coordination between departments. Although it seemed to have worked adequately before, wartime conditions strained it to the breaking point. Patients complained of waiting for hours and hours.

Over at the Hospital, the daily admission quotas were proving flawed, since "emergency" cases were occupying an increasing number of beds, and patients with advance appointments had to wait longer and longer to be admitted. To prevent this, the Administrative Board approved a plan borrowed from Detroit's Harper Hospital. It drew up a list of medical and surgical emergency diagnoses. Only those cases could be admitted ahead of other patients; if a physician felt that a patient with a diagnosis not on the list merited emergency treatment, he could apply to the chief of medicine or surgery for a waiver.

In effect, necessity had compelled the Cleveland Clinic Hospital to institute an early form of utilization review or rationing of health care services. The Clinic's attempt to bring more rationality and order to its operations foreshadowed a more extensive use of management and industrial engineering techniques in the postwar period.

Unfortunately, these measures did not reduce utilization enough to correspond to the shrunken staff levels. Clinic exam rooms were busy from 8 a.m. to 6 p.m. or later. In the Hospital, a night nurse would care for 40 patients virtually unassisted. It was the way things were. "For the duration"; "during the emergency" were the phrases on everyone's lips when referring to the makeshift, unsatisfactory, or difficult arrangements of wartime. Patients, too, mostly took the situation in stride and helped out where they could, as Cleveland newspaperman John C. Davis related.

Recently I told how the demands for doctors for armed service had depleted the ranks of our country doctors. I predicted that country folks would soon flock to city hospitals for treatments and about a week later I made the prediction good by entering the Cleveland Clinic for treatment....I am going to give you a picture of how hospitals are meeting the war manpower emergency.

There was a time when anyone with the price could get into a hospital. If you did not have the cash but were critically ill you'd get in anyhow....

But that was before the war. Your only chance of getting into a hospital today is to have your doctor certify it as a matter of life and death. Entry is more difficult than to an exclusive girl's finishing school. Even after your doctor swears that your only hope of outliving your insurance policy is hospitalization except in cases of great emergency you must wait from four days to two weeks.

I drew a two-bed room with a chap from Indiana, Pa. His affliction had taken away all feeling and much control of his lower limbs. He managed to get around on crutches but was never sure whether his legs were carrying on in the same general direction as his body. His ability to navigate after a fashion was a life saver for bed-bound me. When nurses or nurse's aids were slow answering, he would pile out of bed, mount his crutches, and do the errand. This spirit of helpfulness on the part of patients extended throughout the hospital. It was not unusual to have your light answered by a patient from another room, well enough to be wandering in the hall. I would not have been surprised had Dr. George Crile, head of the Clinic, responded to my bell.

Most of you have read of the hospital work of volunteer Red Cross nurses. They give baths, back rubs, change beds, carry drinking water, take temperatures and give those many small attentions which mean so much to a sick person. They are trained by a Red Cross course and are recruited from housewives and office workers. Pledged to perform 150 hours of work annually, due to the dire shortage many have worked far beyond their quota. One had 350 hours to her credit in less than three months. Each does a three-hour trick daily, housewives during the day and the office workers after their regular jobs.

In addition to the Red Cross volunteers, there's a staff of nurse's aids, young ladies who work a full eight hour shift, augmented by high school volunteers after school and on Saturdays....

Topping the whole complicated system is the crisply efficient professional nurse, limited now to two to a floor. They give hypodermics and medicine and by a deft touch here or a bit of advice there keep the system moving smoothly.

Doctors? Sure, they're still around. They examine an unbelievably large number of patients and do prodigious work in moving them through the hospital....They waste very little time on the 'bedside manner.' Frills are out for the duration and the job is to get you well so that the bed may be available for another sufferer.

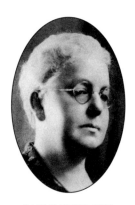

AMY F. ROWLAND

Officially, Miss Rowland's position at the Cleveland Clinic was head of the Editorial Department. But the job title did not adequately describe her role. As secretary, editor, and research assistant, she served as Dr. Crile's right hand for 26 years, from the time she arrived in Cleveland to work at the Office until ill health forced her retirement in 1940 at age 66.

A graduate of Mount Holyoke College, Miss Rowland had wanted to study medicine, but instead became secretary first to a physician in Boston, and then to Dr. Crile. During WWI, she assisted with Dr. Crile's research in France. Preparing his manuscripts for publication had always been one of her primary responsibilities, leading to her appointment as the Clinic's editor-in-charge.

Miss Rowland was also active in numerous civic, philanthropic, and women's organizations. She was a charter member and president of the Cleveland Women's City Club, a director of Alta House social settlement, and a trustee of her alma mater.

Yes, the hospitals are on a wartime production schedule. Nothing counts but turning out a finished product in the shortest possible time. I'll bet cures will exceed the peacetime average.[51]

"We as Nurses Have Lost a Friend"

Mr. Davis was wrong about one thing. Dr. Crile could not have responded to his bell, because he himself was critically ill in the Clinic Hospital at the same time. Within a month he had died, attended to the last by private duty nurses Elizabeth Bidwell and Josephine Belfield (another long-time special nurse at the Clinic). For the past few years Dr. Crile had been spending more time as a patient and less as a physician; he had also gradually withdrawn from active involvement in Foundation affairs. He had resigned the presidency of the institution in 1940, and both he and Dr. Lower had relinquished their seats on the Board of Trustees by early 1942. In December 1939 Dr. Crile had had one eye removed. Dr. Ruedemann performed the enucleation and, in Mrs. Crile's words, "Dear Lou Adams gave the anesthetic. Although she has been through many hard cases with the Chief, I imagine she never has had a harder task; yet how grateful she must have been that her skill and knowledge could save him pain when needed."[52]

A few months later, Amy Rowland, his faithful collaborator, suffered a heart attack and had to give up work. In April, Dr. Crile was hospitalized again, having fractured his left arm and developed bronchitis. Miss Bidwell, who had specialed him after the enucleation, was again called in to serve as his private duty nurse. By November, he was healthy and able to give a session at District No. 4's annual institute for private duty nurses.

In the spring of 1941, Dr. and Mrs. Crile were slightly injured in a plane crash in Florida, and they stayed briefly in a Florida hospital. Agatha Hodgins, retired and living in Coronado Beach, Florida, came to visit, and she and Dr. Crile enjoyed reminiscing at length about the work they had done together and discussing the future prospects of the nurse anesthetist. Miss Hodgins was satisfied with how far the field had come — "The nurse-anesthetist is now accepted, so they no longer hammer at us" — but felt that nurse anesthetists were still continually under pressure to prove their worth. "What I wish is that some institution would put a nurse-anesthetist in charge of the department of anesthesia and allow her to do research." Dr. Crile "agreed with Miss Hodgins in her opinion that now that women are getting such a broad background in their education, the research in anesthesia offered a large field. Personally he felt that women could lick the men any time in that work."[53]

In November 1942 Dr. Crile was admitted to the Cleveland Clinic Hospital with a blood infection. He was at first treated with sulfa drugs, and Mrs. Crile hired Miss Bidwell and Mrs. Belfield for evening and night special nursing (she herself stayed with her husband all day). All this was ultimately of no avail; Dr. Crile died on January 7, 1943, with bacterial endocarditis, cerebral embolism, rheumatic heart disease, and mitral insufficiency given as the cause of death and related conditions.

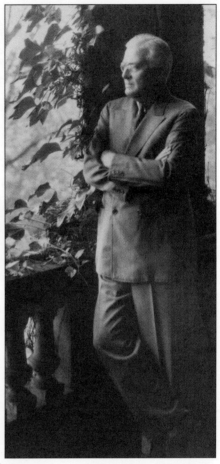

DR. GEORGE CRILE, SR.
In the summer of 1940, photographer Clifford Norton took this portrait of Dr. Crile standing on the loggia of his home. The famous surgeon died two and a half years later, at the age of 79. His family received letters of condolence postmarked from all over the country and the world. Many of them were written by nurses who had memories of working with Dr. Crile, including Linda Sampson, an early St. Luke's Hospital student; Frances Penrose, a former Clinic staff nurse who had moved to east Africa; and many Lakeside Unit nurses, as well the private duty nurses who had cared for him in his final illness.

Josephine Belfield wrote to the younger Dr. Crile, who was at this time with the Clinic Naval Unit in New Zealand:

> It was my privilege to be with "the Chief" these last eight weeks. He was the best patient I ever saw — always cooperative, courteous and considerate. He never for a moment lost his superb optimism and sense of humor....When we had to bother him for those old penicillin IVs he would wake up bright, serene and smiling — with his white hair and pink skin (he never looked ill) there was positively a glow about him that affected me every time. When we apologized for disturbing him he would say, "This is discipline. I am ready." He was a surprise to nurses accustomed to the natural impatience of the average person in the grip of sick-room routine. His personality will always remain an inspiration to us.
>
> As you know, we admired and respected Dr. Crile as a great man — during these last weeks we learned to esteem him as a gallant gentleman.[54]

In her note to Mrs. Crile she added, "Every nurse in the Cleveland Clinic Hospital feels that it is indeed the end of an era and that we as nurses have lost a friend."[55]

However, in those frenetic days in the midst of the war, people had little time for reflection. Doubtless everyone at the Cleveland Clinic agreed with Mrs. Belfield that an era had closed; but in practical terms, Dr. Crile had slipped gradually out of the life of the Clinic, and his passing was overshadowed by long days crammed with work and evenings dominated by war headlines. The wartime routine had become the new routine during the last years of Dr. Crile's life, and it remained so afterwards.

"Trying Years"

With the end of the war, things began to return to normal. But normalcy had changed during those years. Some historians of nursing later called World War II a "watershed" in American nursing. Others observed that while "the nursing profession had made great strides during and as a result of World War I....the far greater strain upon the nursing profession during and after World War II presented a grave problem."[56]

"The war years were trying years and the new period we are entering will be equally so," said Abbie Porter, specifically referring to the situation at the Cleveland Clinic Hospital.[57] Miss Porter had had reason to find the war years trying. As Superintendent of the Hospital, she had five departments reporting to her: Nursing, Anesthesia, Office, Dietary, and Housekeeping. (Other functions, like building maintenance, were managed by the administration of the entire Foundation, and their heads reported, like Miss Porter, directly to Foundation Secretary George Grill and after his departure in 1943 to Foundation President Edward Daoust.) The three largest of these departments, Nursing, Dietary, and Housekeeping, suffered from significant personnel shortages throughout the war.

While dealing with high turnover, lack of trained personnel, and difficulties in finding young employees and male employees, Miss Porter had to keep a hospital running at more than its prewar capacity. Almost as soon as the second floor's 17 beds were closed, at the beginning of 1943, the Administrative Board began to talk about reopening them. Mr. Daoust explained to the Board "that Miss Porter had stated the reason they were closed was because nurses and ward aides were unobtainable under present conditions."[58] The Board raised nurses' salaries in February 1943, and Miss Porter hoped to hire five nurses to reopen the floor by March. But the nurses could not be found.

The shortage of beds had become critical, with a census of 238 patients in a hospital with a bed capacity of 242. The Board ordered Miss Porter to obtain a list of patients by diagnosis, with the hope that some patients could be discharged, but when the Board's Hospital Committee reviewed it, "it was the opinion of the Committee...that not more than 12 of them could possibly be removed from the Hospital....[and] that further efforts to have Staff members discharge patients or refuse to admit them to the Hospital would not solve the problem of the shortage of beds." So the question again came back to finding more nurses. "Mr. Daoust explained some of the difficulties being encountered by Miss Porter. A discussion of the subject ensued and he was directed to express to her the confidence of the Board in her administration of the Hospital." The issue of reopening the beds continued under discussion in the following months.[59]

Although Miss Porter did not serve on the physician-only Administrative Board, she did serve, as of 1944, as secretary of its Hospital Committee. No matter was too small or too large to be referred to Miss Porter. Besides the ever-nagging shortage of nurses and other personnel, she was responsible for everything from planning for the evacuation of the Hospital in case of emergency, to purchasing sterilizers, to determining admission dates for waiting patients; from approving personnel policies to signing off on the building plans for the postwar Hospital expansion. During the difficult days of World War II, she could only promise, in her words, "to meet and handle the affairs of each day as they come and maintain standards where ever possible."[60]

Miss Porter was not the only one to feel the tensions caused by understaffing. The Equipment Room nurse resigned in 1942 after a misunderstanding that occurred when she was called to go to the floors and do dressings — a task not normally considered part of her work — on a day when she had not had time to finish regular duties like counting narcotics and sharpening needles. Sara Jones, Director of Nursing for nine years, stayed at her post for most of the war and then left both the Clinic Hospital (having given several months notice) and the nursing profession in mid-1945.

In Anesthesia, Lou Adams, too, was feeling that her best might not be good enough. "I have been with the Clinic 19 years since the opening of The Clinic Hospital — have always tried to give my undivided attention and loyalty. At any time you feel I am not giving satisfaction and a change would improve the Department I would appreciate an interview." Her feeling of personal loss in the death of Dr. Crile — a man, she said, who had "always placed confidence in me and gave me the incentive to do my best" — seemed to shake her confidence in herself. She closed her 1942 annual report as if in farewell: "The best years of my life have been spent here." However, she neither requested, nor was asked, to resign. Further trials lay ahead for Miss Adams, but she stayed through the war and beyond.[61]

Another of Dr. Crile's old associates, Operating Room Supervisor Emma Barr, did leave her position following the war's end. Her letter of resignation, submitted in July 1946, stated that she wished, if possible, to be transferred to a Hospital job with less responsibility; "otherwise she

AFTER THE WAR
Throughout the difficult years of the war, a core of experienced supervisory personnel like Emma Barr, head of Operating Room nursing (shown here in 1943), remained at their posts. With the return of peace came a new order. Nursing Director Sara Jones resigned in 1945. In 1946, Miss Barr transferred to the less stressful job of head receptionist. For years, she had done a superb job coordinating Dr. Crile, Sr.'s thyroid surgeries in patient rooms. Now conditions had changed. More operations were being performed in the surgical suite, and surgical specialties were becoming more important. She retired in the early 1950s and returned to her home town of Marysville, Ohio, where she helped to organize the operating room facilities at the new Union County Memorial Hospital.

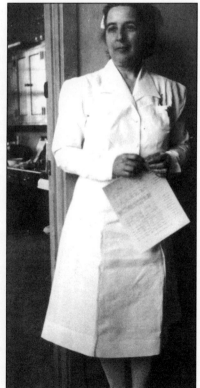

wished to terminate her employment." She was given a position at the main reception desk. Although the wish for "less responsibility" undoubtedly reflected her real feelings, and hinted at the stressful conditions under which she worked, Emma Barr probably did not resign her position altogether of her own accord. In 1944 and again in 1946 surgeons expressed dissatisfaction with "the administration of the surgical floor of the hospital particularly with regard to nurse supervision." The Hospital Committee recommended that a second assistant supervisor, who would work full-time in supervising the specialties, be appointed. Long-time Cleveland Clinic nurse Elizabeth ("Ma") Graber would continue as Assistant Supervisor for general surgery. Although the record gave few details about the events surrounding Miss Barr's departure from the post of Supervisor, the shortages and stresses of the war years, over which no one had any control, may have been a contributing factor. Then, too, she had worked very closely with Dr. Crile, Sr., throughout most of her career, and her ways as a surgical supervisor were perfectly adapted to his methods as a surgical chief. The inevitable changes after his retirement and death, including the increase in specialized services and variety of procedures, created new conditions to which she was perhaps less suited.[62]

After the War

As Miss Porter had anticipated, the postwar years had their own difficulties. In the Operating Room, the number of surgical nurses was increased from 13 to 20 in 1945, as more nurses became available for employment, and as staff surgeons returned from military service. More surgeons meant more operations. More operations meant that not only more operating rooms, but also more beds would have to be opened. More beds meant that still more nurses would have to be hired for the floors.

At the end of 1945, there were 104 nurses on roll, twice as many as the year before. However, a number of these were new cadets, not yet registered, who would need "close supervision."[63] Four undergraduate nurses also remained on the staff. Twenty-four aides and 11 orderlies completed the department's personnel. Not surprisingly, both the number of volunteers and the hours contributed by those remaining dropped substantially after the war ended.

After Miss Jones' resignation, her former assistant, Josephine Hruby, served as acting Director of Nursing until a successor could be found. At the time Miss Jones left, the Administrative Board planned to hire someone to take charge of both Hospital and outpatient Clinic nursing services. There had been no unified nursing service and no director of nursing at the Clinic; a nurse was organizationally part of whatever clinical service she worked for. But when the leading candidate for the combined position decided she preferred remaining in New York, the plan to merge the two nursing services was dropped. Mrs. Hruby, a Western Reserve University School of Nursing graduate and long-time Clinic Hospital nurse, took over the leadership of the Hospital Nursing Department.

Clinic Nursing remained separate, but the position of Nursing Supervisor for the outpatient area was finally created, and Dorothea Bordendorfer, a graduate of Cleveland's St. Luke's Hospital Nursing School and a nurse in the Clinic's Allergy Department, was appointed to the post. Clinic Nursing employees still worked within medical departments assisting physicians as they always had, but there was now a central nursing office to handle administrative matters, giving Clinic nurses a collective identity for the first time.

How Many Nurses?

These nurse administrators, along with Abbie Porter, had to deal with a constantly changing situation. At the beginning of 1946, Mrs. Hruby could say with satisfaction, "The floors, while not staffed fully, are staffed better than they have been for a long time and I hope that we can give better service to both patient and doctor." But while the increased number of nurses and other workers seemed a great advantage to those responsible for the daily operation of the Hospital, those in charge of finance saw it as a mixed blessing. In May 1946, Mr. Daoust "reported that the financial operation of the hospital during the first three months of the year showed it had run at a deficit of nearly $60,000., mainly due to the employment of additional nursing and dietary personnel." The Hospital Committee was instructed to review Hospital operations, with the result that the Administrative Board approved an increase in Hospital room rates and other charges, and that Abbie Porter "was instructed to reduce the personnel in various departments of the hospital, particularly the nursing service," which now included 134 nurses. After the reduction, the number of Hospital nurses stood at 118, including 21 surgical nurses.[64]

While the move may have seemed necessary at the time, it proved shortsighted, as some physicians soon pointed out. By the end of the year, Dr. Walter J. Zeiter, the Foundation's Director of Administration, was reporting that with the recent resignation of seven general duty nurses, "the nursing situation is again becoming critical in the Hospital." "A great deal of surgery is being lost to the Clinic because of lack of Hospital beds," declared Dr. Ruedemann.[65]

With an eye not only to present needs, but to future expansion, Abbie Porter recommended that she be given permission to hire as many graduate nurses as could be obtained. To do this, the Board would have to raise nurses' salaries and, consequently, Hospital rates, both changes already under discussion by the Hospital Committee. Mr. Daoust noted that if Hospital nurses received a pay raise, Clinic nurses would have to be given one also.

In the end, the Board made several changes at the same time. The Hospital had been on a 48-hour work week. As of April 1, 1947, this was reduced to 44 hours "in conformity with the recent practice of other local hospitals."[66] The bonus system was to be eliminated (although, as it turned out, a "surprise" bonus was given at the end of 1947), a shift differential was now being paid, and nurses who preferred to work 48 hours would be paid for the additional time at their regular hourly rates. Nurses continued to receive three weeks of paid vacation, without paid holidays, rather than the two weeks of paid vacation with alternate days off for six holidays recommended by the OSNA.

"Our new rates conform to the latest maximum rates permitted by the schedule of the Cleveland Hospital Council, which we understand is being adhered to by all other hospitals in the Cleveland area. These new rates are higher than those recently recommended by the Ohio State Nurses Association," stated Miss Porter in a letter outlining the new policies to the nursing staff.[67] A beginning nurse on the 7 a.m. to 3 p.m. shift would receive $7.80 per day, or $185.90 per month on a 44-hour week, and $202.80 for 48 hours. After six months the daily pay was $7.90 and after one year, $8.10. A senior nurse received $8.30. Shift differentials were 30 cents a day for the evening shift, and 20 cents daily for the night shift.

Although these measures improved the lot of the individual nurse, they did nothing to solve the "extreme shortage" of graduate nurses. The number of Hospital nurses on roll actually declined to 94 (plus 8 part-time) by the end of 1947, and to 92 (plus 7 part-time and 11 temporary) at the end of 1948. For the first time, nursing administrators mentioned the unwillingness of nurses to rotate and work on weekends as a specific difficulty. Since higher salaries and shorter hours had proven inadequate to attract more nurses, a new benefit, the provision of "suitable living quarters for nurses at reasonable rentals," was added. This had been discussed by the Administrative Board as early as 1945, but not implemented until 1947 and 1948, when the Clinic Annex was remodeled to provide housing for nurses. Also in 1948, the Hospital began laundering nurses' uniforms, a perquisite Mrs. Hruby felt helped improve morale.[68]

Expanding Services...

As the Hospital continued its struggle to maintain an adequate nursing staff in the postwar years, The Cleveland Clinic Foundation as a whole surpassed its prewar levels of activity with expansions of its medical staff, physical plant, and patient services. The quota for fellows was raised from the wartime level of 32 to 80 in late 1945, and again to 90 and then 100 in 1947. Also, since fellows were now much easier to come by, the Board eliminated the extra allowance paid to fellows with dependents, which had been instituted for the sole purpose of attracting more young physicians during the war. In 1942 and 1943 the Administrative Board was already discussing the postwar expansion of the existing clinical departments, and the addition of new services like pediatrics, psychiatry, gynecology, thoracic surgery, and plastic surgery. All of these additions were made in the decade following the war, either as new departments or within existing ones.

Although scarcity of labor and materials and strict government controls on non-defense-related construction made even minor building projects impossible during the war, the Foundation had appointed a Building Plan Committee in 1943. It contracted with Ellerbe & Co. of St. Paul, Minnesota, the architectural and engineering firm that had also been hired at the time of the Clinic's initial construction, to draw up plans for major alterations and additions to the Cleveland Clinic buildings. In 1944, Dr. Robert Dinsmore as Chairman of the Building Plan Committee and Abbie Porter as Hospital Superintendent "in the main" approved the portion of the plans pertaining to Hospital additions.[69] The total bed capacity of the Hospital would increase to 427 through the addition of new wings and remodeling of existing space. A new surgical pavilion would double the number of operating rooms to 16, and include a postoperative recovery area.

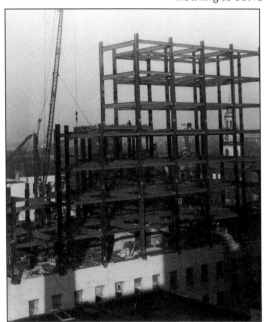

UNDER CONSTRUCTION
As soon as wartime restrictions were eased, the Clinic began much-needed construction projects. In 1945, the framework for seven additional stories went up atop the three floors of the main Clinic building.

Construction was begun soon after the war. When Miss Porter submitted the Hospital's twenty-fifth annual report in early 1949, she proudly pointed out that the Hospital now had 321 beds, compared to 154 in its first year of operation. This was 79 more than the 242 open just a few years back, during the war. However, some of the new beds could not be occupied immediately due to insufficient nursing staff. For example, the new Children's Ward, a separate pediatric unit with space for 25 to 27 patients, was ready for occupancy in December 1947, but did not actually open until November 1948. During 1949, the average daily occupancy in the Hospital was 285, which amounted to 87 percent of the 323 total beds available by the end of the year. The number of Hospital employees on duty on a daily basis averaged 354, out of a total of 430.

...Expanding Roles

As it had during the war, the Cleveland Clinic Hospital continued to look to other workers besides nurses to provide patient care. By 1947, the number of volunteers had dwindled to 13, so they were able to give relatively little assistance. (The use of volunteers was eventually discontinued entirely.) Returning corpsmen, servicemen who had performed patient care tasks in military hospitals, seemed to offer a new source of help. The Clinic Naval Unit had employed more corpsmen than nurses, and Dr. Barney Crile had thought highly of their work. In 1946 the Hospital advertised for corpsmen, and subsequently hired four, who were designated "attendants." Unfortunately, only one of the corpsmen stayed for more than a year. Although at that point he was said to be "doing very well," at the end of two years he also left, "for a better paying position in a factory."[70]

Floor hostesses and nurses' aides, two groups of workers who had become important during the war, remained so. In 1947 the floor hostesses were transferred from the office staff to the Nursing Department. There were generally 12 to 14 full-time hostesses employed at the Cleveland Clinic Hospital in the postwar years.

The upgrading of the aide position continued. The number of full-time aides had increased from 24 in 1945 to 42 in 1949. Due to the difficulty of finding nurses, especially for nights and weekends, the Nursing Department increasingly relied on aides to assist with patient care. Abbie Porter reported in 1948 that despite high turnover and the need for "constant supervision" of the group as a whole, some "excellent aides" had been trained during the past few years. In that year, the Hospital decided to begin an organized training program for aides. This did not initially work out as well as hoped, but another innovation, giving extended duties to the most able women and designating them "senior" aides, was more successful. The senior aides also gave on-the-job training to new aides.[71]

In 1951 the Nursing Department began another formal teaching program for aides, with June Lemmon as instructor. "This program has been of inestimable value to the Nursing Department. In fact, it is difficult to determine how we could have carried on without complete curtailment of service to some parts of the Hospital without it." In 1953, the hospital hired Martha George as the first full-time supervisor of aides. Aides now outnumbered nurses. Eighty-eight of them worked on the floors, and 6 in Central Supply. The registered nursing staff consisted of 44 general staff nurses and 12 head nurses, plus 7 nurses — a director, 2 assistants, and 4 supervisors — in the Nursing Office.[72]

Private duty nurses, who had contributed so significantly to the work of the Cleveland Clinic Hospital throughout the war, continued to be in great demand, as both staff relief and special duty nurses. District No. 4's Bureau of Nursing Service recorded hundreds of calls each month from the Cleveland Clinic Hospital for private duty nurses. For instance, in October 1946, the Bureau filled 266 calls for specials and 3 calls for temporary staff nurses at the Clinic Hospital, a third of the 807 calls that the Bureau filled in Cleveland hospitals and homes that month. Except for University Hospitals, with 122 calls, no other hospital had more than 100 calls filled. In December 1947, the Bureau recorded 370 calls filled, and 124 not filled, at the Clinic Hospital, out of a total of 1,030 filled and 631 unfilled calls.[73]

Private Duty Nursing in the Postwar Years

In 1946, District No. 4 appointed a special committee to study private duty nursing. Laura North, a World War I Lakeside Unit veteran and private duty nurse, chaired the committee. Its recommendations, which the District's Board of Trustees approved, included the following: that the "private duty nurse" should now be known as the "nurse in private practice"; and that the District should discourage the use of group nursing. "Group nursing was a war measure. It was the Private Duty nurse's contribution to the War Effort."[74]

At the same time, the District raised private duty fees again, from $8 a day (to which they had been raised in 1945) to $10 per eight-hour day. Although the $10 fee had been approved by majority vote at a meeting of the Private Duty Section, some private duty nurses had strong feelings against the increase. A petition, on Cleveland Clinic stationery, was submitted to the District Board requesting that the $10 fee be discussed further before being put into effect. The 38 signatures — probably all or mostly those of private duty nurses then on cases at the Cleveland Clinic Hospital — included those of former District Board member Elizabeth Bidwell, future Board member Mary Hennessy Cecconi, and Ella Chown, all private duty nurses who often worked at the Clinic Hospital.

The District's Board took the protest seriously, and the matter was studied and discussed at length. The main argument in support of the raise was that the nurse deserved a good salary in return for her skill, time, and service. Those arguing against the raise feared that if private duty nurses' fees were raised too much, no one would hire them. The private duty nurses' greatest concern was that "'practical nurses' [would] come in and replace the professional nurse" if fees were increased.[75]

In the end, the increase was approved, and the Registry reported receiving no criticism from the hospitals, and no decrease in requests for private duty nurses. What hospital nursing directors did criticize, at a meeting called by the District Board to discuss mutual concerns, was the attempt to discourage group nursing. There were too many unfilled calls for private duty nurses, especially in the evening and at night, and the only way to provide patients with special nurses was to group them.

The District had to agree with this, and so continued to set a fee for group nursing. It also continued to raise that fee until it stood at $8 per patient in an attempt to make group nursing uneconomical. The situation represented a significant dilemma for the Cleveland Clinic Hospital, as Mrs. Hruby noted early in 1948.

> The special nursing service is still inadequate, the demand exceeding the supply. It is a rare occasion when our order for nurses is filled. Since we order more special nurses than any other hospital in the city we are compelled to group or share nurses. This was an emergency war measure and has been discontinued by all hospitals except the Cleveland Clinic....

> ...Approximately 50 per cent of our private duty nurses, by grouping, receive $16 per day. If the nurses were not grouped the patient and family would question the care given the patient. By grouping, the staff nurse's work is decreased to a small degree but not sufficiently to balance the psychological effect of the private nurse's leisure, income and gratuities. This is one of our major problems.[76]

In view of this, the Cleveland Clinic Hospital decided to eliminate group nursing in 1948. Certainly, to a staff nurse, who was earning, on the average, $8 a day and participating in the care of a whole floor of patients, the private duty nurse's fee of $16 a day for the care of two patients must have seemed very high.

The Graduate Nurse in the Hospital

Several times, in 1935, 1943, and 1946, the District had attempted to organize a section for general staff nurses, hoping to develop "general staff mindedness."[77] The 1946 effort seems to have been at least temporarily successful. L. Elizabeth Thompson, a floor supervisor at the Cleveland Clinic Hospital, served as the General Staff Section representative to a District committee. A few years later, Miss Thompson was elected president of the District and then named a vice-president of the state organization. But the section itself stopped meeting due to lack of interest, and a new General Staff Section had to be created in 1953 to prepare for the reorganization of state and district associations mandated by the ANA. Miss Thompson, still on the District Board, made the motion to recreate the section. Since the Cleveland Clinic had led the way in staffing its Hospital with graduate nurses at a time when most major Cleveland hospitals relied on students, it was appropriate that a Cleveland Clinic Hospital nurse took a leading role in giving an official voice to the general staff nurse in the area's professional organization.

By this time area hospital administrators and nursing directors were following national trends and the Cleveland Clinic's local lead, in coming to see graduate nurse staffing as both desirable and necessary. For one thing, hospital nursing schools were not getting sufficient numbers of applicants. Several factors, including demographic and social changes, accounted for this.[78] Many of the young women interested in nursing as a possible career had already been trained in the Cadet Nurse Corps during the war.

Graduate nurse staffing also looked more attractive from a financial perspective. In 1947, Guy Clark, Executive Director of the Cleveland Hospital Council, stated that it cost from $400 to $800 per year, depending on the school, to educate a nurse. Schools were no longer necessarily a source of inexpensive labor; they could be a drain on hospital resources, and there was no guaranteed return on the investment, since nurses might leave the hospital, or even the profession, after their training.

THE FACE OF THE FUTURE
During the postwar years, the issue of licensure for practical nurses was debated in Ohio. While many registered nurses in leadership and management positions supported a greater role for practical nurses in patient care, other R.N.s opposed practical nurse licensure. Private duty nurses, who were numerous and influential in Cleveland nursing, helped lead the opposition, with only temporary success. In the future, practical nurses would play a greater role in nursing care, and private duty nurses a smaller one, even at the Cleveland Clinic Hospital where they had been so important in the past.

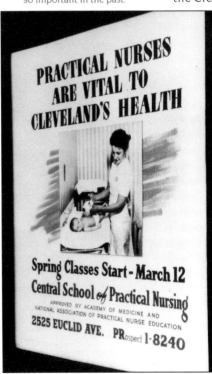

At the same time, private duty nurses maintained that their own field was a specialized branch of nursing, in the same way that public health was, and "not a field that just anyone can drop into." Some, like Elizabeth Bidwell, believed that "by encouraging and demanding special training and qualifications, private duty nursing would be placed on a par with other branches of nursing, where it rightfully belongs." Miss Bidwell recommended that nursing schools "place more emphasis on the training of the nurse for private duty nursing," and suggested that experienced private duty nurses could be engaged to give clinical demonstrations of bedside nursing technique to students.[79]

Private duty nurses interested in setting higher standards for their specialty also supported the suggestion that individuals who had not been active in bedside nursing for a long period of time would benefit by spending several months doing general duty in hospitals before returning to private practice. Offering refresher courses to active private duty nurses and requiring returning nurses to spend some time on general duty could partially alleviate the hospitals' staffing problems, while updating the skills of women in private practice.

However bright the future of hospital staff nursing, private duty nurses still had tremendous influence at the grass-roots level, at least in District No. 4. The substantial market provided by the Cleveland Clinic Hospital for private duty nursing services helped ensure that their numbers would remain high in the Cleveland area, and that their voices would be heard. Within the District organization, private duty nurses had felt "much neglected" in the early years, having had no section of their own until 1924, the same year in which the Cleveland Clinic Hospital opened. Ella Chown had signed her first petition to the District Board in 1926, on an occasion when the Private Duty Section had asked for more representation in District governance.[80]

By 1943, the private duty nurses were being called "the backbone of the District." A public health nurse refused to take over for the District's resigning president because she felt that a private duty nurse should have the position: "No matter where we start; with Public Health, Administration or any others, the private duty nurse is the selling card for the Hospitals and doctors."[81]

The Debate Over Practical Nurses

In some ways the Private Duty Section acted as a progressive force within the District organization. With only occasional dissent among its members, it had always pressed for higher pay and shorter hours for private duty nurses. It had also supported the implementation of standards of education and professional conduct for nurses in private practice. It spoke out against the attacks on nurses' patriotism during World War II.

In other ways the Private Duty Section was a deeply conservative force, fiercely protective of its members' interests. Perhaps the word "populist" would most accurately describe the motives and actions of a group whose members, like American farmers in the late nineteenth century, worked independently, were economically vulnerable during hard times, and sometimes felt "much neglected" by the larger society. During the Depression, the Private Duty Section asked the District Board to discourage out-of-state nurses from coming to the area to find work, and requested that the number of Bureau registrants be limited. But no issue so roused the opposition of private duty nurses, and the entire District, as the training, licensure, and employment of practical nurses.

In the years during and immediately after the Second World War, the Cleveland Clinic Hospital struggled with nurse shortages. In an attempt to cope with the situation, it employed floor hostesses, aides, corpsmen, and volunteers. In the late 1940s, a typical Clinic Hospital floor had a daytime staff of 10 to 12 R.N.s, 4 aides, a hostess, and an orderly, but no L.P.N.s. Licensed practical nurses did not exist in Ohio at this time. There were, and had long been, practical nurses, but as yet there was no licensure for them in the state, and without licensure and

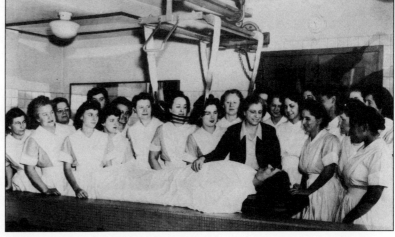

agreement on what the skills of the practical nurse should be, there was no guarantee of what skills a practical nurse would have.

Although the movement to increase the employment of practical nurses did not gain great momentum in the United States until after the Second World War, there had been some attempts to train variously named "subsidiary workers" in the Cleveland area, as elsewhere, before that time. From the beginning, District No. 4, with the Private Duty Section in the vanguard, fought with great tenacity against any formal training or recognition of such workers, especially practical nurses. Even an issue as seemingly trivial as whether to call a particular category of worker "ward helpers," "ward maids," or "nurses' aides" stirred up an argument: it would not do to associate the word "nurse" with anyone other than a registered nurse.[82]

Nurses feared that the general public would not be able to distinguish between a registered nurse and a licensed practical nurse, and that the "insufficient training" they believed would be given to practical nurses would have "tragic consequences" for which registered nurses would bear the blame. They felt that licensing of the practical nurse would "set back the position and rights of the registered nurse, secured in this state only after many years of hard work." The state's Nurse Practice Act, which provided for the registration of nurses in Ohio, had indeed been the result of a long, hard struggle, remembered vividly by older nurses.[83]

This issue of professional reputation affected all registered nurses. But private duty nurses felt uniquely vulnerable, believing that both their professional dignity and their livelihoods were at stake. Some nurse administrators, who were often nurse educators as well, tended to be more positive about practical nurses. Frustrated by their institutions' inability to hire enough staff nurses or enroll enough students, or even to get all of their calls for private duty nurses filled, they saw practical nurses as a solution to their staffing problems. But although the principals, deans, and directors of nursing in Cleveland-area schools

CENTRAL SCHOOL
STUDENTS
The state of Ohio did not license practical nurses until 1956. Before then, however, hospitals were hiring graduates of programs like the ones offered by the Central School of Practical Nursing and the Jane Addams School of Practical Nursing, both of Cleveland. These programs provided clinical instruction for students in affiliated hospitals. Some area hospitals, for instance, Marymount Hospital, set up their own programs. In 1951, the Cleveland Clinic Hospital created a job classification for practical nurses for the first time, although it did not hire anyone immediately.

and hospitals may have had higher status and higher profiles within the local nursing community, they had far fewer numbers than the private duty nurses.

Bills were introduced in the Ohio state legislature in 1949 and in subsequent sessions to amend the Nurse Practice Act and license practical nurses. Licensure for practical nurses had gained the support of the OSNA and some of its districts, at least at the level of the governing boards. However, District No. 4 sent representatives and even a lobbyist, private duty nurse Dorothy Casey, to work against the bills. They also decided to enlist physicians in opposition to the measure. In April 1949 they held a meeting in the Cleveland Clinic staff room, to which physicians from throughout the community were invited. L. Elizabeth Thompson, now a member of the District's Committee on Legislation, presided. However, only a few physicians, Cleveland Clinic staff members Dr. Barney Crile, Jr., Dr. James Kendrick, Dr. William Engel and Dr. A. Carlton Ernstene, attended the meeting.

The bills revising the Nurse Practice Act did not survive the legislative process in 1949, or in the years immediately following. Practical nurses were not licensed in Ohio until 1956. But even before that, hospitals began to turn to practical nurses as a useful and valuable addition to the health care team. In 1951 the Cleveland Clinic Hospital set up a classification for practical nurses; to ensure that applicants would be qualified, they were required to be graduates of a nationally accredited school of practical nursing. Although none were hired immediately, the administration hoped to "recruit twelve to fifteen of this group in the next year or two."[84]

From Special Nurse to Special Care Unit

In some ways, private duty nurses' instincts were not misleading them; a diminishing future lay before them. By 1951, only 20 percent of Ohio R.N.s were working in private duty, compared to the nearly 50 percent working in institutions.[85]

Statistically, the Second World War marked the beginning of the lessened importance of private duty nurses in Cleveland's health care system. In 1941, the District's Bureau of Nursing Service filled 25,087 requests for private duty nurses; it had 999 nurses on its register. Only in 1937 had the Bureau filled more calls (25,489), and between 1936 and 1941 the number of calls never went below 21,000. In 1942 the number dropped sharply, to 18,743, and by 1945 the 561 nurses on the Bureau registry filled only 6,492 calls. After the war the number of calls rose (12,692 in 1950), as did the number of Bureau registrants, but in both cases to little more than half the 1941 levels. By 1957, the Bureau was filling only about 9,000 calls a year, and had only 416 registrants on its rolls. A substantial portion of private duty nursing by registered nurses in the Cleveland area was still done at the Cleveland Clinic Hospital. Although complete hospital-by-hospital statistics do not exist, statistics for those months that are available during the decade 1941-1950 show that from 15 to 36 percent of the calls filled by the Bureau came from the Cleveland Clinic Hospital.[86]

The debate over practical nurses dominated District No. 4's business at intervals over the course of several years, at the same time as the number of calls for private duty nurses decreased. However, competition from practical nurses had relatively little to do with lowering the demand for private duty registered nurses. Several interacting factors contributed to the trend, among them the growing use of hospitalization insurance. At the Cleveland Clinic

Hospital, the proportion of insured patients went from 16 percent covered by all insurers in 1940, to 53 percent of admissions covered by Blue Cross alone in 1952. "The private pay patient is rapidly becoming extinct," reported the Hospital's superintendent.[87]

Patients had done without private duty nurses during the Depression because they could not afford the expense. During the war, patients did without special nurses or shared them because there were not enough nurses to go around. Necessity had taught people that it was possible to rely solely on the care given by the hospital staff. Hospitalization insurance, often paid for by employers, covered this care; it did not typically cover private duty nursing care, which therefore had to be paid out of the pocket of the individual patient. Not until 1958 did John Mannix, as Executive Vice-president of Blue Cross of Northeast Ohio, come to the District with the news that Blue Cross was "considering coverage for Private Duty Nursing Service and Visiting Nurse Home Call Service." He noted that Blue Cross had offered similar coverage since 1954 in Massachusetts, and 1955 in Delaware, and "stressed repeatedly" that coverage had not made a difference in the use of such nursing services.[88]

By this time, an innovation in the way patient care was organized — the development of special care units for postoperative and critically ill patients — was facilitating the transfer of work from private duty special nurses to hospital staff nurses.[89] Nationally, the post-anesthesia care unit, or postoperative recovery room, appeared in military hospitals during the Second World War and spread to civilian facilities during the postwar years. The intensive care unit was introduced slightly later.[90]

At the Cleveland Clinic Hospital, a recovery room and an intensive care unit were both proposed in the late 1940s, with specific reference to their use as alternatives to private duty special nursing. In mid-1948 the Hospital hired a nurse as Recovery Room supervisor, under the administrative direction of the Department of Anesthesiology. "Miss Feran [Mary Therese Feran, a 1946 graduate of St. Vincent Charity Hospital]...cares for the out-patients and for certain of the more serious postoperative patients especially those who have no special nurses. The out-patients are prepared for surgery...and supervised throughout the post-anesthetic period, before being allowed to leave the hospital."[91] The department wished to hire another nurse to work a later shift, to

> 1) Provide immediate postoperative care for the patients operated upon in the afternoon, especially the neurosurgical cases, in whom painstaking attention to blood pressure and respirations is often a life saving matter.

> 2) Lessen the burden of the floor nurses, one of whom must leave her regular duties to attend these patients until consciousness returns.[92]

By 1953 the Recovery Room was staffed from 8 a.m. to 8:30 p.m. by three nurses and a part-time orderly, who cared for 8,343 patients in that year (6,394 postoperative cases, 1,394 "in-and-out," 529 blocks, and 26 for injections of curare and other miscellaneous procedures). The department looked forward to hiring enough personnel to keep the room open continuously from 8 a.m. on Monday to 8 a.m. on Saturday.

Hospital administrators also hoped to open an intensive care unit, which they called a "Constant Care Unit." As of 1949, no such unit had been set up, but, said Mrs. Hruby,

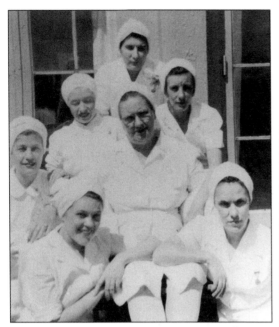

OPERATING ROOM
NURSES, 1940s

Until 1949, operating room nursing
was part of the Department of
Nursing at the Cleveland Clinic
Hospital. In that year, the
Operating Room became a
separate department with Elizabeth
Graber (center) as its acting head.
Before that, Mrs. Graber had served
in positions including general duty
nurse, head nurse, and Assistant
Supervisor of the Operating Room.

The opening of the constant care unit does not
appear to be as important at present. The demand for
private nursing service is not as great and there are
more private duty nurses available. Then again we
need four additional nurses for each constant care
unit, one for each shift and one for relief on days off.[93]

Nursing administrators recognized that opening an
intensive care unit would transfer to Hospital staff nurses
responsibility for patient care services now being provided
by private duty nurses. This transfer was already occurring
in the Recovery Room. The Recovery Room nurse cared
"especially" for postoperative patients who had no special
nurses, and by doing so "lessened the burden" of floor nurses, who had up to that point cared for such patients. The
fact that floor nurses had taken care of postoperative
patients in the absence of private duty nurses shows that
the Hospital Nursing Department was already providing
special care when necessary. Both nursing ethics and
common sense dictated that these patients could not be
neglected. Special care units simply formalized this, and
increased efficiency by concentrating patients, equipment, and nursing personnel with the requisite skills in a designated area of the Hospital. By having
its own employees provide special care, the Hospital helped to create more
demand for it, as more patients now had the option of doing without private
duty special nurses.

The Changing of the Guard

[I will be resigning] effective April 1st, 1949 ending twenty five years with
the Cleveland Clinic Hospital. It has been twenty five vitally interesting
years, each day a challenge.

To the Board of Trustees and to the Clinic Staff, I wish to express my appreciation of the confidence they have placed in me and the fine cooperation
always given. It has been a privilege to have worked in the organization.[94]

So wrote Abbie Porter at the end of her annual report for 1948. After
Charlotte Dunning's brief tenure, Miss Porter had been the Cleveland Clinic
Hospital's only other superintendent. She had worked with Dr. Crile at Lakeside Hospital; served in the First World War; participated in the Cleveland
Clinic's early years of success and prosperity; witnessed the disaster; and guided the Hospital through the difficult years of Depression and war. She had
done everything from consulting with Mrs. Crile on the selection of Hospital
china patterns and stationery, to running a hospital at 94 percent occupancy
with a nursing staff at half-strength. Having brought the Hospital safely
through the war, she could retire feeling she had done her duty.

Along with her tenure ended the Clinic Hospital's tradition of nurse
superintendency — a tradition that had already died out in most Cleveland
hospitals. Following Miss Porter's retirement, the Board of Trustees turned to
laymen as hospital administrators, conforming to a nationwide pattern in which
hospital administration had come to be viewed as a management specialty.[95]

She was immediately succeeded by Maynard Collier. In 1949, under his direction, a Methods Department was set up to study Hospital operations from a management engineering viewpoint. Also, Frances Reiter, a professor of nursing education at Teachers College, Columbia University, was brought in as a consultant to make the first recorded study of the Hospital's nursing service. Miss Reiter made recommendations on staffing levels, initiated a remodeling of the entire sixth floor as an experimental unit for nursing service, and urged "the necessity for reassignment of hospital functions whereby the departments of housekeeping, dietary, pharmacy, etc., operate as serving units to the professional services rendered the patient." With these and other improvements, the nurse would be able to devote more time to bedside care, and the head nurse, with the assistance of the clerk-hostess "to handle routine non-professional duties," would be better able to manage the work of the staff nurses and aides on her floor.[96]

Mr. Collier remained as administrator for only a year and was succeeded by Kenneth Shoos, who stayed for two years before leaving to take over the direction of St. Luke's Hospital. In December of 1952, James G. Harding began his tenure as the Cleveland Clinic Hospital's fifth administrative head.

By 1953 the Hospital had ten departments: Accounting and Admitting; Anesthesiology; Dietary; Housekeeping; Laundry; Maintenance; Methods; Nursing; Operating Room; and Pathology. Two departmental changes had had special significance for nurses.

First, the Operating Room, which had been part of the Nursing Department, became a separate department in 1949. The surgical supervisor's position was upgraded from a supervisor within the Nursing Department to a department head, reporting directly to the Hospital administrator. After Emma Barr's resignation, Susan Budd, a 1921 graduate of White Cross Hospital in Columbus, Ohio, had been hired as Operating Room Supervisor in 1947. She was succeeded by Assistant Supervisor Elizabeth Graber on an interim basis, similar to Josephine Hruby's acting directorship of the Nursing Department. A new permanent head for the Operating Room, Sophia Larsen, assumed her duties at the beginning of 1951. At the end of that year, the department included, in addition to Miss Larsen, 4 head nurses, 17 staff nurses, 8 aides, 3 orderlies, a porter, and a secretary.

Second, what had been the Department of Anesthesia, under Lou Adams, had in 1946 become the Department of Anesthesiology under the direction of Dr. Donald Hale, employing both nurse anesthetists and physician anesthesiologists. Miss Adams had stayed on as Chief Nurse Anesthetist, but she now reported to Dr. Hale rather than to the Hospital superintendent. She had been expecting the change. Back in 1944, she had written,

STAYING ON
In 1946, the Clinic's Department of Anesthesia became the Department of Anesthesiology, with a mixed nurse-physician staff under the direction of Dr. Donald Hale. Lou Adams (shown here in a photograph dating from the late 1940s) supported the change. She stayed on as Chief Anesthetist until her retirement in 1952.

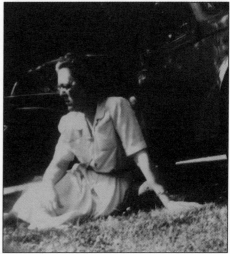

In many ways I feel that it has been a very trying year but we have tried to give the best service possible. In June of this year I will have been with the Clinic 21 years. I have had the feeling this year that you might desire Medical anesthetists. I offer this suggestion for your consideration. There are many changes I would like to make but with the present conditions they could not be carried out....

I can assure you of my continued interest and support as long as my health holds out.[97]

She was probably aware that the Administrative Board had been discussing the hiring of a "male anesthetist." Along with the other medical specialty departments being started, the Board hoped to create a physician-headed Department of Anesthesiology as soon as possible.[98] In the summer of 1945, with the interview process for physician anesthesiologists imminent, the Administrative Board directed Mr. Daoust to discuss the subject with Miss Adams. The war years had not been easy for her, with the increased work load and the difficulties of maintaining an adequate staff, along with the death of her beloved chief, Dr. Crile. Perhaps genuinely relieved to relinquish some responsibility, she accepted the change with grace.

> With the war over, I would appreciate it if you could select a medical anesthetist to take over the department. This has been under consideration for two or three years, and with the new building, the increase in work and the planning for the new surgery, I feel that the change would be beneficial for all concerned....I can assure you of my continued interest and support as of the past 22 years. It is a pleasure that we are able, now, to greet the old members of the surgical staff, back after three years' absence. It has been a year of many changes and I anticipate less complications with the coming year.[99]

When Dr. Hale's appointment was confirmed in early 1946, the Administrative Board approved Dr. Ruedemann's proposal that "the surgical staff give a dinner for Miss Lou Adams on her sixtieth birthday in recognition of her years of loyal service."[100]

The increased presence of physician anesthesiologists on hospital staffs was a national trend. Physicians who administered anesthesia were now fully qualified specialists, rather than the surgical interns of Dr. Crile's day. The Cleveland Clinic continued to employ nurse anesthetists as well, unlike many hospitals, which converted to physician-only anesthesia services. A few blocks away, at University Hospitals, the pioneering school for nurse anesthetists founded by Agatha Hodgins was closed, as nurses were phased out of the department there.

The End of an Era

Miss Adams retired on July 1, 1952, at age 66, with 28 years of service. Along with her retired Andrew Eanes, Maintenance Service Supervisor, also with 28 years of service; and Lillian Grundies and Financial Secretary Mary Slattery, each with 31 years of service at the Clinic, and more years before that at the Office of Drs. Bunts, Crile, and Lower. The Foundation had instituted a mandatory retirement age of 65, and so these long-time employees all retired together. As had the death of Dr. Crile, these retirements marked the end of an era.

Lillian Grundies had left her position as Chief Nurse on the surgery corridor of the Clinic long before this. When the Clinic's purchasing agent, Emily Perram, married and resigned her job in 1937, Miss Grundies — who at that time had been head of the Equipment Room for more than five years — was asked to take her place. She remained in charge of purchasing until she retired. The assignment proved to be another difficult one during World War II, since she had to work around shortages, rationing, and government

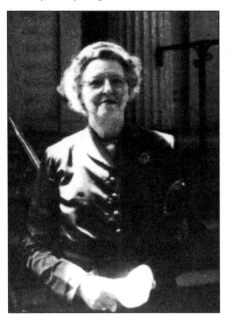

YEARS OF
LOYAL SERVICE
Between 1946 and 1952, four nurses with 112 years of service among them left key positions at the Cleveland Clinic: Hospital Superintendent Abbie Porter (shown here shortly before her retirement in 1949), Chief Anesthetist Lou Adams, Surgical Supervisor Emma Barr, and Purchasing Agent Lillian Grundies. Miss Grundies had been with the institution since its founding in 1921; the other three arrived with the Hospital's opening in 1924.

priorities to obtain the supplies and equipment needed at the Cleveland Clinic. Dr. William L. Proudfit later recalled Miss Grundies as he had known her during those years.

> She had been a nurse, but Doctors Crile and Lower thought that she should be the purchasing agent for the expanding Clinic, a position to which she did not aspire and for which she had absolutely no training. Miss Grundies had a razor-sharp mind, a retentive memory, and a good sense of values, so she met the need quickly. She had no pretense about her, but no one could fail to be impressed on first meeting her. Most often she would be at her desk using two telephones, one tucked between her head and her right shoulder, the other held in her left hand, and she was making notes....Miss Grundies was courteous, but it required no great insight to realize that she was a busy woman. Despite the pressures on her, she was always anxious to do a favor for someone who could not help her in any way, such as one of the young physicians-in-training. She never seemed aware that she was doing a favor.[101]

She had just turned 65 in the year she retired; she died in October 1969, at age 82. She had no full obituary, only brief death notices, in the *Cleveland Press* and the *Plain Dealer*. The November issue of the Cleveland Clinic's *Newsletter* carried a paragraph in memoriam. The only special honor Lillian Grundies claimed was burial in Arlington National Cemetery, a privilege she had earned some 50 years before by her service with the Lakeside Unit.

Lillian Grundies, Lou Adams, Abbie Porter, Emma Barr — the "first generation" of Cleveland Clinic nurses — all left the Clinic between 1946 and 1952. If the Second World War was a watershed for nursing, it was a watershed for The Cleveland Clinic Foundation as well. The founding years were over. Dr. Crile had died during the war; Dr. Lower had retired from any active role in Clinic business in the early 1940s, and died in 1948. After a quarter century of leadership by nurse superintendents, the Clinic Hospital had turned to management specialists for administrative direction.

The administration of the Nursing Department itself was also in a transitional period. Sara Jones had left in 1945. Since then, Josephine Hruby had been serving as acting Director of Nursing. As it turned out, Mrs. Hruby's "caretaker" directorship lasted six years, far exceeding the tenure of her successor, Marie V. Dowler, who arrived in late 1951 and remained for only a year. In January of 1953 Mabel F. Selfe assumed the post of Director of Nursing.

Coming of Age — the Cleveland Clinic at Mid-century

The immediate postwar period was therefore an unsettled one as measured by turnover in leadership. Susan Budd and Elizabeth Graber as operating room supervisors, Josephine Hruby and Marie Dowler as nursing directors, and Maynard Collier and Kenneth Shoos as hospital administrators — all had brief tenures, or were appointed on a temporary basis. The beginning of 1953 ushered in an era of stability corresponding to (and in fact extending beyond) the era of "peace and prosperity" experienced by the nation under President Dwight D. Eisenhower. Sophia Larsen, Mabel Selfe, and James Harding — all came to the Cleveland Clinic within the space of two years and would remain in their respective positions for at least a decade each.

In the years following the war, young Americans completed their educations, married, moved to the suburbs, started their families, and settled into their jobs, or, in the case of many women, settled back out of their jobs and into the home. During the same period, the Cleveland Clinic, with the passing of its founders, settled into its institutional maturity and the normalcy of postwar life.

Soon after his appointment, Administrator James Harding stated his vision for the Hospital: "The year 1953 should find us all working together with the attitude that nothing we are doing is beyond investigation. Our goal should be to provide the best possible care with the least possible cost. If we do this, we have fulfilled our purpose for existence."[102]

By 1953, many changes in the day-to-day routine and environment had taken place at the Cleveland Clinic and its Hospital. In 1948 a children's ward had opened, under the charge of Fairview Park Hospital graduate Georgine Steigerwald. At this time, about 70 percent of the Hospital's nurses were married, compared to none in 1925. The "Pillow-Tone Radio System," installed in all patient rooms in 1949, gave patients their own radios for the first time. And the Hospital was considering buying its first television set, for the lobby. Cubicle curtains had been placed in all rooms and wards. "Ice cuberators" had been installed on every floor, so that a porter no longer had to distribute ice from the central ice-making plant. In 1950 a nurses' station, on 6 East, was air-conditioned for the first time. (The only other air-conditioning in the Hospital was in the operating suite.) In 1951 the Hospital went on a 40-hour work week, "a revolutionary step for the hospital field in this community," according to the administrator.[103]

In the outpatient Clinic, Mary Walding, who had succeeded Dorothea Bordendorfer in 1948, was now serving as Nursing Supervisor, responsible for administering Clinic Nursing. By 1953, the basic outlines of the modern nursing care structure were taking shape in the Cleveland Clinic Hospital. In the Hospital, before the Second World War, a single Department of Nursing had existed, including the personnel of both the nursing floors and the Operating Room. All nursing care outside of the Operating Room had been given by general duty nurses, assisted by a handful of ward maids and orderlies, and supplemented by a large contingent of private duty nurses. The only important separation in function within Hospital Nursing was between general duty and Operating Room work.

By the time Mabel Selfe arrived in 1953, the Operating Room function had been split off, so that nurses now served in two departments (three, including the nurse anesthetists in the Department of Anesthesiology). Nurses were now beginning to staff special care units; a Recovery Room had been set up and a Constant Care Unit was proposed. On the general nursing floors, things had also changed. An expanded staff of nursing employees in several job classifications — aides, senior aides, orderlies, and hostess-clerks, with practical nurses soon to come — assisted, and in fact outnumbered, registered nurses. They all now served together, doing the work that, not so many years ago, registered nurses had done almost alone.

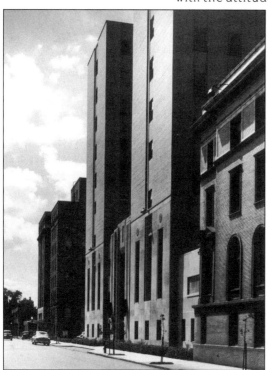

THE CLEVELAND CLINIC, 1949
By the middle of the twentieth century, the basic outlines of the modern nursing structure were taking shape in the Cleveland Clinic and its Hospital, just as the skyline of the Cleveland Clinic campus was taking on a new appearance. In this photograph by A. R. Thiel, looking south on East 93rd Street toward Carnegie, the twin towers added to the 1931 Clinic building (center) in 1945 dwarf the original 1921 Clinic building (foreground). The old Research and Hospital buildings are seen just beyond the remodeled Clinic.

4

Managing to Change

Bigness must never be a substitute for quality of care!
This is the never-ending struggle our hospital faces as we expand to
keep step with medical progress. The patient must be "number one"
always or voluntary hospitals will lose their reason for existence.
— James Harding,
  Administrator, Cleveland Clinic Hospital,
  1957 Annual Report

Peaceful Change

Following the eventful years of World War II and its immediate aftermath, the 1950s and 1960s were a time of relative peace and stability in the history of Cleveland Clinic nursing. Under a new Hospital administration, the fundamental changes of the previous decade — the hiring of auxiliary nursing personnel to work with registered nurses, and the development of special nursing units in addition to general medical-surgical floors — were consolidated and gradually extended. Other nursing programs, notably education and recruitment, that had existed before the 1950s on an informal or limited basis now expanded in scope and importance.

During the 1950s, the projected hiring of practical nurses became a reality. Other Nursing Department personnel categories that had developed during the war became firmly established, although with some changes in name by the 1960s. "Aides" became "nursing assistants"; "hostesses" were first designated "ward clerks" and then "unit secretaries." All Nursing Department personnel were expected to meet increasingly higher standards of performance in technical or managerial skills. In-service education helped them meet those standards.

The Hospital's patient care areas, traditionally referred to as "floors" or "wards," became known as "nursing divisions" or "nursing units." The new names made clear what had been true all along: that a hospital was a place where seriously ill patients received *nursing* care. By now, bed shortages and oversight by third-party payors were discouraging the use of inpatient facilities for all but the sickest people. "In-and-out" (ambulatory) surgery eliminated overnight stays for more and more patients. Only those patients who really needed nursing care were admitted to hospitals or stayed there following surgery.

The Cleveland Clinic Hospital's germinal special care areas — the Recovery Room and the Constant Care Room — grew in size, with the latter subdividing into several distinct nursing units. By the end of the 1960s, Surgical Intensive Care, Medical Intensive Care, and Cardiovascular Intensive Care Units existed to accommodate patients needing intensive monitoring and care. Within a

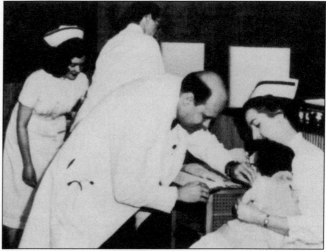

OPERATION LOLLIPOP
Poliomyelitis made headlines in the 1950s — first because of its high incidence, and then because of the new vaccine developed to prevent it. In 1957, the Cleveland Clinic offered free polio inoculations to children on Saturday mornings — with lollipops afterwards. Clinic physicians and nurses volunteered their time to the program.

few more years, a Coronary Care Unit and a Neurology/Neurosurgical Intensive Care Unit were added.

As the delivery of health care, following scientific advances, grew in complexity, so did the tasks performed by Cleveland Clinic nursing personnel. Olive Cannon, R.N., began her career at the Clinic in 1929, holding the "Crile lamp" while the famous surgeon operated in patient rooms. In the 1950s she was head nurse of a unit, responsible for training and leading a whole cadre of workers, from young beginning nurses to experienced nursing assistants. Antibiotics, unheard of at the time Miss Cannon started nursing, were now an everyday part of treating patients.

Older private duty nurses remembered caring for typhoid patients by bathing them every three to four hours, in beds that could not be raised or lowered. They remembered when postoperative cases had "hardly moved a muscle"; nurses, with little or no auxiliary staff assistance, had had to do everything for these patients. Ella Chown, R.N., still doing private duty at the Cleveland Clinic Hospital and University Hospitals in 1956, commented on the changes in her work: "The new drugs perform wonders but also keep nurses on their toes, watching reactions." [1]

General medical-surgical units like the one headed by Olive Cannon were still the norm at the Cleveland Clinic Hospital in the 1950s, but "specialized," "departmentalized, or "closed" units were being proposed as the ideal. The overwhelming demand for beds to accommodate the patients of Clinic physicians delayed their development for a time. However, the specialization of nursing units, and with it, the specialization of nurses, was inevitable. By the end of the 1960s, it was becoming the rule rather than the exception for patients of particular medical specialties to be concentrated on corresponding specialized nursing units.

Nurses in the ambulatory Clinic, on the other hand, had worked within specialized medical departments from the very beginning. The addition of new departments in the postwar period had increased opportunities for specialization there even before the 1950s. However, float nurses, oriented to work in a variety of Clinic departments, also played a key role in the ambulatory area.

A Continuing Shortage

The core personnel categories of the Hospital Nursing Department — registered and practical nurses, assistants, and secretaries — remained the same after the early 1950s. They would be joined on the nursing units by more and more ancillary health workers, including clinical corpsmen, administrative service coordinators, physical therapists, occupational therapists, and inhalation therapists. Often, the reason given for adding such workers was to "ease the burden of the nurse" or "get nurses back to nursing." Essentially, the Clinic Hospital administration was aiming to conserve that scarce and valuable resource: nurses.[2]

The end of the Second World War did not bring an end to the nationwide hospital nursing shortage, even though a number of nurses did return to the hospitals where they had worked before the war. For instance, Lillian Mullaly, R.N., had left her job as assistant night supervisor at the Clinic Hospital to join the Army Nurse Corps during the war. In 1946, she returned as evening supervisor, a position she held until retiring in 1967.

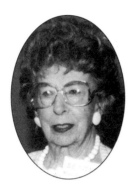

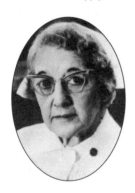

LONG-TIME NURSES
Olive Cannon (above) and Ethel Reichwein (below) were among the Cleveland Clinic nurses still active in the 1950s who had witnessed Dr. Crile performing thyroid operations in patient rooms. Each had, as a young staff nurse, stood on a chair and held the "Crile lamp" throughout the surgery. Miss Cannon later became a head nurse; Miss Reichwein went on to work in Central Supply.

Some nurses remained in the armed services, having found military nursing less restrictive, and sometimes more remunerative, than their prewar work in civilian hospitals. Others, taking advantage of the educational financing offered under the G. I. Bill, went back to school. Mary Gruber, R.N., one of the two Cleveland Clinic nurses who had joined the Fourth General Hospital unit, enrolled at Ohio State University after the war. A large number of returning nurses chose homemaking and motherhood over hospital careers.

The nursing shortage, after the acute crisis years of World War II, and the disappointing postwar recovery, showed all signs of becoming a chronic condition before the 1950s were well under way. "The words 'shortage of nurses' are now in the category of 'death and taxes' as inevitable, but we intend to ignore it and work toward the best utilization of those people who are available," declared Cleveland Clinic Hospital Administrator James Harding in 1956.[3]

During the next 20 years, American medical institutions, including the Cleveland Clinic, would intensify their recruitment efforts among young women. They would also seek to employ nurses from overseas, either through exchange programs or on a permanent basis. And finally, they would find it necessary to look to groups of people previously underutilized, ignored, or even disdained as potential nurses: men; married women and mothers; and African-Americans and other minorities.

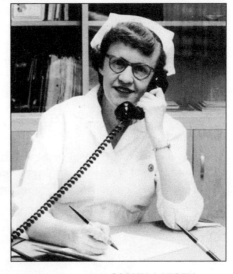

SOPHIA LARSEN
Miss Larsen came to the Cleveland Clinic as Operating Room Supervisor in 1951. During her tenure, which lasted until 1962, the new 21-room operating suite opened, a program for training surgical technicians was started, and Operating Room nursing was organized into specialized services. Nurses came to consider specialized practice as a hallmark of operating room nursing at the Cleveland Clinic.

The Cleveland Clinic Hospital in 1953

In 1953, the Cleveland Clinic Hospital was inspected for the first time by the Joint Commission for the Accreditation of Hospitals and granted "Full Approval" status. The new team responsible for the Hospital's administration and patient care activities — Mr. Harding, Operating Room Supervisor Sophia Larsen, R.N., and Director of Nursing Mabel Selfe, R.N., B.S.N. — could now look to the future, confident that the organization they were guiding met current standards.

At the time, the Hospital had 357 beds and was experiencing a relative lull in the cycle of construction and expansion that became a Cleveland Clinic fact of life in the second half of the twentieth century. At the end of 1953, the Nursing Department had 30 part-time and 183 full-time employees: 7 administrators and supervisors, 12 head nurses, 44 general staff nurses, 94 aides, 14 hostesses, 3 messengers, and 9 orderlies. Although a classification for practical nurses had been set up, the Hospital still had none on roll. The Operating Room employed 23 nurses, 3 technicians, 7 aides, 5 orderlies, a porter, and a secretary/hostess. Clinic surgeons performed 10,539 inpatient operations in 1953, assisted by 3 staff anesthesiologists, 3 fellows, and 9 nurse anesthetists. The Recovery Room, under the medical direction of Anesthesiology, and staffed from 8 a.m. to 8:30 p.m. by 3 nurses and a part-time orderly, cared for 8,343 patients during the year.

Operating Room Nursing

Under Sophia Larsen, the Operating Room Department was organized so that five head nurses reported to her. Head nurse I covered general surgery; head nurse II assisted Miss Larsen and had three assistant head nurses reporting to her, who covered general surgery and the gynecology, chest, urology, and dental services. Head nurse III covered orthopaedic surgery and also had responsibility for "expendable supplies" and call rotation. Head nurse IV covered neurosurgery and supervised in the evenings. Head nurse V covered otolaryngology and ophthalmology. Staff nurses reported to their respective head nurses or assistant head nurses. Aides, who reported directly to Miss Larsen, were assigned to the linen room, sterilizing room, instrument room, glove and suture room, and supply room, where they handled "routine work and preparations for each days physical operative needs."[4]

Each service had a separate inventory of instruments and supplies for which the nurses on the service were responsible. By modern standards, the major equipment needs of the early 1950s were modest. In 1952, for example, the Operating Room Department's major purchases consisted of: five laparotomy instrument sets; two portable "Castle" operating room lights; a "Shampaigne" operating room table; and two small model O-4 Bovie coagulation units. Even the Bovies would have been considered high technology items at some hospitals. Standard practice in many operating rooms at this time was for bleeding to be clipped with a hemostat and then tied with catgut, rather than "bovied."

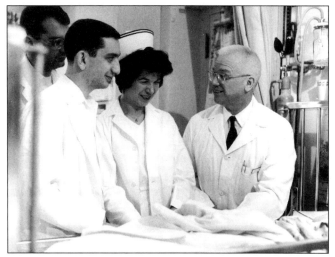

AT THE BEDSIDE
Clinic staff physicians and fellows depended on nurses' round-the-clock presence to monitor changes in patients' conditions. As post-anesthesia and intensive care units developed in the 1950s and 1960s, this might mean one nurse for every two patients. Here, a nurse accompanies Dr. Stanley O. Hoerr (right) and fellow doctors on their rounds.

The Operating Room was open for scheduled surgeries from 7 a.m. to 7 p.m. Monday through Friday (Saturday morning surgery was eliminated when the Hospital went to a 40-hour week in 1951). The nursing staff was "staggered" into three assignments: 7 a.m. to 3:30 p.m., 8 a.m. to 4:30 p.m., and 10:30 a.m. to 7 p.m. Operating room nurses were also subject to call for emergency surgery.

Operating room nurses worked closely with the Clinic's staff surgeons. Relations were still very formal at this time. Nurses did not address surgeons by their first names, but called them "Dr." The quiet atmosphere of any room where Dr. Stanley O. Hoerr (Chairman of the Division of Surgery from 1957 to 1971) presided as surgeon left a lasting impression on nurses who worked with him. They remembered him saying, "The operating room is a cathedral."[5]

But Sophia Larsen was very clear about where nurses' prime responsibility lay. When she asked a nurse, "Who do you work for?", the answer she wanted was not, "The surgeon," but, "The patient."[6]

The Manager in the Hospital

The Hospital's administrative structure was still quite simple in 1953. Ten departments, including Nursing and the Operating Room, reported to Hospital Administrator Harding. Mr. Harding, who had no assistants, reported to Foundation Executive Director (from 1948 to 1955) Clarence M. Taylor. Mr. Taylor, as a retired executive vice president of a major industrial concern, had brought a new perspective to the administration of the Foundation.

Although having only one administrator for a three-hundred-plus-bed hospital may appear incredibly "top-light," the creation of a Methods Department in 1949 signaled the growing importance of management techniques at the Cleveland Clinic and its Hospital.[7] In fact, the Clinic's Methods Department was the first management engineering department in a health care institution nationwide. In 1965, a new evening administrator position was added, and the duties of the incumbent also included work on methods projects. James Harding, as a professional administrator, instituted and encouraged the application of time studies, workspace layouts, and other industrial engineering concepts to hospital activities; he also brought in outside consultants to study broader organizational issues.

As the Hospital's pivotal, and largest, department, Nursing came in for its share of analysis. The 1951 study by nurse-consultant Frances Reiter, R.N., had been the first formal analysis of the institution's nursing organization and procedures. Numerous studies and reports, performed by consultants and Hospital employees alike, followed over the years. In 1952 the Cleveland Hospital Council's methods program, in which the Cleveland Clinic Hospital participated, investigated the amount of "paperwork involved in operating a nursing division."[8]

In 1953 Earl Frederick, the Clinic Hospital's one-man Methods Department, studied activity on the nursing divisions. He concluded that "an increased amount of the graduate nurse's time could be devoted to providing bedside care to the patient if a reclassification of the duties performed by personnel associated at the nursing station was made."[9]

His more important recommendations included having the division hostess spend less time performing minor services for patients in their rooms and more time at the nursing station doing routine paperwork and answering calls, freeing nurses (head nurses in particular) from these latter tasks. He suggested making more use of aides to take routine temperature, pulse, and respirations (TPRs), and allowing aides to participate in shift reports. He recommended creating a more extensive messenger service to transport forms, requisitions, prescriptions, and specimens between the nursing divisions and other Hospital and Clinic areas to decrease the amount of time nursing personnel spent away from the divisions. He also recommended that red and black fountain pen sets be purchased to replace the old-fashioned dip pens and inkwells being used to chart TPR graphics.

Mabel Selfe and the Nursing Department put all of these ideas into practice. The total salaries of nursing personnel made up a significant portion of the Hospital's budget, and nurses were in short supply. Their time had to be used wisely.[10]

In addition to Hospital-wide studies of nursing, Clinic industrial engineers also analyzed more specific activities that involved nursing personnel. Central Supply was a favorite area for study. As a technical or production-type activity, it lent itself more easily to a type of analysis originated for use on the factory floor. On the whole, the Methods Department seems to have been wise enough to avoid making recommendations in the area of nursing practice. It generally refrained from advising nurses how to efficiently administer medications or change dressings, concentrating instead on areas more easily judged by laypersons, such as paperwork, supplies and equipment, and nursing station layout.

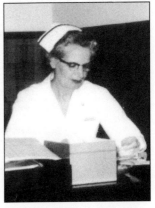

MABEL F. SELFE
In 1953, Miss Selfe, a 1935 graduate of the Battle Creek College School of Nursing, was appointed Director of Nursing at the Cleveland Clinic Hospital. She came to Cleveland from Mansfield General Hospital, where she had been Assistant Superintendent. During her 14 years as head of the Nursing Department, the Hospital opened its first intensive care units and also began converting general medical-surgical nursing units to departmentalized units. The Nursing Department hired a large number of practical nurses, and began implementing team nursing. Miss Selfe spent the year preceding her 1968 retirement on the Hospital's general administrative staff.

The Cleveland Clinic and Nurse Education

Education was one of the three components (along with patient care and research) of the Cleveland Clinic's stated mission. However, although the Clinic had an extensive program of physician education, its offerings in the area of nurse education had generally been very limited. A "postgraduate" course, a few weeks long, had been available to graduate nurses in the 1920s. Except during times of severe nursing shortages, primarily the Second World War, student nurses had not been hired. Cleveland Clinic nurses were expected to come to the job ready-prepared. This expectation, although never entirely eliminated, underwent considerable and lasting modification in the 1950s.

As early as 1946, Abbie Porter was looking forward to beginning a program of in-service education. "The first of January we will have on our staff a nurse qualified to teach. A program is being outlined and I trust with the aid of the staff we can start classes with an interesting and educational value." In 1949, Josephine Hruby, too, expected to institute a regular schedule of classes to be given by the Foundation's medical staff: "We are planning a series of lectures for nurses to be given monthly by our doctors. This will stimulate interest and aid in a better understanding and care of the patient."[11]

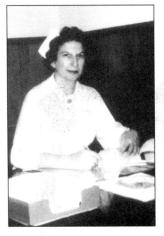

INEZ SALERNO
Also in 1953, Miss Salerno (above, at her desk, and below, at a nurses' station in 1960) was hired as Assistant Director of Nursing. Initially responsible for nurse education, her duties grew to include patient care, staffing, and recruitment as well.

Marie Dowler, R.N., during her brief tenure as the Hospital's Director of Nursing, pointed to effective education and adequate supervision as the department's two key needs, in view of the high turnover rate and the low ratio of nurses to aides at the Cleveland Clinic Hospital. According to her statistics, aides gave 1.3 hours of care per patient per day, whereas registered nurses gave only .7 hours. She believed that such a ratio could provide the patient with acceptable care if "a well organized educational and supervisory program were in effect....The professional nursing staff is not quantitatively or qualitatively prepared to direct and supervise this large ancillary group."[12] In addition, Miss Dowler believed that better orientation and teaching would help boost the nurse's confidence and satisfaction with her job, leading to a lower turnover rate and an increased number of nurses on staff.

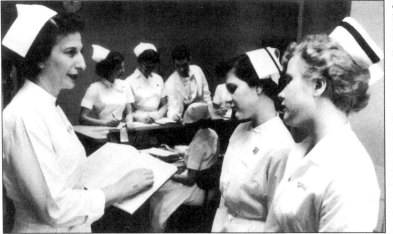

The nurses' aide training course started by June Lemmon in 1951, and praised by Miss Dowler in her annual report, was the one really well-established teaching program for Nursing Department personnel in the early 1950s. When Martha George, R.N., was hired as the full-time supervisor of aides in 1953, one of her chief responsibilities was teaching. In that year, seven groups of aides were trained and began work as junior aides; 33 of the 48 trainees were still on roll at the end of December. In 1954, 11 junior aides took additional class work and were promoted to senior aide status.

In 1953 Inez Salerno, R.N., was hired as Assistant Director of Nursing and directed to institute an orientation program and an in-service program "which was workable in fact and not just on paper."[13] New employees would receive a tour of the facilities, a review of Hospital policies, and orientation to their own units. In-service education for nurses past the orientation period would consist of two classes each month, alternating lectures by medical staff members with nursing workshops. Private duty nurses were also invited, as were aides when the content of the class was relevant to their work. Regular monthly meetings for supervisors, hostesses, and aides would round out the new educational program.

Also in 1953, the Hospital began offering tuition aid at Western Reserve University's Frances Payne Bolton School of Nursing for all nurses wishing to work toward a bachelor's or master's degree in nursing. The aim was twofold: to attract young nurses to the staff, and to prepare nurses for "larger responsibilities."[14]

The following year, the Cleveland Clinic expanded its nurse education program yet again, to a point just one step short of opening its own school. Through the Bunts Institute, the Foundation's educational division, the Department of Nursing began an affiliation with St. John College's School of Nursing.[15] St. John College was operated by the Roman Catholic diocese of Cleveland, and its nursing school, Cleveland's second college-level nurse education program, had begun offering a B.S. in nursing in 1947.[16] St. John was affiliated with a number of other area hospitals as well, and initially the affiliation with the Clinic covered pediatric nursing only. After the first year, medical-surgical nursing was added. Nursing students, accompanied by a St. John clinical instructor, came to the Clinic Hospital five half days a week to receive their clinical experience.

Nurse Recruitment

The Department of Nursing had two assistant director posts at this time. Josephine Hruby, who had remained on the nursing administrative staff after Mabel Selfe assumed the department's directorship, served as Assistant Director in charge of Central Supply, orderlies, and private duty nurses. Miss Salerno, originally hired as Assistant Director for Education, continued to be responsible for that area. Her duties were expanded to include oversight of patient care, staffing, and eventually nurse recruitment as well.

Until the 1950s, the Cleveland Clinic had no formal program of nurse recruitment. The Foundation's Personnel Department, which hired nurses for both Clinic and Hospital positions, handled recruitment on an informal basis. By 1959 the Hospital Nursing Department was directing its own intensified nurse recruitment effort. Operating room nurses were also recruited through the Nursing Department. Advertisements prepared by the public relations firm Edward Howard and Associates, including a full-page ad in the American Journal of Nursing, and "nursing representation" by Miss Salerno were cited as two key elements in the Hospital's growing nurse recruitment program.[17] However, of the seven unrealized goals listed by the Nursing Department in 1959, five involved recruiting, including the hospital's need for male R.N.s.

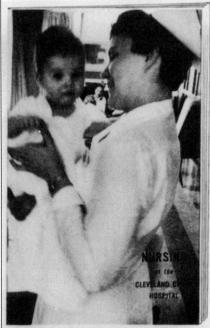

PAMPHLET TELLS ABOUT NURSING AT CLINIC HOSPITAL

The ink is scarcely dry on a new pamphlet describing, for prospective recruits, the life of a nurse at the Cleveland Clinic Hospital.

Illustrated with candid photographs of many of the facets of a nurse's job, the booklet is expected to be rather widely distributed.

Copies — for you or a friend — can be obtained from the personnel office.

A SUCCESSFUL APPEAL Under Miss Salerno's direction, an intensive recruitment effort, which included advertisements, brochures, and visits to nursing schools, doubled the Hospital's general duty staff between 1959 and 1961, from 87 to 170 R.N.s. The brochure shown here dates from 1957.

By 1960, recruitment efforts were having more success. The Hospital employed or rehired 102 registered nurses in that year, bringing the total number of general staff nurses in the Nursing Department to 127, a net increase of 40.

Some needs remained unfulfilled. For example, the Hospital was still running ads for a "Registered Man Nurse." On the other hand, it was able to expand the new Constant Care Unit, staffing it with its own nurses rather than private duty nurses, as had been the case initially. Hospital Administrator Harding was enthusiastic. "We are approaching the [recruitment] goal set several years ago, which at that time seemed out of reach."[18] By the end of 1961, with 170 full-time general staff nurses on roll, he could declare the goal reached. In two short years, the Nursing Department had doubled its R.N. staff — no mean feat at a time when most Cleveland hospitals were struggling to maintain adequate staff levels. Mr. Harding cited several reasons for the success in hiring more nurses: the advertising campaign, the good salaries offered, the tuition aid program, and the availability of subsidized housing in the Bolton Square Hotel.

Nurse Housing

There had always been a substantial population of nurses living in the many small apartment buildings in the neighborhood surrounding the Clinic. Some were Foundation employees. Lou Adams, for example, had lived in the Bolton Square Hotel long before it became an official nurses' residence for the Clinic. Many others were private duty nurses who did most of their work at the Clinic Hospital and at nearby University and Mt. Sinai Hospitals.

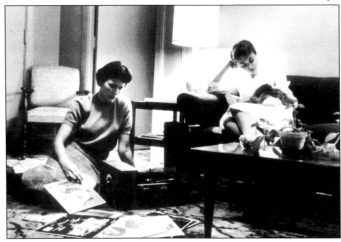

NURSES' HOUSING, 1960
The Cleveland Clinic remodeled an annex building to house nurses in the late 1940s. As of 1957, nurse housing was moved to the nearby Bolton Square Hotel. The hotel was not run like a student dormitory, with strict curfews and lights-out rules, as a recruitment brochure made sure to point out: "Every nurse has the same privacy she would in any large apartment building."

Not until the late 1940s did the Foundation take an active role in providing housing for registered nurses, when it remodeled an annex building for the purpose. In 1957, the Clinic began housing nurses in the Bolton Square Hotel as well. At the end of that year, 30 nurses were living in apartments in the hotel, with 25 nurses still in the nurses' residence in the annex. In the same year 80 house staff physicians were living on the Hospital's eighth and ninth floors. All nurses moved to the Bolton Square Hotel in 1959, so that the annex could be used exclusively for house staff living quarters. "The nurses seem to enjoy the apartment living at the Hotel, although placing compatible people in apartments is difficult," remarked Mr. Harding. (In later years the Hospital refrained from "forcing" roommates on nurses who did not want them, although this cut down on the number of nurses who could live in the hotel.)[19]

By the 1950s, the old belief that the "country girl" made the best nurse was disappearing. However, a fair number of American nurses still came from nonurban backgrounds, partly because nursing offered a way for young women who could not afford college tuition to continue their education beyond high school and prepare for a career. As the nursing shortage wore on, the Clinic had to look beyond Cleveland and its suburbs for new hires. In 1964 the Nursing Department recruited 110 nurses "from mainly outside greater Cleveland....We hope to make Cleveland more attractive to those we recruit by trying to institute recreational and entertainment programs for them. Also, the improvement of the neighborhood surrounding the Clinic will certainly help, since most of the girls are from small towns and are not accustomed to the problems of the cities."[20] For these out-of-town nurses, employer-provided housing was an especially useful benefit.

In Cleveland, the urban unrest of the 1960s culminated in the Hough riots of 1966, on the east side of the city where the Clinic was located. This increased uneasiness about the surrounding neighborhood's attractiveness. The nearness of the disturbances, and the stationing of National Guard troops around the Clinic campus, gave the impression of a fortress under siege. A nurse who was making a telephone call in the Bolton Square Hotel during the riots said that the person at the other end of the line claimed to hear gunshots in the background.

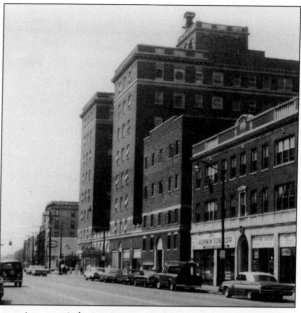

BOLTON SQUARE HOTEL
The Bolton Square Hotel (the tall building in the center of this 1963 photograph) was located on Carnegie Avenue, near the Clinic campus. In the 1960s, the Clinic also began leasing units in off-campus apartment buildings for rental to nurses at subsidized rates. By 1969 well over a third of Cleveland Clinic R.N.s were living in subsidized housing. Monthly rentals ranged from $40 to $80.

The Hospital administrators responsible for nurse housing, mainly Assistant Administrator James Zucker, had to increase their efforts. They began offering social and recreational activities for nurses, like cocktail parties and skiing lessons, under the "unofficial leadership" of young Mr. Zucker. A more substantial step was the leasing of apartments for nurse housing at off-campus locations, first at Horizon House, about a 30-minute drive east of the Clinic in Euclid, Ohio, next at Crystal Towers in nearby East Cleveland, and later at Emerick Manor, "of English Tudor architecture and located in a country setting" on the eastern edge of the suburb Warrensville Heights. Nurses continued to live in the Bolton Square Hotel, which was connected to the Hospital by a second floor-passageway, as well.[21]

At Horizon House in 1968 the subsidy paid by the Foundation averaged out to $43.14 per nurse per month. (This was including outlay for utilities and furniture; actual rent subsidies were $21.74 per nurse per month. In that year, the monthly starting salary for a nurse with no experience was $600.) By 1969 the program had become so popular that 118 of 300 Cleveland Clinic nurses, including operating room and ambulatory nurses, who were also eligible for the program, were living in Foundation-subsidized housing. Both Crystal Towers and Horizon House had waiting lists. At Crystal Towers, nurses paid monthly rentals of $65; at Horizon House, $55. Rents at Bolton Square varied from $40 to $80, depending on the type of apartment and how many nurses shared it.

The provision of housing for nurses has sometimes been regarded as a form of hospital control over nurses that extended into their private lives, a paternalistic tool to ensure that nurses conformed to house rules — for example, curfews and restrictions on visits from men — in their hours both on- and off-duty. This was perhaps true in the case of hospitals that had staffs made up mostly of young students, particularly during earlier time periods. The situation at the Cleveland Clinic in the 1950s and 1960s was very different. Administrators and nurses each viewed the value of nurse housing in a purely practical light. The former saw subsidized housing as an important tool for attracting and retaining registered nurses to their staff. Nurses saw it as a perquisite or employee benefit that, in the case of the Bolton Square Hotel, reduced commuting time to almost nothing.

"It was great," declared an operating room nurse who lived there in the early 1960s and worked one of the staggered shifts beginning at 10:30 in the morning. "Every night was like a Saturday night. You could go to bed late and sleep in every morning because you were just across the street." For the Foundation's graduate nursing staff, curfews and house rules were unnecessary, undesirable, and probably unenforceable. In recruitment literature, the Nursing Department emphasized that even Bolton Square was "not a dormitory set-up; every nurse has the same privacy she would in any large apartment building."[22]

Affiliation or A School of Our Own?

ST. JOHN COLLEGE
NURSING STUDENTS
The Cleveland Clinic never had a nursing school of its own. In 1954 the Clinic formed an affiliation with a nursing school, that of Cleveland's St. John College. Students first came for clinical instruction in pediatric nursing (upper photo), and then medical-surgical nursing as well. The distinctive checked blouse of their uniform made them easy to spot on the units or in the dining area (lower photo).

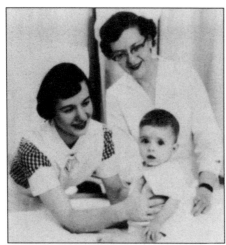

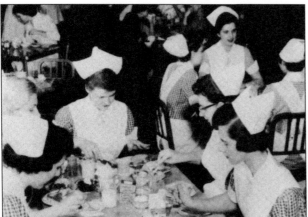

Tuition aid and the St. John College affiliation were regarded partly as recruitment and retention measures. In 1955, Mabel Selfe stated that the Clinic Hospital had hired the majority of the previous year's St. John nursing graduates. By 1958 there were 15 St. John graduates on the staff, including 3 in supervisory positions, out of the 100 nurses who had been through the affiliated program.

The affiliation "in effect gives us a nursing school," declared James Harding. However, he went on to say: "During the next two years, administration must study the possibility of expanding our clinical affiliation perhaps with our own sponsored school even though St. John College does provide us with capable students and graduates. This is a tremendous step and will only be recommended as the only alternative." Indeed, during 1957 an "intensive investigation" of the possibility of opening a school had already "convinced administration and the Hospital Committee that our role for the present at least should be offering clinical experience to existing schools. However, this is a problem which administration must constantly investigate."[23]

The amount of work contributed by the students was not a consideration at that time. Initially, the St. John students came to the Clinic Hospital for "observation only." The Hospital kept track of the number of hours worked by the students — for instance, 21,395 in 1960 — but these hours must have included a good deal of time spent in observation. Besides its recruitment value, administrators believed the program helped keep staff nurses "on their toes" while they were serving as mentors for students. Also, there was a general feeling that the enthusiasm of the young women "improve[d] the Nursing atmosphere" and was, in the words of a physician interviewed by the *Cleveland Clinic Newsletter*, "Good for everyone's morale." "That appraisal isn't frivolous," the *Newsletter* went on, in a vein typical of media writing about nurses at the time. "Everyone likes a pretty face. And the girls from St. John are nice-looking girls. Almost without exception, since they started to come here, the Clinic staff with whom they work has found these young women alert, and pleasant to work with....Their checker-bloused uniform has become a heart-warming sight throughout the institution."[24]

But whatever the intangible advantages of the affiliation with St. John College, recruitment outweighed them in the balance. By the early 1960s, Hospital administration was beginning to re-examine costs and benefits of the relationship. "One of the basic reasons for our affiliation, in our opinion, is recruitment after graduation," and in more recent years this had "not been fruitful," especially in view of "the conference rooms, etc." that had to be set aside for the use of the students."[25]

In 1963, the College had 173 nursing students enrolled in its freshman through senior classes, who came to the Clinic Hospital for their clinical experience. The Clinic employed only 9 students from the class of 1964, and, lamented Miss Selfe, "the prospect for recruits from the '65 class is not quite as bright, as Sister Edith reported that many in the class have already made commitments — some to matrimony."[26] Nonetheless, a 1965 study strongly recommended continuing the affiliation because of its potential, if not its actual, recruitment value. The Hospital followed this advice. It also continued to resist the idea of opening its own nursing school.

"Though hospital schools still provide 80 per cent of the nurses now employed, it is obvious that the future definitely will be for training to be conducted in a college with the hospital providing the clinical experience, as we are doing. This means we must set aside conference rooms on each floor for instructors, etc., but this is far less costly than building a nursing school that would become part of a college in the future."[27] Mabel Selfe may have been looking toward the future when she made this statement, but the resolve not to open a nursing school was also completely consistent with her department's past. Historically, the Cleveland Clinic had depended on graduate nurses to provide care for its patients, and it would continue to do so.

Practical Nurses:
"Increasingly Important to the Health Care Team"

The Cleveland Clinic Hospital did not provide clinical experience only to registered nurse students. As early as 1955, it was looking to affiliate with some local school of practical nursing as well. The Clinic Hospital Nursing Department created its first seven practical nurse positions in 1954. The women who filled these positions had first worked at the Hospital as aides, and through ability and hard work, had gained promotion from junior to senior aide, and then to practical nurse.

Unlike the graduates of formal programs, the Clinic-trained practical nurses had no school caps to wear. In 1958, Miss Selfe put getting caps for them on her "wish list" of things to do in the coming year. They did receive their caps in 1959, and also insignia to be worn on their sleeves, identifying them as practical nurses.

In 1954, the designation "L.P.N." (licensed practical nurse) still did not exist in Ohio. However, in the following year, proponents of licensure for practical

IN THE 1950s
During the 1950s, Muzak was piped into the operating rooms. In 1954, the inventory of the Anesthesiology Department included a single combination EKG/EEG machine. Mechanical syringe and glassware washers were installed in Central Supply and the laboratories and blood bank. Patient wrist identification bands were trialed in 1955. The Pharmacy began furnishing the units with emergency drug trays and new, disposable IV tubing. Nursing standards of care were established in 1956. The average length of stay in the Hospital was 9.9 days. The Nursing Department's capital equipment budget for 1957 was $6,530. In 1958, the first inhalation therapist was employed, as a member of the Nursing Department. In 1959, a system for prepackaging syringes was put into use in Central Supply. An institution-wide Infections Committee was formed. The year's annual report listed a nurse's publication for the first time: *"Bedside Self-Medication,"* by Marie Parnell, Supervisor of Obstetrics, which appeared in the October issue of the *American Journal of Nursing.*

nurses finally achieved their goal when a new Nurse Practice Act for the state was signed into law on July 11, 1955. The new law regulated licensure of both registered and practical nurses on a permissive basis, and also provided for annual renewal of nursing licenses in the state for the first time. Since licensure was permissive, hospitals might employ both L.P.N.s and unlicensed practical nurses, as the Clinic Hospital did in the 1950s. However, just as the Clinic and its Hospital had for years hired licensed registered nurses only, the practical nurse staff soon became made up mostly, and eventually entirely, of L.P.N.s. Not until 1967 did amendments to the Nurse Practice Act make licensure mandatory in Ohio for both groups. All R.N.s practicing in the state were to be licensed as of January 1, 1968. Practical nurses would have until April 1, 1971, to obtain their licenses.[28]

The Clinic Hospital-trained practical nurses were joined by graduates of Cleveland's Jane Addams and Central Schools of Practical Nursing in 1955. Through a concentrated recruitment and hiring effort on the part of the Clinic Hospital, the number of practical nurses on its roll grew substantially each year, to a total of 67 by the beginning of 1959. Graduates of hospital-based programs (for instance that of Marymount Hospital, a Catholic hospital located in a Cleveland suburb) were considered especially valuable additions to the staff.

Cleveland Clinic Hospital nursing regulations did not originally allow practical nurses to give medications or treatments — "as some hospitals have been forced to do," noted Mr. Harding. But they assumed some of the duties of both nurses and aides. For example, they took TPRs, a task which had been delegated to aides in the recent past. A number of the new practical nurses were assigned to the pediatric area. One of them later recalled Miss Selfe wanting to "flood" pediatrics with practical nurses, so that they would be able to hold and cuddle the children. The Hospital also needed practical nurses for its obstetrics unit, opened in 1956.[29]

During subsequent years, Clinic Hospital administrators found that practical nurses were "becoming increasingly important to the patient care team."[30] In 1965 the Clinic finally formed an affiliation with the practical nursing program at Jane Addams High School. By the terms of the agreement, 15 members of each Jane Addams class would come to the Clinic Hospital for their eight months of clinical experience. These students would be paid $12.40 a day while on duty.

The outpatient Clinic areas, too, were employing practical nurses in the 1950s. For instance, Elizabeth Minnick, L.P.N., a 1954 graduate of the Central School of Practical Nursing, was hired by Clinic Nursing in February of 1957. She worked in the General Surgery Department headed by Dr. Barney Crile, and took charge of that department's nursing service in 1958. As of 1962, she was permitted to give subcutaneous and intramuscular injections.

The Surgical Technical Aide Program

In the Operating Room Department, Sophia Larsen had also developed an important role for practical nurses. In 1957, a six-month postgraduate course in operating room technique for practical nurses was set up. The three members of the first class, all graduates of the Central School of Practical Nursing, entered the Clinic's Surgical Technical Aide Program in the spring of 1958. Two of the three graduated and were employed by the Cleveland Clinic Hospital "to assist the professional nurse on the first level of operating room nursing." Two more Central School graduates registered for the course in the fall, and applicants for the spring 1959 course came from the Central, Jane Addams, Lakewood Hospital, and Mercedian (in Scranton, Pennsylvania) Schools of Practical Nursing. Technical aides trained by the program were enabled "to scrub and circulate, dependent on their individual aptitudes." On the basis of a two-to-one ratio of registered to practical nurses, the Operating Room could now "maintain a much-improved nurse coverage."[31]

One perhaps unexpected consequence of the Surgical Technical Aide Program was the pressure the Hospital came under to create an educational program open to all qualified applicants. The Operating Room Department had instituted the program solely to fill its own need for skilled workers; it had not intended or wished to become a school per se. However, the program continued to receive inquiries from both individuals and other institutions. When the National Association of Practical Nurse Education (NAPNE) approved the program after an accreditation visit in December 1960, its letter stated that to maintain accreditation, the Hospital would have to accept outside applicants as well as its own employees.

As of 1964, there were three L.P.N. graduates of the technical aide course employed in the Clinic Hospital Operating Room. Despite the program's apparent success, it was terminated in 1968, the reason being given that there were not enough qualified applicants. However, the Operating Room Department immediately replaced it with a new training course "adapted for our own hospital, that expanded the field of qualified applicants."[32] This new course, although not accredited by NAPNE because it accepted not only practical nurses but other applicants as well, maintained the same educational standards as the previous program.

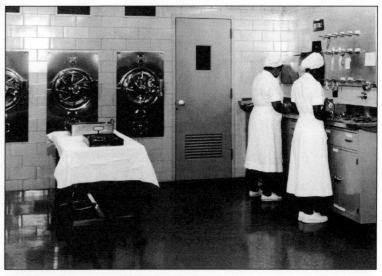

SURGICAL AIDES
In 1958 the Cleveland Clinic Hospital Operating Room Department began training practical nurses as surgical technical aides. Graduates of the six-month program were able to fill the scrub nurse role under the supervision of an R.N. circulating nurse, or even, in some cases, to circulate. Technical aides also cleaned and prepared instruments and equipment in the sterilizing room (as in the photo), and the setup and cleanup rooms.

Nurse or Technician?

An important consideration in implementing the technical aide course had to do with changes in nursing education. "Unless it reverses, the trend is to de-emphasize operating room training during the nursing school years. Therefore, perhaps the only answer is to train special technicians as we have been doing."[33]

In earlier years, at least certainly at the Cleveland Clinic — described by one nurse as "a pretty surgical place" — operating room nurses, as specialists, had been considered among the elite of their profession.[34] In hospitals staffed mainly by students, the operating room service was one of the few areas where graduate nurses might be employed. But in subsequent years, as the technological sophistication of the operating room grew, and as new models of care delivery like total patient care began to replace functional nursing in general staff areas, operating room nurses began to feel that they were being looked upon as "mere" technicians. Because they were responsible for patients over relatively brief periods of time, the operating room nurses' role might appear to be less significant and involve less judgment than that of the staff on the nursing units.

Operating room nurses were quick to respond that just the opposite point could be made. As Patricia Sommer, R.N., Assistant Supervisor of the Clinic Hospital's Operating Room, wrote in 1970:

> Many critics of operating-room nursing state that there is not enough patient contact. It is true that the period of time spent with the individual patient is short, but the patient needs support as he is about to undergo what may be the single most important experience of his life. At this time, the operating room nurse has a grave responsibility....By her own calmness and sureness, the nurse inspires the patient's confidence in all the operating room personnel.[35]

An assertive personality could be an asset for an operating room nurse, since she had to act as surrogate and advocate for patients when they were sedated or unconscious. She positioned the patient on the operating table; she made sure that the correct instruments were at hand; and, when necessary, she spoke up for the patient — for instance, she might need to insist that a surgeon change gowns between procedures.

This does not mean that relationships between surgeons and operating room nurses were adversarial. Indeed, working together in teams as they did, all day long, often under pressure, they naturally developed camaraderie. "You usually worked very closely with both your nursing colleagues and your physician colleagues." The surgeons depended on these nurses to manage the work of the operating rooms, in the same way that physicians depended on nurses to manage work in the Clinic departments, and on the Hospital nursing units: "Although the surgeon is in charge of the room where he performs surgery, he cannot be present eight or more hours a day to supervise and direct all that goes on. Because of her education, experience, and commitment, the professional nurse assumes the responsibility of supervision, decision making, and direct care."[36]

The Registered Nurse As Manager

By the late 1950s, registered nurses were working with numerous other employees to provide patient care in all areas of the Foundation: outpatient Clinic departments, Hospital nursing units, and operating rooms. And just as professional managers became an integral part of the Hospital's administration during these years, management responsibilities became integral to the role of the registered nurse.

Over the years, the image of what a nurse needed to be, and know, had acquired multiple facets. Physicians like Frank Bunts had considered womanly character and compassion to be the key attributes of the nurse; nurses like Isabel Hampton Robb had pointed out the importance of education in clinical subjects. The development of medical technologies had increased the need for technical skills; and now nurses were being asked to become leaders and managers as well.

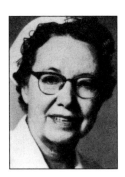

LILLIAN MULLALY

Miss Mullaly was the Nursing Department's evening supervisor for more than twenty years. In this position, she had responsibility for all nursing activities during the evening shift. The nursing supervisor also acted as the Hospital's evening administrator until 1965. A graduate of the St. Elizabeth Hospital School of Nursing in Youngstown, Ohio, Miss Mullaly did industrial and private duty nursing before joining the Cleveland Clinic Hospital nursing staff in 1937. She served with the U.S. Army Nurse Corps in the Second World War, and was appointed evening nursing supervisor upon her return to the Hospital in 1946. She retired from that position in 1967.

Although nurses had always had managerial responsibilities, these had fallen mostly to supervisors and head nurses, rather than to staff nurses. The student nurses who in the past had made up a large part of many hospital staffs had had very limited opportunity for independent decision-making. Private duty nurses, who worked independently, had managed their own work but had little if any responsibility for supervising others. Now, every staff nurse had to be able to train and guide the other personnel who worked with her, and also to liaise with the growing number of hospital departments involved directly or indirectly with patient care.

In point of fact, registered nurses at the Clinic Hospital were not at this time becoming an ever-smaller minority in the Nursing Department. The great change actually had taken place earlier, during the Second World War, when auxiliary workers had come to outnumber nurses on the floors of the Hospital. During the period between 1953 and 1970, the percentage of R.N.s in the Hospital Nursing Department tended to fluctuate rather than to show any steady trend. Overall, the percentage certainly did not decline, and it generally was higher in the 1960s than in the 1950s. For instance, in 1953, the Hospital's 56 registered nurses made up 32 percent of the Nursing Department's personnel, a figure typical of the 1950s. In each of the years 1960, 1961, 1966 and 1970, registered nurses comprised more than 40 percent of the department.

If supervising non-R.N. personnel was the criterion, Clinic Hospital nurses had needed management training at least as much during the Second World War as they did during the following decades, but in those frenetic years, no one had had time to stop and think about it. Also, people had assumed, or at least hoped, that the nursing shortage was a temporary effect of the war. Peace, it was believed, would bring nurses back to perform all duties related to patient care, as they had in the 1930s and before. It took a few years for everyone to realize that nursing care could no longer be provided exclusively by registered nurses, and that practical nurses, aides, and other kinds of health workers could serve as long-term, valuable additions to the health care team. With this realization, and with the relative calm of peacetime, came a considerable amount of attention to "leadership development" for registered nurses.

During her year as the Clinic Hospital's Director of Nursing, Marie Dowler had been the first to point out that in a situation in which non-R.N. personnel provided nearly twice as much patient care, measured in hours, as did R.N.s, registered nurses had to be prepared to supervise. A first step in this direction was the tuition aid program begun in 1953. Beyond the program's recruitment value, Hospital and nursing administrators also expected that the education nurses received through its means would prepare them for "larger responsibilities."[37] Mr. Harding voiced the hope that in-service training, which at this time was still relatively limited and focused mostly on clinical topics, could be expanded to further the same goal: "'Executive Development'."

NIGHT NURSES' DAY OUT
From 1937 on, when the Nursing Department went to a straight eight-hour working day for nurses, the inpatient nursing units were covered by three shifts. This photograph shows nurses from the Cleveland Clinic Hospital's third shift during the 1950s. Elizabeth Hartman (front, just to right of center, and also in the 1973 photograph below) brought her little daughter to this gathering; a night secretary (right) is holding her.

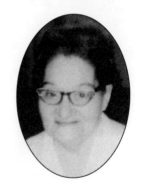

In the future our promotion policy should be based on promotion from within to qualified girls who constantly try to improve. The nurse who doesn't improve herself must, of necessity, find that she is slipping backwards and has no place of responsibility on a growing team.[38]

In other words, the Hospital had a responsibility to provide educational opportunities to the nurse. The nurse had a responsibility to take advantage of those opportunities and in turn would be rewarded with the chance to advance her position at the Hospital.

The Clinic Hospital at this point made a conscious decision to promote from within, and, in the coming years, put this policy into practice. In 1958, Miss Selfe reported: "We were able to promote from within our Assistant Head Nurse group to fill a Head Nurse vacancy, and from our staff group to fill Assistant Head Nurse positions. All of these nurses have or are taking advantage of our tuition-free courses at Frances Payne Bolton School of Nursing."[39] In the following year, six more staff nurses were promoted to assistant head nurse, and two assistant head nurses to head nurse status.

Miss Selfe also suggested that the tuition aid program could be supplemented by bringing an instructor to the Hospital to teach "Ward Management" to nurses who did not wish to attend university classes.[40] However, in-service instruction lagged behind tuition aid in providing management training for a number of years. This was perhaps due to the fact that Inez Salerno, who was in charge of in-service, had several additional responsibilities, including recruitment. She was giving this activity an increasing amount of time, as evidenced by the Hospital's stunning success in filling its "out-of-reach" staffing quota in 1961.

Growth and Change

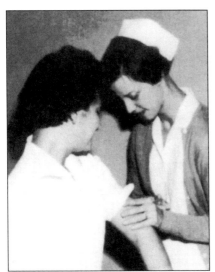

GIVING IMMUNIZATIONS
Nurses in the outpatient Clinic were often called upon to give injections, both immunizations and medications. Clinic nurse Marcia Luke (right) was part of the team that immunized Clinic and Hospital employees against Asian flu in 1957.

Before the completion of a new south wing in 1955 and 1956, the Cleveland Clinic Hospital had 357 beds. The Nursing Department had 225 full-time and 16 part-time employees, including 87 full-time registered nurses, 11 practical nurses, and 89 aides. Six years later, in 1961, it had 468 beds and 410 full-time employees, including 197 registered nurses, 80 practical nurses, and 87 aides. Including part-time and temporary positions, the total number of Nursing Department employees was 452, almost one per bed. In 1966, with another 100 beds added for a total of 554, the Hospital had 191 registered nurses, 94 practical nurses, and 94 aides on roll. In 1970, 578 full-time Nursing Department employees, including 267 registered nurses, 136 practical nurses, and 101 aides worked in a 610-bed Clinic Hospital.

But growth, and change, could not be measured by size alone. During this time, the Clinic opened — and then closed — a Department of Obstetrics. It completely remodeled its operating suite. Ohio's first heart transplant was performed in the Clinic's self-contained Cardiovascular Unit. In 1966 Medicare began providing health insurance for all Americans over age 65. The Cleveland Clinic hired its first social worker and appointed a chaplain. Within the Nursing Department, the first African-American nurses were hired. Team nursing began to replace functional nursing, and "closed" or "specialized" nursing units became the rule rather than the exception. Increasing complexity and increasing diversity characterized this period for the Cleveland Clinic, its Hospital, and its nurses.

Clinic Nursing

The nurses who worked in the outpatient areas of the Clinic remained, as they always had been, far less numerous than Hospital nurses. After a tenure of nearly a decade, Mary Walding, R.N., the Clinic's second Supervisor of Nursing, was succeeded by Jessie Nadine Schwartz, R.N., in 1957. A new era of managerial stability began with the promotion of Corinne Hofstetter, R.N., to the position in 1959. Miss Hofstetter was a graduate of the Mt. Sinai Hospital nursing school, and had worked for two years in the Clinic's Plastic Surgery Department.

At this time, Clinic and Hospital Nursing were still entirely separate. For instance, Clinic nurses were not invited to educational programs for Hospital nurses. It was possible for nurses to transfer from Clinic to Hospital Nursing, but not the other way around. If a Hospital nurse wished to work in the outpatient Clinic, she had to resign her position at the Clinic Hospital first. The Clinic Nursing supervisor had no official connection to the Hospital's Nursing administration. Over the years, she reported to various Clinic administrators

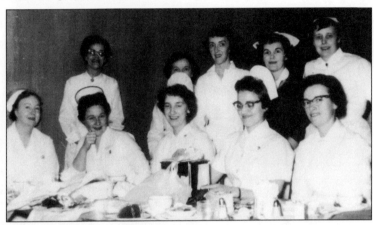

— to Dr. Zeiter, then to the director of personnel, and then to a Clinic administrator (who also had the Clinic receptionists and secretaries reporting to him).[41]

In the late 1950s, Clinic nursing personnel consisted of R.N.s, L.P.N.s, nursing assistants, and a few technicians. There was no formal role of "head nurse" at the time, since in most areas a single R.N. worked together with L.P.N.s and nursing assistants and naturally acted as the leader. For instance, an R.N., an L.P.N., and a nursing assistant constituted the entire nursing staff on the corridor where the eight physicians of the General Surgery, Colorectal Surgery, Plastic Surgery (all at Desk 60) and Gynecology (Desk 71) Departments had their offices. The R.N. was officially assigned to the Plastic Surgery Department, where the chief of service preferred to work with an R.N. The L.P.N. was assigned to General Surgery, because Dr. Barney Crile preferred being assisted by L.P.N.s. The nursing assistant worked wherever she was needed, cleaning exam rooms, sharpening needles, washing equipment, and assisting to prepare patients for examination. The R.N. also had to give medications for all of the physicians on the floor, since L.P.N.s were not permitted to do so at this time.

As the number of R.N.s working in the various departments of the Clinic grew, it became necessary to have someone designated as the accountable person in each area. That person was first called the charge nurse, and later, the head nurse. In 1960, 52 registered and practical nurses were employed in Clinic Nursing. They worked in 21 clinical areas and also in the Emergency Department.

> The head nurse in each area assigns the duties of her staff and is responsible for training her aides....Clinic nurses can...take considerable initiative because of their permanent assignment to a few doctors in a single area of clinic service. They know their doctors and they know their specialty; they are expected to know what tests and preliminary examinations are required and to make them.[42]

CLINIC NURSES
In 1961, Clinic nurses were still a small enough group that everyone knew everyone. About 50 registered and practical nurses, along with nursing assistants, cared for the 220,000 ambulatory patients who visited Clinic physicians each year. The Clinic nursing staff included: (left to right, front row) Betty Minnick, Corinne Hofstetter, Romona Muchow, Anne McCracken, Antoinette Norick, (back row) Kay Scruggs, Rose Moran, Ethel McLaughlin, Tedi King, and Jo Dawley.

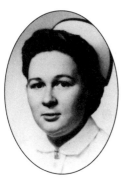

The relative autonomy of Clinic nursing practice ruled out the brand-new graduate as a staff member. Clinic nurses were required to have a minimum of one year of general duty experience.

The duties of Clinic nurses varied according to the departments to which they were assigned. For instance, a registered nurse in the Allergy Department gave injections and helped the technicians in the laboratory prepare extracts for skin testing. At Desk 91 — Neurosurgery, Pulmonary, and Thoracic Surgery — one R.N. and one L.P.N. assisted eight staff physicians. The R.N. prepared the patient and assisted the physicians in performing outpatient surgical procedures, did routine dressing changes, took vital signs and blood pressures, and made sure that surgical instruments were cleaned and set up for autoclaving. The duties of the head nurse on Desk 71, Gynecology, at one point included doing pelvic exams and pap smears for all female admissions to the Hospital. In all areas, nursing personnel were responsible for making sure that exam rooms were cleaned and set up for receiving the next patient.

In addition to the nurses working in specific Clinic departments, float nurses were assigned out of the supervisor's office to assist in whatever area they were needed. Since float nurses had to be familiar with all Clinic departments, they needed as much as a year's worth of training. Miss Hofstetter asked that each float nurse stay at her job for at least two years after being hired. She often relied on float nurses to assist in orienting new employees. When Miss Hofstetter herself had begun work at the Clinic, there had been no one to orient her — she was the only nurse in Plastic Surgery, her predecessor had already left, and Clinic Nursing had no overall orientation program. As Supervisor, she remembered how she had felt as a new employee, "with no one to show me anything," and decided to set up an orientation program for new nursing personnel.[43] Later on, she implemented an in-service program as well.

The supervisor of Clinic Nursing could select her own float nurses, but personnel for clinical departments had to be approved by their respective physician department heads. Miss Hofstetter did the initial interviewing, made sure nursing credentials were in order, inquired about any special skills or experience a nurse might have that would especially suit her for a particular department, and tried to find individuals whose personalities would suit the style of the physicians with whom they would be working. When a physician and a nurse had good rapport, the department worked smoothly. A nurse would "read her doctor," for instance making sure that no aggravations would occur in the office to unsettle him when he returned there after a difficult surgery; a physician would "go to bat" for his nurse if he felt she was being treated unfairly by anyone.[44] On busy days, some physicians might help clean exam rooms if there were patients waiting and no one else available to do the job; others would never do this. It depended on the department and on the individual physicians involved. The one-to-one relationship of nurse and physician was a key aspect of Clinic nursing practice.

In some ways, working in a Clinic outpatient department was similar to working in a private physician's office, except that, instead of just one doctor (as was generally the case in medical offices at the time), the nurse was responsible to several. Also, being part of a large institution meant that additional support services were available. Lab technicians drew blood for tests; Central Service provided sterile supplies; other supplies and medicines could be ordered from the storeroom and the Clinic Pharmacy rather than outside vendors. There were secretaries and receptionists assigned to each desk; and nurses who had worked in doctors' offices were especially delighted when being interviewed for Clinic positions to hear that they would not have to do insurance forms. The Clinic's insurance office handled that.

The most important difference was that the Clinic, because of its status as a tertiary referral center, had a different patient load from the average doctor's office. Clinic physicians performed advanced procedures and prescribed new medications. As one nursing assistant later said, "What was unique to the Cleveland Clinic was the variety of pathologies that were treated on a daily basis. During the four years I was there, I saw many things on such a regular basis that I did not realize how rare they really were, until much later."[45]

The Cardiac Catheterization Laboratory

The Cardiac Catheterization Laboratory was one especially significant area in which Clinic nurses worked. Dr. F. Mason Sones, Jr., the director of the laboratory, did the world's first coronary artery catheterizations. His pioneering work was one of the most important factors in developing an internationally known program in cardiology and cardiovascular surgery at the Cleveland Clinic. Vae Lucile Van Derwyst, R.N., was initially the only nurse assisting Dr. Sones (who for all his brilliance, was, according to accounts of others, not an easy man with whom to work). She worked in the department for 35

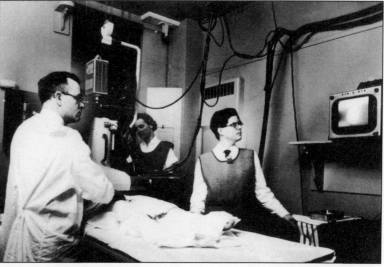

CARDIAC CATHETERIZATION This early photograph of the Cardiac Catheterization Laboratory shows Vae Lucile Van Derwyst (center) and Dr. F. Mason Sones, Jr. (left) at work during a catheterization procedure in 1958. As nurse in the Pediatric Cardiology Department headed by Dr. Sones, Miss Van Derwyst was present at the world's first coronary artery catheterization. She became the first nurse to work in the field of cardiac catheterization, and headed the new laboratory's nursing staff, which grew from one to more than forty members. The nurses she instructed spread knowledge of this new nursing field throughout the U.S. and the world.

years, first as a staff nurse and then as its Nursing Supervisor. By developing this new area of nursing practice, and training other nurses in the care of cardiac catheterization patients, she played a role similar to that of Agatha Hodgins in the early years of nurse anesthesia. Nurses came from all over the country to be instructed by Miss Van Derwyst, and were then able in turn to instruct other nurses, further expanding the field.

Miss Van Derwyst recounted the development of the cardiac catheterization program at the Cleveland Clinic:

> I began work at CCF in January 1952. It was a new department ... specializing in Pediatric Cardiology .... Our patients were infants and small children with cardiac problems. Most of these patients had surgery done by Donald Effler, M.D. Methods for Cardiac Catheterization and Cardiac Surgery were very crude in comparison to the sophisticated equipment and methods used today. There was no intensive care for these patients and because it was difficult to find nurses experienced in caring for these tiny, critically ill patients, Drs. Sones and Effler often 'specialled' them through the first night after surgery.[46]

Miss Van Derwyst was present when Dr. Sones did the first coronary arteri-ography. After that milestone, she remembered, adults became our primary patient load and our department grew from one laboratory to six, from one physician to over fifteen and from a nursing staff of one to over forty.

Our patients came from everywhere, Asia, South America, Europe and all fifty states in the USA. Our fellow doctors came from everywhere also.[47]

Eventually, having grown so much, the Cardiac Catheterization Lab became a separate nursing department under Miss Van Derwyst's supervision.

A New Look: The Operating Suite

SURGICAL PAVILION, 1955
The Cleveland Clinic opened a new surgical pavilion on the second floor of the Hospital in 1955. It included 21 operating rooms and one large setup room. Each room was equipped with: a table, two stools, two IV poles, four platforms, a ring stand, two

In 1955, at the suggestion of Operating Room Supervisor Sophia Larsen, an Operating Room Committee was set up, on which she and Mr. Harding served with several surgeons. It became a permanent subcommittee of the Surgical Committee in 1956. The Operating Room Committee was involved in making decisions in areas such as the purchase of equipment and supplies and the setting of operating room rates. In 1956 the rate for the most expensive class of operation — including laparotomies and thyroid and brain operations — increased twice, from $35 to $45 to $55.

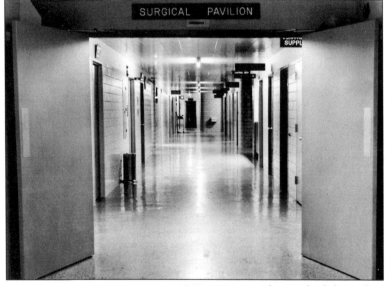

Also in 1955, the Hospital's operating suite moved from its old location on the seventh floor to a brand-new 21-room facility on the second floor of the new south wing of the Hospital. This was part of the general expansion of the Hospital and Clinic that had been planned for the postwar period by the Building Plan Committee, appointed in 1943 and headed by Dr. Robert Dinsmore. A long-time Clinic surgeon, and Chief of the Division of Surgery from 1949 to 1957, Dr. Dinsmore had been confident that there would be a need for such a large number of operating rooms.

The new suite remained in use with remarkably little alteration until the

sponge pails, a portable light and an overhead light, and a Bovie coagulation unit. The setup room received twelve instrument tables. In 1955 the Operating Room Department had 47 employees, of whom 36 were registered nurses. More than ten thousand operations were performed that year. At this time, approximately two-thirds of the Hospital's patients were surgical.

1980s. Nurses who worked there during the 1960s could precisely remember, decades later, which surgical specialties had used which rooms. Rooms 1 and 2 were genitourinary surgery, 3 through 5 cystoscopy, 6 and 7 neurosurgery, 8 and 9 plastic surgery, 10 and 11 orthopaedics, 12 and 13 ophthalmology and neurosurgery, 14 and 15 general surgery, 16 and 17 chest surgery, 18 and 19 otolaryngology (ENT), and 20 and 21, colorectal surgery. The suite featured one central scrub room, a single instrument cleanup room, and a single large setup room, which nurses also clearly remembered. "All those cases in this one setup room, it was unreal." "But it worked!" "Neuro was first and ortho was next and I never had enough room." "ENT was in the back and we'd crash into everybody coming out."[48]

To staff the new operating rooms, Operating Room Department nursing positions were eventually reorganized into 10 service areas, each headed by a head nurse or supervisor: general surgery and gynecology; general surgery and plastic surgery; general surgery and dental surgery; neurosurgery;

ophthalmology; chest and heart surgery; arteriovascular surgery; orthopaedics; otolaryngology; and urology. In 1955 the number of registered nurses on the Operating Room staff averaged 33, although this number dipped to 22 in the following year.

New nurses spent two weeks in orientation and were then assigned to whichever service needed them. They could transfer to another service when a vacancy opened. Later, nurses had a week of orientation on each service. Although operating room nurses worked as specialists, they were also assigned to cases on other services in order to gain experience. They had to cover for other specialties and were expected to be able to function in each. "There wasn't any call until 11 o'clock, so we had to finish up all the other services after our service got finished. You could work on four or five different services in one day," and sometimes end up going home at one or two in the morning.[49]

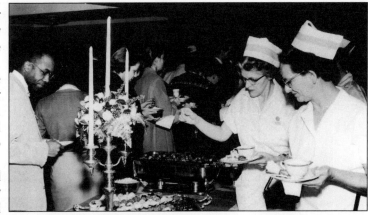

CHRISTMAS, 1957
Each year, Cleveland Clinic employees celebrated Christmas at a holiday party. The annual event included refreshments and music.

Operating room nurses who also had experience at other hospitals frequently characterized working at the Cleveland Clinic as "special." A nurse recalled that when she had scrubbed a particular procedure with a Clinic surgeon, it had lasted about 30 minutes. The same procedure took eight hours at a hospital where she later worked. On the neurosurgical service, craniotomies were done on an almost daily basis, whereas elsewhere, they might be done once a month. "I didn't even want to do neuro after doing it at the Clinic," said one nurse. "The work was more interesting and challenging, not just routine appendectomies," said another.[50]

Continuum of Care

The old part of the Hospital's second floor, which had been closed or used as office space during the war, was remodeled at about the same time as the new wing was being built. The Clinic Hospital's Recovery Room and Central Supply Room moved to the second floor in 1955, the same year the new operating suite opened.

The Recovery Room, after its relocation to Room 224, had 12 beds and cared for "In and Out," or ambulatory surgery patients, as well as inpatients. The Nursing Department had administrative responsibility for its staff, although the area was still under the clinical direction of Anesthesiology. The Hospital's intravenous service, started in 1958 "to alleviate work performed by Fellow doctors and to give more prompt service," was also jointly directed by the Nursing and Anesthesiology Departments and operated out of the Recovery Room.[51] By 1965 two nurses were administering all IVs between the hours of 8 a.m. and 8:30 p.m.

In early 1957 the Constant (Intensive) Care Unit, under discussion since the late 1940s, opened in Rooms 225 (for postoperative open-heart patients) and 226 (for general surgical constant care), so that patients could have "concentrated nursing care with expert medical care and special equipment immediately available."[52] The new unit was managed by the Recovery Room head nurse.

At the other end of the care spectrum, a Convalescent Unit for patients needing "minimal" nursing care also opened in 1957. Together with the regular Hospital nursing units, the new Constant Care and Convalescent Units made it possible for the Clinic Hospital to provide "three stages of care": intensive, acute, and subacute. Patients could move from one stage of nursing care to another, in accordance with the progressive patient care (PPC) model just coming into vogue in the hospital industry.[53]

Private Duty Nurses and Constant Care

The Constant Care Unit had originally been proposed in order to decrease the need for private duty nurses, who were both scarce and expensive for the patient ($45, and rising, for 24 hours of care). However, when the unit's two rooms first opened, they were staffed by private duty nurses "paid directly by the patient," since the Clinic Hospital did not have enough nurses of its own.[54] Mr. Harding and Miss Selfe had visited the offices of District No. 4 to ask for help, as the District's general secretary related.

> [They] came...asking the cooperation of District No. 4 in conducting a "pilot study" for the nursing care by private duty nurses in a "constant care" room they have equipped for six cardiac patients. These are the "open heart" and "mitro" [mitral] patients.
>
> They will need two to three private duty nurses around the clock. The plan is that the first day following surgery, the nurse has one patient only, the second day she is assigned the second patient, and will continue with these...assignments for a period of time and not over one week, when the nurse will be expected to contact the Bureau to register off duty from the "constant care" room, and if she so wishes to register in for another case.
>
> The private duty nurse, who has had the opportunity to work in this room is very much pleased with the complete set-up and close proximity to the patients. They state they are not as tired when going off duty. This sharing the patients does not make them cover any more territory for supplies and equipment for their care.
>
> It was my privilege to see this "constant care" room, which really has the equipment one would find distributed in a well equipped hospital.
>
> It is hoped, after the study is completed, that this may be the beginning of a better distribution of private practice nurses, through a more centralized unit for sharing nurse care, thus distributing these services to a larger group of patients.
>
> Only private duty nurses, who are working with the Cleveland Clinic will be asked to cooperate in this program.
>
> It is very gratifying to go over the list of private duty nurses, who work at the Clinic, to find a large number of them are willing to accept of the heart cases. The main objection has been they thought there would be a danger of having to work in this room indefinitely.[55]

The District's Board of Trustees approved the project. But very early on, in the spring of 1957, the private duty nurses working in the unit voiced concerns about an "impossible" situation: "such as being assigned to two patients, both of whom require continuous attention, no Head Nurse, no written orders, necessity of leaving the room to have IV solutions mixed, etc." At the same time, Miss Selfe was suggesting changes: "It would be desirable to have the constant care unit staffed with hospital personnel rather than private duty

nurses and also to offer this service to medical as well as surgical patients."
Mr. Harding had always hoped to attract the private duty nurses working in the
Constant Care Unit to the hospital staff, rather than continuing to call them on
a per diem basis as independent contractors.[56]

By the beginning of 1958, the District's Private Duty Section was complain-
ing that private duty nurses were being unfairly barred from practicing in
special care units:

> Registered Private duty nurses when engaged
> by a patient should accompany the patient
> wherever he goes in the hospital except ...oper-
> ating rooms. The long established practice of
> the hospital in permitting the registered private
> duty nurse to practice throughout the hospital
> precludes the right of the hospital to exclude
> them from continuing to practice in Recovery
> Rooms, Constant Care Rooms, or throughout
> the hospital.[57]

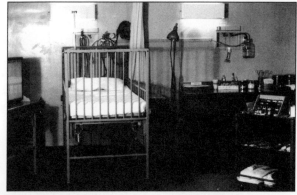

The Section members may have been referring to the
Clinic Hospital, historically their largest market, where,
in 1958, St. John College graduates hired by
the Hospital replaced private duty nurses in
the "Heart Room" (the Constant Care Unit's
Room 225). However, excluding private duty
nurses from such units was common practice,
not just in Cleveland but in the rest of the
country as well.[58]

In 1960 private duty nurses were also
replaced in Room 226, when the Clinic Hospital, reaping the benefits of its successful
recruitment program, was able to transfer 24
R.N.s and staff the entire Constant Care Unit
(now expanded to an additional room, 228)
with its own nurses. The number of Clinic

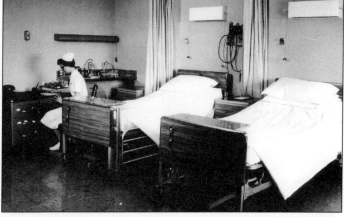

Hospital patients cared for by private duty nurses continued to decrease during
the 1960s, from 20.6 per day at the beginning of 1961 to 17.1 a year later.

Private duty nurses would continue to special Clinic Hospital patients — in
fact, in 1965 a consultant's report recommended that the Hospital start its
own registry — but in proportionately far fewer cases than during the early
years. In 1962 staff nurses replaced private duty nurses in the dialysis unit.
When the Hospital expanded its intensive care facilities in 1966, a further
decrease in the number of special nurses needed was projected.

By this time, veteran private duty nurses like Flora Short, who had entered
nursing school in the 1910s, had ended their careers. Miss Short had nursed
the patients of two generations of Cleveland Clinic physicians, beginning in
the days of Dr. Crile's thyroidectomies. During the 1950s, her cases included
ileostomy and colostomy patients of Dr. Rupert Turnbull, femoral and aortic
graft patients for Dr. Alfred Humphries, lung and heart surgical patients for Dr.
Donald Effler, and patients on Dr. Willem Kolff's artificial kidney. Since private
duty rates had doubled after World War II, she was able to work fewer days for a
higher income. She retired in 1956, after nearly 40 years in nursing.

CONSTANT CARE ROOMS
In the 1950s, intensive care at the
Cleveland Clinic Hospital began
in these rooms, together known as
the Constant Care Unit. Room
225, the "Heart Room," had six
beds and admitted postoperative
open-heart patients; Room 226
provided constant, or intensive,
care to other types of surgical
patients, and to some medical
patients as well. Desks were
furnished so nurses could do
paperwork without leaving the
room. The Recovery Room's head
nurse, Isabelle Chauby Laude,
also supervised the new Constant
Care Unit, becoming the first nurse
in charge of intensive
care at the Hospital.

The Greater Cleveland Nurses' Association (formerly District No. 4) closed its registry in 1974. Commercial registries and temporary agencies continued to provide nurses and auxiliary health workers to care for Cleveland-area patients.

Intensive Care in the 1960s

By the early 1960s, the physical facilities of the Clinic Hospital's whole second-floor area had been further improved, promoting continuity of care. Surgical patients could be moved "from the Operating Room to Recovery and Constant Care away from the public gaze behind two sets of electric eye doors. Also, Constant Care and Recovery space can be used interchangeably as the need arises."[59] In 1961 the Constant Care Unit had 22 beds and a nursing staff of 39. During that year the nurses cared for 1,395 patients, mostly from the vascular, thoracic, open-heart, and neurosurgical services.

A separate, six-bed Medical Constant Care Unit opened on 3 Central in 1964, with the most up-to-date hospital amenities: wall-mounted oxygen and blood pressure units at each bedside. The other major equipment purchased for the unit consisted of a defibrillator and cart, a Bennett machine, a "direct writing" EKG, a telethermometer, an electric toothbrush, a standing scale, and an IV cart.[60] (In the same year, the hospital's first intensive care Isolette was purchased for the pediatric nursing unit.)

The original Constant Care Unit now officially became the Surgical Constant Care Unit. Although the Constant Care Unit had admitted some medical patients, it had always been predominantly a surgical intensive care unit. Even in these critical care settings, nurses not only cared for patients, but also taught patients to care for themselves. "The Nursing Staff [of the Surgical Constant Care Unit] is continually working on methods of instructing patients in self-care. A plastic tube is being used to teach patients with tracheostomies to do their own tracheostomy care."[61]

Nurses who worked in the Hospital's intensive care units in the 1960s looked back from the perspective of the 1990s and marveled about "the technology that we didn't have then." Needles for IV therapy were hard and sharp, so that patients could not move their arms freely. "You'd get a lot of infiltrate and you'd see people's arms just sloughed off." There were no infusion pumps for automatically monitoring the rate of infusion, so that nurses were titrating constantly to be sure that the correct amount of solution was administered.[62]

There were no invasive lines to measure central venous pressure. Intensive care nurses used "a pole, like a big yardstick, that had a carpenter's level in it, with the little bubble. When the patient came back from open heart surgery, you had to know how to level off for your central venous pressure." The admitting nurse visually determined where the apex would be. She "drew a line on the patient's chest with an ink pen...and that was the mark for the rest of the day."[63]

Patients who needed to be kept hypothermic, like some neurosurgery patients, were placed on an ice mattress. Nurses applied lanolin cold cream all over these patients to protect their skins, and ended up with their hands blue from the cold.

Nurses also had clear memories of individual patients, even down to the particular bed spaces they occupied. Some patients remained in the Clinic Hospital intensive care units for months but never recovered, causing nurses sometimes to feel that "you couldn't see anybody getting well, but you'd see people die."[64]

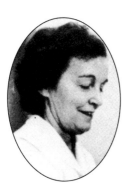

ROSE MORAN

Miss Moran, a registered nurse who worked in the Orthopaedic Department, began her career at the Clinic in 1937. To her, the rewards of more than 25 years of nursing in the Clinic's outpatient area included meeting people of many nationalities from all walks of life, and seeing surgical patients both before and after hospitalization.

There were success stories, too. One man was defibrillated over two hundred times. In this case, even though it was generally a physician's task, nurses received permission to defibrillate the patient, "because you just couldn't be calling a resident" all the time. Although the patient's chest was burned, doctors refused to give up. The man was young, and new advances in open-heart surgery gave hope. The patient lived, and eventually returned home: "He did — it was a miracle — he left and went home."[65]

At this time, ancillary health care workers were still less common than they were later. "Every job that wasn't done by somebody else — and there weren't that many that were done by other people — was done by nursing." "You were the physical therapist, you were the respiratory therapist, you were the one who put the patients on the Bennett breather every hour." Nurses had mixed feelings when comparing those days to a later period: "Thinking back, it was so crude, before the high technology, and the invasive lines, and the things that we have now — but, nursing, you had your hands on that patient."[66]

Nursing Organization: Present and Future Needs

During the 1960s, management techniques and skills were being more systematically applied to the delivery of health care. "Change the organization, change the result," declared management consultants; better organization could produce better health care. In practice, this theory probably had about as much truth in it as did any other generalization — sometimes it worked, sometimes it did not. But for better, for worse, or for a little of both, changes in departmental organization were not just diagrams that men on governing boards and women in nursing offices drew on paper. They had real, tangible effects on the everyday working lives of nurses and their fellow employees.

In 1965 the Cleveland Clinic's Board of Trustees — "because of the complexity of organization [of the large department] and the nationwide shortage of nurses" — gave the Hospital permission to hire the management consulting firm Cresap, McCormick and Paget to study the Nursing Department. Their assignment was to "review and evaluate the organizational arrangements and operations of the Nursing Services Department, to determine whether they are adequate to meet present and future needs." In a cover letter to Hospital Administrator Harding, the firm declared: "We believe one of the Hospital's objectives should be to maintain a reputation for nursing care commensurate with the Foundation's reputation for medical care, graduate medical education and research."[67]

The Cresap study helped shape the Clinic Hospital Nursing Department for years afterward. The consultants reviewed the department's current functioning and then made recommendations for the future. Administrative responsibility within the department, and the place of the department within the Hospital's administrative structure; the way in which patients were assigned to nursing units, and nursing employees were assigned work — these were among the most important areas in which Cresap, McCormick suggested changes. A number of the consultants' recommendations were based on programs and innovations already under way at the time the study was made, initiated in the era of "peace and prosperity" presided over by Mabel Selfe and James Harding.

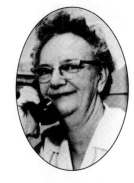

EDNA SHEADY
For many years, Miss Sheady worked on the 3 to 11 shift in the Cleveland Clinic Hospital. Born in Canada, she received her nursing education at St. Joseph's Hospital in Guelph, Ontario. She began her career as an R.N. in 1929, and was employed at University Hospitals of Cleveland before coming to the Clinic in 1938. She celebrated her 25th year at the Hospital in 1963.

Administrative Responsibility

Administrative responsibility was a predictable subject of a management consultant's study. The direction in which the Cresap study pointed the Hospital Nursing Department had a substantial impact on the place of nursing within the Foundation as a whole, and on the administrative attention given to services (such as in-service education) provided to nurses.

To begin with, the study looked at the existing administrative structure: a Director of Nursing, an Assistant Director, eight Nurse Supervisors, two Assistant Nurse Supervisors, and three Instructors. According to the interviews the consultants conducted, lines of authority and communication at middle levels of the department were ineffective, even though, at the top level, Mabel Selfe's door was open to all nurses.

Solving the communication problem was probably beyond the ability of any study. Cresap, McCormick's recommendations focused instead on the lines of authority: "responsibility - along with commensurate authority for its exercise - should be delegated by the administrative head of nursing services, and, in turn, by other nursing services administrators and supervisors to the lowest level practicable." Change should start at the top. The position of Director of Nursing should be "elevated in the Hospital organization to the post of Assistant Administrator and given the title of Assistant Administrator - Director of Nursing Services....The stature in the Hospital organization accorded by the position and title of Assistant Administrator would aid substantially in the exercise of the duties involved." Although Miss Selfe already worked closely with Mr. Harding, the new title would make formal and permanent the Director of Nursing's position as "a member of the Hospital management team at the policy formulation and decision-making level."[68]

Secondly, there should be three Assistant Directors of Nursing: one for Patient Care, one for Continuing Education, and one for Recruitment. This would strengthen the in-service and orientation programs.

The Assistant Director for Patient Care would have day-to-day operational responsibility for all bedside nursing in the Hospital. Six Clinical Supervisors would report to her. Each of these supervisors would be assigned a number of nursing units — where possible, all of the units on a single floor — and would be responsible for staffing, scheduling, budget management, and routine administrative decision-making in her area. (Three evening and two night supervisors would handle administrative duties on the off-shifts, but their decision-making powers would not be as wide as those of the Clinical Supervisors.)

Essentially, this was an expansion of the traditional role of the floor supervisor. During the 1950s and early 1960s, as hospital additions were built and the number of beds per floor increased, floor supervisor positions had been created as needed (the threshold level was considered to be about 110 to 120 beds), to "better coordinate patient care."[69] The first floor supervisor was hired in 1954, to be responsible for the third floor. As of 1962, there were three supervisors for the general medical-surgical floors. The Clinic Hospital also had nursing supervisors for specialized areas — pediatrics and obstetrics — by the late 1950s.

By the 1960s, Hospital administrators had recognized that the large Nursing Department, with five hundred employees and a growing number of

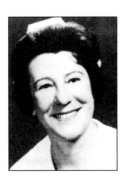

ISABELLE MULLER
Miss Muller was Assistant Administrator-Director of Nursing at the Cleveland Clinic Hospital from 1967 to 1971, the year in which the Department of Nursing was decentralized. A graduate of the Roosevelt Hospital School of Nursing, and of Teachers College, Columbia University (B.A. and M.A.), she served in the U.S. Army Nurse Corps during World War II. Before coming to the Clinic, Miss Muller was Assistant Director of the East Orange General Hospital in New Jersey.

specialized services, was like many departments in one. The consultants also recognized this, and specified that each proposed Clinical Supervisor should be an individual qualified to serve as a director of nursing in a one- to two-hundred-bed hospital.

Cresap, McCormick had recommended that the Director of Nursing be placed on the Assistant Administrator level within the Hospital to strengthen the Nursing Department's organizational position. However, the delegation of substantial amounts of authority to the Clinical Supervisors introduced a decentralizing tendency. The Hospital's annual report for 1966 expressed the hope that "we are on our way to the ultimate organization where the department is run by various clinical supervisors acting independently but in a coordinated organization."[70] The attempt to achieve this "ultimate organization" led to the abolition of the Director of Nursing position and the temporary disappearance of Nursing as a unified Hospital department in the 1970s.

Most of the Cresap report's major recommendations on administrative reorganization were carried out in the years immediately following the report's publication. After Mabel Selfe reached mandatory retirement age, a new Director of Hospital Nursing, Isabelle Muller, R.N., M.A., was hired in 1967. Her title, as suggested by the report, was Hospital Assistant Administrator as well as Director of Nursing.

The number of assistant directors grew from one to three. Jacqueline Heed, R.N., M.S.N., joined the Hospital in 1966 as Assistant Director for Continuing Education. Miss Heed, an experienced nurse educator, was responsible for planning and implementing a wide-ranging, systematic continuing education program. In 1968 Ruth Elmenthaler, R.N., M.S.N., was hired to fill the new position of Assistant Director for Patient Care, and Nortrud Schindzielorz, R.N., became the Assistant Director for Recruitment, completing the new management team.

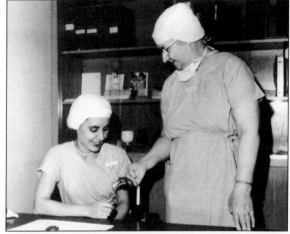

MARTHA HOFFMAN
AND MA GRABER
After nearly forty years at the Cleveland Clinic Hospital, Elizabeth Pratt Graber (right) retired in 1966. "Just about everyone in the place knows 'Ma' Graber," commented the Clinic's *Newsletter.* Mrs. Graber had headed the Operating Room Department twice, as Acting Supervisor before Miss Larsen's arrival, and as Supervisor from 1962 to 1966. Her successor, Martha Hoffman (left), had joined the Operating Room in 1962, after a short stint in the Cardiac Catheterization Laboratory. Mrs. Hoffman served as Operating Room Supervisor for 7 years

Cresap, McCormick did not study ambulatory nursing and operating room nursing, areas outside the Hospital Nursing Department. Clinic Nursing was enjoying its own period of administrative stability at this point. The situation in the Operating Room Department in the 1960s, however, was similar to that of the immediate post-World War II years, with frequent changes in leadership. Sophia Larsen departed suddenly in 1962, reportedly after she had refused to change department rules on mandatory maternity leave to please a surgeon. Elizabeth Graber, R.N., now a 35-year veteran of the Hospital, again stepped into the breach, serving as head of the department until her retirement in 1966. Martha Hoffman, R.N., who had done a short stint in Clinic Nursing (in the Cardiac Catheterization Laboratory) before transferring to the Operating Room, became the next Supervisor of the Operating Room Department.

Central Sterile Supply

Central Sterile Supply had always been part of the Hospital Nursing Department, originally under the name "Equipment Room." More recently, it had been completely reorganized in 1963. Its head nurse now had full responsibility for the service, rather than reporting to a supervisor. A complete delivery system to the nursing units was instituted so that unit personnel would not have to interrupt their patient care duties to make trips to Central Supply. In addition, the service took over all preparation and packaging of gloves and syringes for the entire Cleveland Clinic — the outpatient Clinic as well as the Nursing Department, the Operating Room, and the Pharmacy — using automated equipment. As of 1956 Central Supply had had responsibility for the Hospital's pool of orderlies. During the 1950s, fewer R.N.s and more aides were assigned to Central Supply. In 1965, 2 R.N.s, 23 aides, and 32 orderlies made up the staff.

Cresap, McCormick singled out Central Supply and its head nurse — Eleanor Reilly, R.N., B.S.N. — for special praise. "The central sterile supply unit in the Cleveland Clinic Hospital is a well-managed and effective operation, with continuing efforts for further improvement. The head nurse in charge deserves substantial credit for the sound operation of the unit." The report recommended removing Central Supply, as a technical unit that served the entire Clinic, from the Hospital Nursing Department. It suggested that the new Central Sterile Supply Department could provide "a valuable service" by monitoring the appearance of disposable supplies on the market and continually comparing their cost to that of reprocessing supplies in the department. It also recommended assigning orderlies to nursing floors, where they actually did most of their work, rather than pooling them in Central Supply.[71]

The Hospital did make Central Service (as it became known) an independent department. Some of the consultants' other recommendations were adopted as well. "We are now awaiting the arrival of disposable needles," reported Eleanor Reilly in 1966. "This will eliminate many man hours spent on re-sharpening needles."[72] During subsequent years, the cost of preparing reusable gloves was continually measured against the price of disposable gloves. For instance, in 1967, reprocessing cost 14 cents a pair, compared to a purchase price of 22 to 25 cents for disposables. Disposables finally won out and replaced reusable gloves throughout the institution in 1971. Disposable syringes replaced most washable glass syringes in 1967.

For the time being, most orderlies remained in the Central Service pool, from where they were sent as needed to the units. Miss Reilly felt that this situation was not fair to the men.

> I think the usefulness of the pool concept has reached its end.... More and more men are being employed by the nursing department as "ward aides." These men are given assignments just as the women aides. However the orderlies are still being called to care for patients in these areas - the situation has become a very demoralizing factor resulting in very unhappy orderlies who feel that they are doing scut work. Many of the orderlies would rather be part of the nursing team at the bedside where they would have a better feeling of fulfillment.... The men are just tired of being "second class citizens."[73]

She recommended that the day and evening shift orderlies be transferred to the Nursing Department immediately. The job description and title of the orderlies did eventually change, so that there was not so much overlap between their duties and those of Nursing Department employees.

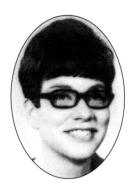

ELEANOR REILLY

The Cleveland Clinic's Central Service Department was originally part of the Hospital Nursing Department. Known in the early years as the "Equipment Room," it was the area where gloves, dressings, syringes, and other supplies and equipment were prepared for use. In 1965, Central Sterile Supply, as it was then called, had 58 employees, including 23 aides and the 32 members of the Hospital's orderly pool. Miss Reilly was the head nurse. In that year, Central Supply, which served the outpatient areas, the Operating Room, and the Pharmacy, as well as Hospital Nursing, was made an independent department, with Miss Reilly as Supervisor. She directed Central Service for the next three decades, and also directed the Operating Room Department in 1973-1974. New packaging and sterilization methods, enormous growth in the use of disposables, and increased attention to infection control during this period made for substantial changes in the work of Central Service. In addition to guiding her own department, Miss Reilly made numerous overseas visits to share knowledge with hospitals and colleagues in other countries.

Special Care and Specialized Units

Innovations in the way patients were assigned to their beds were already under way at the Clinic Hospital when the Cresap study was made. Special care or intensive care units had been created to group critically ill patients together under the care of Hospital staff nurses, decreasing the need for special nurses. Clinic physicians and surgeons were recommending the creation of specialized or departmentalized units as well, in which patients would be grouped by diagnosis — that is, orthopaedic patients on one unit, cardiac patients on another, and so forth. As special care units and specialized units replaced general medical-surgical units, the Clinic Hospital Nursing Department made changes in the way nursing personnel were assigned to units, and in the way work was assigned to personnel within those units.

Special care units were well-established by the time the Cresap, McCormick study was made. The Recovery Room served as a way station rather than a permanent stop for the patient within the hospital. In the Surgical and Medical Constant

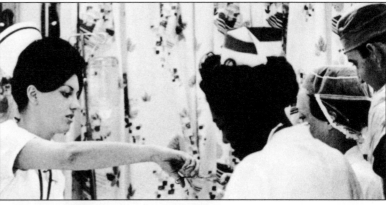

RECOVERY ROOM
Opened in 1948, the Hospital's Recovery Room quickly became an integral part of the patient care continuum. Under the medical direction of the Department of Anesthesiology, and the administrative direction of the Department of Nursing, the Recovery Room was caring for more than 12,000 patients annually by the mid-1960s. The Intravenous Therapy Team nurses, who handled IV starts throughout the Hospital and Clinic beginning in 1958, were also based in the Recovery Room.

Care Units, critically ill patients received "constant,"or "intensive," nursing care: approximately 13 or 14 hours per patient per day at this time. Patients on a general medical-surgical unit typically received 3 to 4 hours of nursing care a day, and patients in the Convalescent Care Unit received fewer hours of nursing care.

Specialization, or departmentalization, of nursing units had gotten off to a shakier start. The Clinic Hospital had not traditionally grouped patients by clinical service. Most of the departmentalized nursing units in the Hospital at this time had come about as a result of the postwar addition of new medical departments at the Clinic: Pediatrics, Obstetrics, and Psychiatry. A Hospital nursing unit devoted to pediatric patients had opened in 1948. In 1956, expecting to do its part in delivering the babies of the boom years, the Cleveland Clinic opened an obstetrical nursing unit for the first time. Labor, delivery, and patient rooms, as well as a nursery, were located on the Hospital's sixth floor. In 1961, a psychiatric nursing unit was created.

The creation of specialized floors or units to separate patients by services within the general medical-surgical area had been proposed at least as far back as 1949, but not really tried out until 1957. In that year, following a request by the physicians on the Hospital Committee, the attempt was made to place medical and surgical patients on separate floors. Even this modest experiment failed, and was quickly aborted, due largely to the Hospital's near one hundred percent occupancy rate and the consequent continual need to transfer patients from one area to another. Also, although the Hospital's patient load was about 30 to 35 percent medical and 65 to 70 percent surgical at this time, many patients had both medical and surgical diagnoses. However, later in the year, 14 beds on the 4 South nursing division were allocated to

Dermatology "as a trial of partial departmentalization. This trial was successful....Partial departmentalization can be made to work to the advantage of doctor and patient, but full scale departmentalization, we believe, is impractical for out type of institution unless we either accept empty beds, which is expensive, or much transferring of patients, which causes patient dissatisfaction."[74]

The situation had not changed much by the time Cresap, McCormick looked at it. Dermatology still had 12 beds on 4 South. On 5 Central, Urology now had 16 beds and Gastroenterology, 18. But except for the Constant Care Units and the pediatric, obstetric, and psychiatric units, the rest of the Hospital's beds — 305 out of a total of 490 — were divided among 10 general medical-surgical units.

There are few, if any, hospitals in the country operating at such a consistently high level of utilization as the Cleveland Clinic Hospital. The ability to maintain a high level of occupancy is in part attributable to the group

Obstetrics at the Clinic, 1956-1966

The Cleveland Clinic did not have a Department of Obstetrics until 1956. The obstetrics unit which opened on the Hospital's sixth floor incorporated the innovative ideas of Dr. Howard P. Taylor, head of the new department. The unit had a standard nursery, but also small four-bed nurseries (photo at left) situated between semi-private rooms. This promoted the "rooming in" concept: with help and teaching from nurses, mothers could immediately begin to care

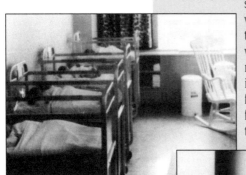

for their babies. Dr. Taylor also encouraged the participation of fathers (below and at right), including them in prepartum hospital tours and permitting them to watch the delivery. (This was so unusual at the time that the state had to grant a waiver to allow non-medical personnel in the delivery room.) With the baby boom waning and demand growing for care in other specialties, the Clinic closed the department in 1966. Twenty-nine years later the Clinic opened a Department of Birthing Services, which included nurse-midwives.

practice of the Clinic medical staff; however, a substantial measure of credit is due the Hospital administration for its organizational and administrative achievements in overcoming the complexities and pressures of such high utilization in order to operate the Hospital successfully.[75]

Credit was also due to the hard work of nursing personnel and other employees. The average occupancy level for medical-surgical beds was 99.8 percent, "a maximum attainable level."[76] The consultants noted that if more specialty nursing units were established, as the Cleveland Clinic planned, the Hospital almost certainly could not continue to maintain such a high occupancy rate.

One of the reasons for the move toward departmentalized nursing units was to promote specialization of nursing practice. A feature of the plan for departmentalization was to have the head nurse make rounds with physicians on a regular and frequent basis "so that she becomes more familiar with the patient's problem and the thinking of the doctor." Just as the ever-growing body of medical knowledge was compelling physicians to specialize, so nurses would have to become experts in the care of the particular types of cases admitted to their units: "By departmentalization of patients by services, the nurses become more knowledgeable about the nursing needs of specific patients. Eventually, perhaps, all medical and surgical specialties can have their own nursing divisions, since only in this way can nurses be expected to gain the necessary expertise required by each physician specialty."[77]

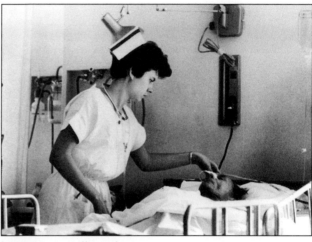

INTENSIVE CARE, 1963
During the 1960s, the number of patients admitted to the Constant Care Unit increased substantially. In 1964 the Clinic opened the first separate Medical Constant Care Unit in the region, increasing the Hospital's intensive care bed capacity from 22 to 28. The original unit, now devoted entirely to surgical patients, remained one of the nation's largest such units. These areas, which together cared for 10 percent of the Hospital's patient census, had been the first units in the Hospital to have wall-mounted oxygen and blood pressure sets for each bed. An EKG machine, a defibrillator, and a Bennett breathing machine constituted the major part of the Medical unit's high-tech equipment when it opened.

Team Nursing and the Closed Unit

With or without departmentalization, nursing would have to be reorganized at the unit level. The current fashion in nursing care delivery at the time was team nursing, a concept developed in the early 1950s "in response to the shortage of registered nurses and the need to utilize several categories of ancillary staff ...to provide nursing care." Mabel Selfe had suggested as early as 1955 that "a modified form of the 'Team Method'" could be instituted at the Clinic Hospital in order to "bring the R.N.'s in closer contact with the patient." Like departmentalization, team nursing was slow to take hold at the Clinic Hospital. Not until 1963 did the first two units — pediatrics and psychiatry, which were also departmentalized units — implement team nursing. The following year the new Medical Constant Care Unit started up under the team system, and a general medical-surgical unit, 5 South, switched from functional nursing to team nursing. Miss Selfe hired a St. John College instructor to plan the organization of the unit and orient the staff.[78]

When the Cresap, McCormick consultants made their site visit in 1965, they described both the old and new arrangements on the units:

> Except for 5 South, the organization of the nursing units is generally along traditional, or functional, lines - that is, graduate [registered] and auxiliary [practical nurses and aides] nurses are assigned to work in specific nursing units for a period of time and, within the units, are assigned to specific tasks or functions. In such an arrangement, where there are two

graduate nurses on duty, one may be designated as medication nurse and one as treatment, or general, nurse; auxiliary nurses are usually assigned to a block of beds or rooms, usually without regard to the number or condition of the patients.

The 5 South unit is organized under the team nursing concept. This unit is under the direction of a head nurse, who has 24-hour responsibility for the operation of the unit and the nursing care of patients admitted to it. On the day shift, there are three teams organized to care for a total of 32 patients; each team consists of a staff nurse-team leader having one or more auxiliary nurses reporting to her and working under her direction. The evening shift has two teams, each consisting of a staff nurse-team leader and one or more auxiliary nurses; the night shift has one team. Teams are assigned to provide all of the nursing care of specific patients; the number of patients per team varies according to their condition and the level of nursing care required.[79]

Under the functional system, Clinic Hospital head nurses did not have around-the-clock responsibility for their units. The Hospital's 16 assistant head nurses, who generally served as charge nurses on the units during the evening and night shifts, were not assigned to specific units, but rotated among units and shifts.

Staff registered nurses also generally rotated among units and shifts. Nurses could choose to work permanently on evening or night shifts when positions came open, "but if they prefer day shift, they take this assignment with the understanding that they must take their turn in working on the evening and/or night shifts." Most nurses preferred the day shift. This meant that three or four times during a year, a day nurse would work a five-week stint on one of the other shifts, often on a different unit, so that rotation among shifts also resulted in a rotation of personnel among units. "Thus, there is a constant need for nurses, head nurses and auxiliary nurses to adjust to new or less familiar people and, perhaps, to work in units involving types of clinical nursing which they do not enjoy."[80]

Although practical nurses, aides, and ward clerks had to cope with a changing parade of registered nurses, they had permanent assignments to specific units and shifts. More than half of the ward clerks worked on the first shift, but many units had afternoon clerks as well, whose hours generally began at noon and substantially overlapped those of the first shift. There was no night clerical coverage on the units.

As an exception to the rotation system for staff nurses, the Hospital's specialized units, like the obstetric unit, and also the team unit on 5 South, functioned as "closed" units. All personnel, including registered nurses, were permanently assigned to the unit, with the unit's head nurse arranging any shift rotation necessary. (The Assistant Director of Nursing planned rotation schedules for the rest of the hospital.) The head nurses on closed units tended to have more 24-hour responsibility for their units than did their counterparts on open units.

A typical general medical-surgical unit, like 4 West, with 35 beds, had budgeted positions for a head nurse, an assistant head nurse, five staff nurses, seven licensed practical nurses, six aides, and two ward clerks. Orderlies came from the pool in Central Sterile Supply.

Changes on the Units

The Cresap, McCormick report placed particular emphasis on improving the nursing unit's cohesiveness and efficiency. First, it recommended that the head nurse position be strengthened. "Most head nurses, according to members of the medical staff who were interviewed, are the key persons with whom physicians communicate and on whom they depend in arranging for the proper care of patients," and they therefore should have 24-hour responsibility, "and authority," for their units. To effectively shoulder this responsibility, head nurses should be trained in "sound techniques of supervision."[81]

Second, each unit should have an assistant head nurse permanently assigned to it, particularly on the evening shift — "when the nursing units are often especially busy because of late admissions, physicians' rounds, evening medications and treatments, visiting hours and relatives' inquiries" — and preferably on the night shift as well.[82]

Third, the units should make better use of ward clerks to "relieve head nurses and other nursing personnel from routine clerical, telephone and receptionist chores to permit maximum time to be given to the direct nursing care of

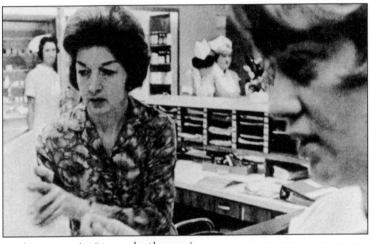

patients." Ward clerks — renamed "nursing unit secretaries" to make the position "more attractive" — should be assigned to units on regular evening shifts and on weekends, as well as weekdays, and should receive more extensive formal training.[83]

Fourth, written care plans should be prepared, under the head nurse's direction, for each patient admitted to the nursing unit. Fifth, team nursing should be instituted on as many units as possible: "Most nurses currently on the Hospital staff who were interviewed expressed a desire to have team nursing in their units. In addition, nurses graduating from most nursing education institutions nowadays are led to expect or to seek out hospitals with team nursing in effect." Finally, partly to implement team nursing, and partly to improve morale, rotation should be discontinued, and all units should convert to the "closed unit" model of permanent assignment already in effect for auxiliary nursing personnel. Nurses should, "whenever possible," choose the unit and shift to which they would be permanently assigned.[84]

Some, but not all, of these recommendations were put into practice over the next few years. Nurses were given the chance to choose their assignments; however, choices naturally did not always match available positions, and so "whenever possible" was far from always. Rotation of registered nurses decreased, but was not eliminated. In fact, by 1969, L.P.N.s were being hired with the understanding that they, too, would rotate. Team nursing continued to be an elusive ideal. Although it gradually found its way onto more units, on other units it was still a goal or an experiment, rather than an achievement, well into the 1970s. The same was true of written nursing care plans.

WARD SECRETARY, 1969
The "floor hostess" position created during the World War II nursing shortage had developed into a job description including a wide range of clerical duties, such as transcribing physicians' orders and filling out requisitions for laboratory studies. Known successively as "ward clerks," "ward secretaries," "division secretaries," and "unit secretaries," they had become an indispensable part of each nursing unit's staff on the day and evening shifts by the late 1960s.

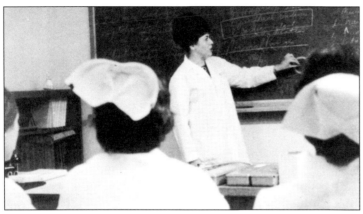

NURSING EDUCATION, 1970
Jacqueline Heed (above, at the blackboard), a nursing instructor at St. John College, was appointed Assistant Director for Continuing Education in 1966. Under her direction, continuing education for nursing personnel included orientation, skill training, leadership development, and staff development, both centralized and decentralized. To upgrade skills of support personnel, she instituted a senior nurses' aide training course, and started a new course for ward secretaries.

Starting in 1967, ward clerks, now designated ward secretaries, went through a training program enabling them "to carry out specific clerical and semi-managerial functions formerly done by the professional nursing staff, thus freeing the nurses to do nursing."[85] In particular, they learned to transcribe doctor's orders. Also, the hours of secretarial coverage were extended to 10:30 p.m. by changing the time at which the evening secretaries went on duty. However, weekend coverage was not instituted until 1972.

In 1968, 12 additional assistant head nurses were hired — an improvement, but still not nearly a large enough number to permit their permanent assignment to all units. Progress in strengthening the head nurse's role was not easily documented, but two programs being implemented at this time did have positive results for head nurses.

In 1969 the director of nursing commended the Continuing Education office, headed by Assistant Director Jacqueline Heed, for an "outstanding contribution": its new "Leadership Development" program for all of the Hospital's registered nurses. Clinic and Central Supply supervisory personnel were also invited to participate. All registered nurses would attend a one-day session; separate five-day courses were designed for supervisors and assistant head nurses. The most intensive training was reserved for head nurses, who attended a seven-day session. "The Head Nurses seemed to grow personally and to be very responsive in each session. There are follow-up sessions monthly with this group and they are attending these with enthusiasm. Their comments and suggestions are constructive," reported Miss Muller.[86]

A program of increased departmentalization also tended to strengthen the role of the head nurse. In 1967, at the Hospital Committee's request, departmentalization was begun on all but five of the nursing units. Mr. Harding observed that grouping patients of the same clinical service on the same nursing unit had sparked "renewed interest" among the head nurses. They began to plan weekly conferences with their units' personnel and "enlisted the assistance of the physicians," promoting teamwork among all those who worked together on a departmentalized unit.[87]

"A Lot of Camaraderie"

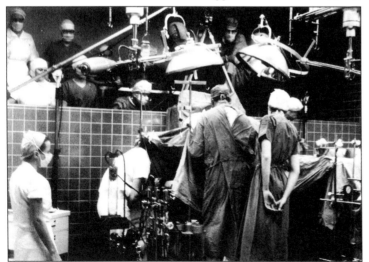

HEART SURGERY, 1958
Between 1955 and 1967, cardiac surgery was performed in the Hospital's second-floor operating pavilion. In 1967, a separate Cardiovascular Unit, with its own operating suite and intensive care and stepdown units, opened on the sixth floor of the Hospital where the obstetrics unit had been.

Clinic Hospital operating room nurses had been assigned to specialized surgical services since the early 1950s. Teamwork was especially important in the operating

170

room, where, during a surgical procedure, nurses generally worked in tandem in the complementary roles of scrub nurse and circulating nurse. The scrub nurse set up the table for surgery with the necessary instruments, which she passed to the surgeons during the procedure. Since she had to maintain "the integrity of the sterile field throughout the operation," and had to be at hand to anticipate the surgeons' needs, she could not go far from the table to obtain additional supplies or instruments. She could not take used instruments to be cleaned, or answer or make telephone calls. These were duties of the circulating nurse, who was also responsible for "maintain[ing] a safe and comfortable environment in the room."[88]

During the 1950s and 1960s, circulating nurses often worked more than one room at a time. A neurosurgical nurse might circulate two craniotomy procedures. A nurse on the vascular service might "do two aneurysm rooms and an angio room, or the amputation room." One nurse remembered circulating four rooms at a time. Most nurses felt that the overall atmosphere was one of cooperation. "There was a lot of camaraderie. If somebody needed help, they just had to go out the door and grab somebody....Or if somebody saw you racing around doing something, they'd just come in and offer."[89]

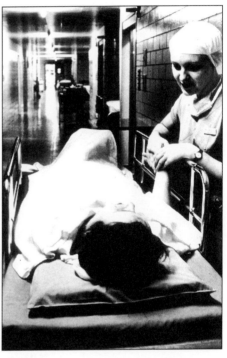

Sometimes nurses had to stay at their posts in difficult circumstances. For instance, a nurse and surgeon on one service were dealing with a situation that included a waiting patient in one operating room, a case in progress in the next, and a bleeding patient in the Recovery Room. The nurse came out of a room into the hallway. Moving quickly, she "turned left but looked right," collided with an operating room table, and was knocked to her knees, breathless and almost unconscious. The operating surgeon came out "in his bloody gloves and gown" and saw her "sliding down the wall." Not knowing what had happened, he ordered her to get up. "I'm still working!" she thought immediately, aware of the waiting patients. She had fractured a rib and separated intercostal cartilages, but got up and scrubbed for procedures the rest of the day.[90]

REASSURANCE
An operating room nurse holds a patient's hand as they wait in the hallway of the operating pavilion, offering support at this critical time. During the surgery ahead, she is responsible for seeing that all conditions and activities in the operating room are organized around the patient's welfare.

Nurses had praise for Clinic surgeons of the era, many of whom were renowned in their fields. "I've never worked with such a group of people who were so respectful, and so eager to teach, and treated you like you were someone, instead of just someone who was their handmaiden." Dr. Rupert Turnbull, an internationally known colorectal surgeon, was described by nurses as "so much of a gentleman": a man who, at the end of the day, would go out of his way to thank each individual who had worked with him in the operating room.[91] Another nurse recalled that Dr. René Favaloro, who originated the saphenous vein bypass graft and performed the Clinic's first heart transplant, was modest about his own role as a cardiothoracic surgeon. Like Dr. Frank Bunts a half century before, he reserved praise for nurses, "without whose aid" open-heart patients would not recover. He pointed out that the nurses who took care of patients after surgery made sure that the surgeon's work was not wasted.[92]

Cleveland Clinic nurses needed to be able to do more than follow a routine. Innovations in surgery required nurses to be innovative in the operating suite, as well as on the nursing unit afterward. Operating room nurses frequently found themselves involved in do-it-yourself projects during those years, whether they were adapting to new procedures, accommodating surgeons' likes and dislikes, or "manufacturing" commonly used supplies. "We even made our own hats!" declared one nurse.[93]

Since disposables were not yet in widespread use, many items had to be cleaned and sterilized for reuse by operating room nurses, technicians, and aides. Black rubber suction tubing was emptied of blood, cleaned, and wrapped around old adhesive tape cans to be autoclaved. Putting cystoscopes in the "formaldehyde cabinets" after they had been soaked was an especially distasteful job: "I still have a mental block about cysto instruments —I hated that room."[94]

For surgeons who did not like prepackaged gauze, operating room personnel made up oiled gauze. They melted Vaseline, and sterilized beeswax. On a routine basis, nurses warmed their own saline, which came in glass bottles with rubber stoppers. "You just got it cold out of the cupboard, and we had hot plates....You had to pump the tops to release the vacuum because you were heating it, and then you'd put it on to cook while you were starting your rooms."[95] The temptation was great to speed the process by turning up the heat, and nurses would occasionally return to see stoppers popping off and the ceiling dripping with boiling hot saline.

When a "bone bank" for bone plugs harvested from cadavers was started at the Clinic, operating room personnel had to figure out what kind of containers to use for sterilization. Jelly jars were considered as an option. In the days before synthetic grafts were available for vascular surgery, the Clinic had a human artery bank, and the arterial sections, too, had to be stored in glass containers.

As increasingly delicate instruments came to be employed for eye operations, the packaging then in use would not protect them from damage during sterilization. The head nurse on the ophthalmology service devised more suitable plastic containers with lids: "damage of the equipment was nil, and sterilized instrumentation was readily available." In many cases, the Maintenance Department was called in to help make or adapt operating room equipment. "They used to make all kinds of instruments for us. They would come up and we would tell them, and they would make it for us."[96]

On the whole, surgical procedures took longer because the preparation was different, and equipment, although not plentiful by the standards of a later day, could be cumbersome. "I remember when opening on a cardiac case was 84 hemostats, every single case was 84 hemostats, which they buzzed off with the Bovies....And that old heart-lung machine, it would take them a whole day to set it up, almost, and almost a full day to tear down....And they had those big glass oxygenators."[97]

Clinic Hospital operating room nurses also had favorite items of equipment. For instance, they used large overhead Mayfield tables, instead of smaller Mayo stands and back tables, to accommodate the large amount of instrumentation needed for major cases. "They were the best tables," many nurses agreed.[98]

Growing Diversity

As had been true of the nurses of the Lakeside Unit, Cleveland Clinic nursing personnel were in the early years nearly all white, native-born, single women. The situation had not changed much by the time the Second World War ended, except that the number of married women had increased significantly. But even in the mid-1960s, the Cresap report was still recommending that the Hospital Nursing Department could increase its staff by "attracting and employing effectively, on a part time basis," women who had left nursing to marry and raise families.[99] Wives and mothers who had education and experience could not be ignored as potential staff members at a time when the Clinic's demand for nurses was growing, amidst a national shortage.

The Cleveland Clinic had not generally employed men as nurses, although men had served in nursing assistant and orderly positions from the Clinic's beginning. Men were actually preferred as nursing personnel in limited areas, primarily in positions that involved patient transport, mechanical equipment, or care of male patients. Edward Rogers, for example, worked from 1922 to 1964 as a valued assistant in the Clinic's Urology Department. Dr. Barney Crile described his abilities as outstanding: "He treated the patients more expertly than the average doctor could have. He satisfied them with his personal attention, his understanding, his humor, and his skill."[100]

In general, however, Clinic physicians were still reluctant to approve the hiring of male nurses to work in the outpatient areas, because men could not serve as "chaperons" during examination of female patients. (There was also a fear, it was said, that male nurses would be mistaken for physicians.) On the other hand, in the Hospital, nursing administrators expressed specific interest in hiring male R.N.s in the late 1950s, but again, for the usual limited range of positions: "for our male wards, and possibly one in charge of the Orderly program." In 1967, Central Service workers assigned to the newly specialized nursing units included "a senior orderly in charge of orthopedic equipment and one who cares for the male urological patients."[101]

In the period immediately following the Second World War, overt racial segregation was still common in the United States, and Cleveland, and the health care industry, were no exceptions. The African-American population of Cleveland had grown steadily during the twentieth century, concentrated on the east side of the city within easy reach of the Cleveland Clinic.

The Clinic had not initially employed a large number of African-Americans, however. In the 1920s and 1930s, most nurses were of northern European extraction, although this was beginning to change as the daughters of the great wave of eastern and southern European immigration reached adulthood. A large number of women with eastern European surnames did work on the Clinic's cleaning staff. (On into the 1960s, the Hospital librarian kept books in the Hungarian language on hand for members of the housekeeping staff.) African-Americans were most likely to work as porters or in the kitchen in the early years.

In the 1940s the Hospital segregated both patient rooms and employee locker rooms. In 1943 Abbie Porter noted that "during the past year we have

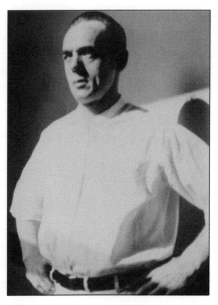

EDDIE ROGERS
During the 1960s and 1970s, men gradually gained a greater role in patient care at the Clinic and Hospital, as nursing assistants, clinical corpsmen, and increasingly as R.N.s. However, at least a few men had worked in nursing areas at the Cleveland Clinic from the beginning. One of the most outstanding was Edward Rogers (shown here circa 1925), an assistant in the Urology Department from 1922 to 1964. A native of Ireland, he served in the U.S. Army during World War I, and joined the Clinic only a year after its founding, when he was 27. Known both for his sense of fun and his devotion to patients, Eddie Rogers had become "almost an institution" at the Clinic by the time he retired in 1964.

admitted more colored patients. This constitutes a real problem as we segregate them and are many times forced to give them a private room." In 1944 the Administrative Board approved "the assignment of a 4-bed ward on the third floor for colored women and a 4-bed ward on the fourth floor of the Hospital for colored men."[102]

The proportion of African-American employees also grew during the Second World War. In 1942 "all colored men were given space in one locker room,"and "colored maids," who had been sharing a crowded locker room with the rest of the Hospital's 60 to 70 maids, were also moved to a separate area.[103] In 1945 a house on East 90th Street was converted into locker space for African-American employees, with porters and male kitchen workers on the first floor, and dietary and housekeeping maids on the second.

As other departments took over the jobs formerly done by nursing personnel, African-Americans gradually came closer to providing direct patient care. Older employees and "colored maids" were trained to dust patient rooms in 1943, a task that had formerly been done by nurses' aides. In 1950 the head of the Nursing Department suggested that hiring African-Americans as nursing personnel was a possibility.

> Our auxiliary help has dropped considerably (more than 25%). This, I believe can be attributed to industrial demands and will create a hardship for the hospitals. I feel that with select people, negro if necessary, we can...train them on the floors.[104]

Nationwide, the next 20 years were eventful ones. In 1954, the United States Supreme Court declared that segregated public schooling violated the Constitution; Dr. Martin Luther King, Jr., led a historic battle for civil rights, and was assassinated in 1968; Carl B. Stokes was elected as Cleveland's first African-American mayor in 1967.

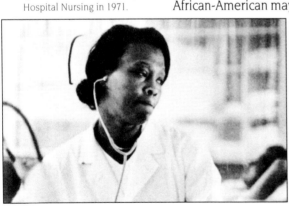

ALMA DAVIS
Health care, like much of American society, was still segregated in the post-World War II years. During the first thirty years of the Clinic's history, African-American employees could be found only in support departments like Dietary and Housekeeping. The Cleveland Clinic Hospital began hiring African-American R.N.s, L.P.N.s, and nursing assistants in the 1950s. By the 1960s, African-American women were working as head nurses in the Hospital. Alma Davis, head nurse in Hemodialysis, was appointed one of seven clinical directors responsible for administering Hospital Nursing in 1971.

Over those same 20 years, African-Americans were hired in all areas of Cleveland Clinic nursing, not only as aides, as had been suggested in 1950, but as registered and licensed practical nurses as well. The push to hire practical nurses for the Hospital in the 1950s, under Mabel Selfe's direction, was perhaps the key event. The addition of a large number of practical nurses at that time, both black and white, gave African-American women an increased role in providing patient care at the Clinic Hospital. (However, as of 1957, there were still no African-American nursing personnel at all working in the outpatient Clinic.)

Since licensed practical nursing was a new field, it was more open to African-Americans than registered nursing. Cleveland City Hospital (later MetroHealth Medical Center) had been the first Cleveland hospital to admit African-American students to its R.N. diploma program, in 1930. On the national level, the Nurse Cadet Corps, which was pledged to admit students without regard to race, gave African-Americans increased opportunities to become R.N.s during the 1940s.

In 1951, OSNA District No. 4 hotly debated the issue of admitting African-American nurses to its membership. Cleveland's African-American registered nurses had in the past joined the local affiliate of the National Association of

Colored Graduate Nurses (NACGN), but after the Buckeye Graduate Nurses Association (the state organization for African-American nurses) was dissolved in 1950, and the ANA absorbed the NACGN in 1951, African-American nurses had to join the District if they wished to belong to a professional organization.[105] To ensure that their applications would not be routinely turned down, the District Board of Trustees assumed control over the admission of new members, up to this point a prerogative of the District membership at large. Rose Peebles, the former president of the Cleveland African-American nurses' organization, was the first African-American R.N. admitted to District No. 4 under the new system.

The Cleveland Clinic Foundation began hiring African-American registered nurses in the mid-1950s, first in the Hospital and then eventually in the Clinic. By the 1960s African-American nurses were attaining positions as head nurses: Alma Davis in Hemodialysis, Loretta Prince in Pediatrics, and Josephine Smith in the Operating Room.

In the United States, the nursing shortage of the 1950s also caused the health care industry to turn to other countries for nurses. In Cleveland, two English nurses arrived at City Hospital in 1954; in the next year Mt. Sinai Hospital began "importing" nurses from Great Britain.[106] In 1954 the Clinic Hospital began to participate in the ANA-sponsored exchange visitors' program, receiving one nurse from England and one nurse from the Netherlands. The number of exchange nurses increased over the next several years, to three in 1957 and six in 1958. In 1959, several nurse anesthetists came to the Clinic Hospital through the program, easing the perennial shortage in that area.

At this point, most nurses immigrating to the United States were coming from northern Europe — for example, several nurses from Germany joined the Cleveland Clinic staff during the 1950s and 1960s. Changes in United States immigration law in 1965 meant that an increasing number of nurses would come from other areas of the world as well, particularly from countries like the Philippines where nurses received education in English.

Friends and Family

"It was just like a family." "All my best friends were here." "You helped each other out." "Everyone knew everyone." Many nurses who worked at the Cleveland Clinic in the 1950s and 1960s described their experience in words like these in later years.[107]

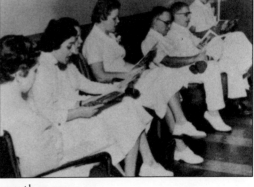

In the 1950s and 1960s — even though nurses may not have regarded any physician or administrator as a "father" (in the way Lakeside Unit members had regarded Dr. Crile), and even though they looked at Clinic-subsidized housing more as a financial benefit than as "home" — there was still a family atmosphere at the Cleveland Clinic. However, the "family" was even then growing extremely large and more diverse in a number of ways.

The change could not be measured by size alone. The numbers of patients, physicians, nurses, and other employees grew, but it was not just a matter of departments growing larger. New departments were being added, and all health care work was becoming more specialized. In 1970, the 610-bed Clinic Hospital had, in addition to its largest department, Nursing, the following departments

A SIMPLER TIME
In 1951, Cleveland Clinic staff physicians, fellows, nurses, and other employees gathered to rehearse before singing Christmas carols to Hospital patients. At that time, the institution had 840 employees, only 100 more than in 1941; the number would nearly double in each of the next two decades. Long-time employees looked back with regret: "It's different now from the way it was then," said most.

and programs: Administration; Admitting/Business Offices; Administrative Service Coordinators; Clinical Corpsmen; Inhalation Therapy/Chest Physiotherapy; Hemodialysis; Radiology; Physical Therapy; Operating Pavilion; Anesthesia; Pharmacy; Central Service; Dietary; Laundry; Housekeeping; Social Work; Pastoral Care; Laboratories; and Methods Improvement.

Nurses and porters, pharmacists and bookkeepers; workers in the kitchen, the laundry, the administrative offices — these employees were now joined by inhalation therapists, occupational therapists, cardiac perfusionists, hemodialysis technicians, social workers, a chaplain, and even a librarian.[108] Occupational and inhalation therapists, among others, actually started out as Hospital Nursing Department employees, but eventually split off into separate departments.

A similar situation occurred in Clinic Nursing, which had initial administrative responsibility for employees such as EKG, EEG, and pulmonary function technicians. New workers were hired by the Clinic nursing supervisor and

Enterostomal Therapy

The field of enterostomal therapy (ET) was founded at the Cleveland Clinic in 1958, when the famed colorectal surgeon Dr. Rupert Turnbull hired Norma Gill as the world's first enterostomal therapist. Mrs. Gill herself was not a nurse, but nurses quickly entered the field.

Enterostomal therapists worked to rehabilitate individuals who had undergone surgery that removed parts of their intestines or their bladders and created stomas, openings for elimination of wastes. An article in the Cleveland Clinic Hospital nursing publication *Under Your Cap* explained the idea behind the new field. "In rehabilitation surgery, you must spend time with patients," stated Dr. Turnbull. The enteros-

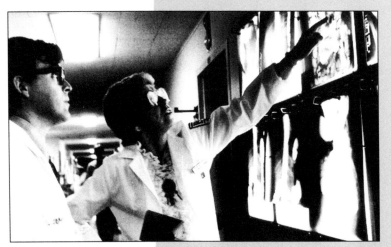

Norma Gill (right), first enterostomal therapist, in 1979

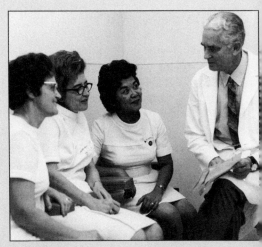

Dr. Turnbull (right), with Mrs. Gill (center) and two of her students, 1969

trained on the job by co-workers. Such areas started out with only a few employees, but later expanded into entire new departments or programs. For example, in 1958, Norma Gill was hired by Dr. Turnbull as the country's first enterostomal therapist. Although not a registered nurse, Mrs. Gill reported to Clinic Nursing for administrative purposes. The program grew to include additional therapists, some of whom were nurses, and also the world's first school of enterostomal therapy, established by Dr. Turnbull and Mrs. Gill.

Some of the Cleveland Clinic's new workers, for example, inhalation therapists and cardiac perfusionists, specialized in handling the new technical procedures and new equipment that were becoming integral to the delivery of health care. Others, like social workers and the chaplain, provided counseling, practical advice, and spiritual support to patients and their families. Technology was advancing, but so was awareness of patients' emotional and psychological needs. Nurses had to maintain a foothold in both camps, keeping up with the technical complexities of modern medical care while promoting their

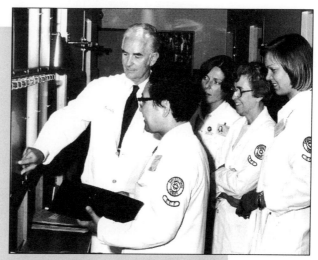

tomal therapist was educated to spend that time to the best possible effect, playing "not only an instructive role, but also a supportive one."

The Clinic's School of Enterostomal Therapy, established by Dr. Turnbull and Mrs. Gill in 1962, was the world's first. Most of the program's students were nurses, who came from all over North America and from other countries as well. In 1976, the school graduated its 200th student. By this time, the Clinic's ET staff numbered five: Mrs. Gill as program coordinator, registered nurses Joan Kerr (program chairman) and Rose McNeil, and L.P.N.s Marilyn Spencer and Pat Hill.

Therapists made preoperative visits, taught patients self-care after surgery, and followed their progress during outpatient check-ups. Twenty years later, the program continued teaching new therapists at the Rupert E. Turnbull School of Enterostomal Therapy, and provid-

A Japanese surgeon (foreground), the first physician to enter the Clinic's ET program, with Dr. Turnbull; registered nurse Joan Kerr, ET Program Director; Mrs. Gill; and another trainee, a German nurse, 1976

ing care to Cleveland Clinic patients. In a 1994 article in *Cleveland Clinic Nurse*, registered nurse Paula Erwin-Toth, Manager of ET Nursing and Director of ET Education, quoted the words of a recovering patient to his surgeon: "You may have saved my life, but it was the ET nurse who made it a life worth living."

patients' mental and emotional well-being. Nurses also had to work with, communicate with, and just plain get along with co-workers from other departments, both old and new.

Conflict and Cooperation

The Nursing and Dietary Departments, for instance, sometimes had difficulty in coordinating their work, at least in the postwar decades. In the simple but important task of routine food service to Hospital patients, the point where Dietary's responsibility ended and Nursing's began was not entirely clear. Passing trays to patients had originally been the job of nursing personnel, but was now handled by food service workers. Private duty nurses had traditionally made sure that patients were ready to eat and had the correct meals, and they fed those patients who were unable to feed themselves. But since fewer patients now had special nurses, the task of coordinating meal service fell to unit personnel.

The increased centralization of food preparation also affected meal delivery. Floor kitchens had been eliminated when a new centralized kitchen system, judged state-of-the-art by the food service industry, came on-line in 1956. The sheer distance between kitchen and unit made communications, not to mention keeping food hot, more difficult than before. The new system freed nursing personnel from tasks like preparing patients' breakfasts, but it complicated other things, like getting food for patients who were admitted to a unit too late to receive regular meal service. Not until the late 1960s did the placing of microwave ovens and refrigerators for food on the nursing units help make late tray service easier.

In 1956, the Director of the Dietary Department suggested that by making dietary serving teams entirely responsible for meals, "even to getting patients ready to eat," the patients would be assured of prompt service of hot food. When, in the course of the next few years, therapeutic dietitians were first stationed on each floor, and then "transferred the major part of their activities" to the nursing units, interdepartmental coordination seemed to improve. "This has been particularly helpful in enabling [dietitians] to work more closely with nursing," and also with physicians, and "to have closer contact with the patients and to handle problems more quickly before they become magnified."[109] But by 1967, the dietitians, whose primary responsibility was working with patients on special diets, did not really have time to check tray service as well, and so checking had to be done by delivery personnel. Margaret Foust, Director of the Dietary Department since 1957, felt that this was not an ideal situation.

> Checking of patients for tray delivery does not seem to me to belong in the dietary department. Dietary personnel do not have the medical knowledge of a patient's condition to even guess whether the patient should be eating - it is very frustrating when checking rooms to be barging in on doctors and patients in the process of examinations or changing dressings etc., however, a complete thorough room tray check cannot be accomplished unless you check each room and behind each curtain and closed door. Sometimes this becomes a very embarrassing situation for the patient as well as the person checking rooms. It seems to me much more advisable for someone in the medical end to do this checking.[110]

The problems of coordination between Nursing and Dietary were probably inherent in the system, rather than the fault of any one person or group of people. It seemed more efficient for the Nursing Department to turn full responsibility for meal service over to the Dietary Department, and it seemed more efficient for the Dietary Department to prepare food in a centralized kitchen. At the same time, however, this specialized division of labor also meant that the nursing unit had less direct control over food service to its patients.

One of the new departments that had to develop a collaborative relationship with the Nursing Department was Social Work. The Cleveland Clinic Foundation did not employ a social worker until 1966, when Medicare went into effect. It seems astonishing that a large urban medical center could have done without a social work department for so many years, until the atypical history of the Cleveland Clinic Hospital is considered.

Although the Cleveland Clinic had always provided a certain amount of uncompensated care, it did not trace its origins to the social welfare movement. Referring to the Clinic Hospital as a "hotel for the sick," the institution's founders had envisaged its patients as coming primarily from the middle class, and thus not in need of the kind of referral service — to community or charitable agencies for social or financial assistance — that the typical public or voluntary hospital provided through its social workers. Also, as a practical matter, the fact that many patients were from out of town would have made it difficult for a Cleveland-based social worker to refer them to the appropriate agencies.

By the 1960s, as medical treatment and the health care system grew more complex, Cleveland Clinic patients needed the kind of help that someone trained in social service work could give. To take one specific example, patients receiving chronic renal dialysis — an area of treatment in which the Clinic was a leader, running one of the first and largest programs in the country — struggled with chronic medical expenses and emotional strains as well as disease. To help these patients and their families, a kidney dialysis team grew up in the late 1960s which included physicians, nurses, and a social worker.

As sicker and sicker patients were treated and released from hospitals, convalescent patients were increasingly likely to need transfer to nursing homes or home health care, rather than simple discharge. As early as 1960, the Clinic Hospital began looking for a social worker. "During the year, we shall try to locate a trained Social Worker who understands the special problems of our type of Hospital. It has become obvious that this is a definite need for our institution; however, only if we are fortunate enough to find such a person, will we establish a Social Service Department."[111]

Not until 1966 was the Hospital's first social worker, Joan Hober, hired, primarily to assist with discharge planning. She also counseled patients and their families, generally at the family's or attending physician's request. She pointed out one of the reasons why even an institution like the Cleveland Clinic could no longer do without a social work department: "So many of our patients are middle-class and although educated, they are, for the most part, unaware of existing agencies and resources available to them."[112]

Miss Hober quickly recognized the need to involve nurses in her work. "Of particular interest is the increased number of nurses who have referred cases.

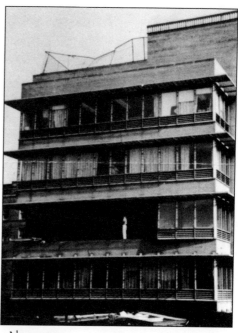

TORNADO DAMAGE, 1962
On August 20, 1962, a tornado touched down on the Cleveland Clinic campus, tearing off portions of the Hospital's H-building solariums. Fortunately, there were no injuries to patients or employees. The following winter was no better. A severe snowstorm hit northeastern Ohio, temporarily making the roads all but impassable. On the worst day, only two of the outpatient nurses were able to get to work; they floated the entire Clinic, possible because few patients showed up for their appointments.

Hemodialysis

The Cleveland Clinic was a leader in hemodialysis. Dr. Willem Kolff, head of the Department of Artificial Organs (lower photo, standing at left with his team), invented the artificial kidney in the Netherlands during WWII, and perfected its use during his tenure at the Cleveland Clinic.

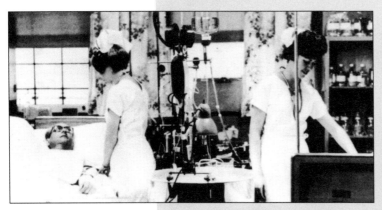

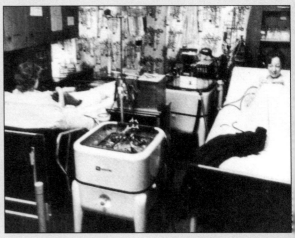

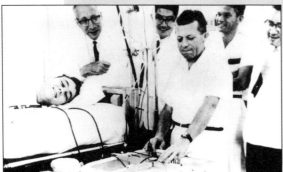

The compact machine he developed in the 1960s (upper right photo) made hemodialysis accessible to more patients across the country and the world. At the Cleveland Clinic, a new five-bed Hemodialysis unit opened on 6 North, tripling the Hospital's dialysis services (upper photos). A head nurse, an R.N., two dialysis technicians, and a supervisor staffed the unit.

This is an area which we have tried to develop, believing that nurses are frequently in a position to become more quickly aware of a problem or impending difficulty than other staff members who are not in as close contact with the patient." In 1970, the nurses on 4 South requested that the social workers (by now three in number) help them in their planning for the leukemia patients hospitalized on the unit, "who, because of their need for frequent hospitalization and expensive medications, have overwhelming financial and social problems." The Social Work Department participated in the Cleveland Clinic's School of Enterostomal Therapy by giving lectures on medical social work to the students.[113]

Shifting the Burden?

In the late 1960s, the Hospital implemented two more new programs, the clinical corpsman and Administrative Service Coordinator programs, specifically to help "take the burden off the nurse."

The clinical corpsman's appearance on the scene was perhaps the most visible impact of the Vietnam War upon the Cleveland Clinic. In 1967, Hospital administration began "to develop a nucleus of highly trained ex-military

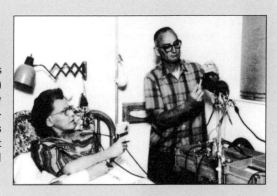

A teaching unit on the Hospital's second floor (shown here in 1969) prepared patients and family members to carry out home dialysis. Nurses were key members of a multidisciplinary team that offered care, instruction, and support to dialysis patients.

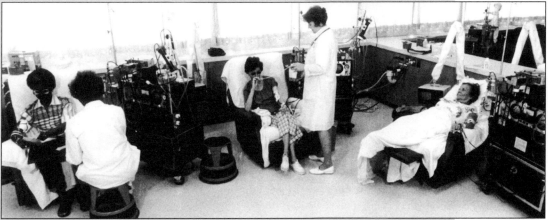

The opening of the outpatient West Side Dialysis Center (shown here in 1979), staffed by nurses and technicians, helped accommodate the increasing number of dialysis patients.

corpsmen as a means to assist our professional staff" in technical areas like cardiovascular intensive care, kidney dialysis, and inhalation therapy. In particular, "these young men supplemented the work of the Intensive Care nurses" by performing some of the technical tasks integral to the critical care setting, which might otherwise have been done by nurses.[114]

The Cleveland Clinic Hospital had started a similar program before. Immediately following the Second World War, its administrators had taken advantage of the availability of ex-servicemen trained as medics, hiring them to supplement the critically short-handed nursing staff. This program soon came to an end through attrition. Administrators of the 1960s, seeing a special niche for the corpsmen opening out of the growing need for technically skilled personnel, hired veterans not just as additional hands but as "formidable resources," with "the capacity to learn a variety of techniques rapidly."[115]

The word "corpsman" was itself telling. The program gave men an opportunity to work on the nursing unit at a time when male R.N.s and L.P.N.s were still relatively rare. Unless corpsmen attended nursing school — which some eventually did — they did not become nurses. But, by "supplementing" the work of nurses, they gained the opportunity to make careers in patient care.

The Continuing Education instructors in the Nursing Department, who conducted part of the corpsmen's training, found that "the gentlemen were very interested, attentive, intelligent and a pleasure to teach."[116]

On the whole, this second trial of clinical corpsmen was considerably more successful than the first, although it, too, had its problems. Administrators and physicians became concerned that the program had "developed a Physicians Assistant tinge," and tried to steer it back toward its original direction: "a patient care emphasis, concentrating on the Intensive Care areas."[117] Despite this, by 1970 Mr. Harding was wondering if the corpsmen might not be better transferred to the Clinic to assist the medical staff there.

The Administrative Services Coordinator program began in 1968, the year after the first clinical corpsmen were hired. This program aimed to release nurses, in particular head nurses, from the job of coordinating work with the now numerous hospital service departments, and to alleviate or prevent problems like the ones between Dietary and Nursing. The Hospital had already, in 1965, hired an evening administrator for a similar purpose at the supervisory level, to assume the after-hours administrative responsibility that had previously fallen to the lot of the evening nursing supervisor. To fill the coordinator positions, the Hospital again looked to the military medical corps for recruits.

> For several years we have worked to implement the "Ward Manager" concept used by a few hospitals, wherein a person trained in administrative techniques relieves the head nurse of problems in connection with other departments which in turn gives her more time to supervise the direct patient care activities of nurses, practical nurses, and aides. We were fortunate in having Mr. Cook develop this program, and two young men recently discharged from the Army Medical Administrative Corps have been hired. In order to allay the suspicions of nurses against the term "manager" we call these men "Administrative Services Coordinators."[118]

The administration was perhaps too pessimistic in predicting that nurses would be suspicious of these new helpers. Isabelle Muller stated that the coordinators were "well received" on 3 South and 5 South, the first units where they were introduced. James Harding agreed. "While several large hospitals throughout the country are using a similar approach, we know of no place where nursing has accepted these men as well as in this hospital."[119]

By 1970, 13 coordinators — all men — were on roll, supervised by the first individual hired under the program, Joseph Lazorchak. The day men were each assigned one to three nursing units, and the three evening coordinators worked one, two, or three floors. "I find myself becoming increasingly more dependent upon them for implementation and surveillance of new procedures and administrative decisions," declared Hospital Assistant Administrator Gilbert Cook, who oversaw the program. In that year, the coordinators took on the specific charge of coordinating the work of the Admitting Department and the patient care units to expedite admissions, discharges, and transfers, and they assumed responsibility for maintaining the floor stock of parenteral solutions. The program also served as a hatchery for embryo managers. "The program is a fertile area to fill supervisory positions in other areas as they occur," wrote Mr. Lazorchak in 1971. He himself was planning to enter graduate school in hospital administration.[120]

However well-intentioned and effective both the coordinator and clinical corpsmen programs may have been, it was possible to see them as threats to the status of nurses within the organization, and to opportunities for career development for nurses. "Getting back to the bedside" might also be interpreted to mean giving up administrative power and losing touch with technology, if other employees were to take over from nurses in these areas. And since for some years all employees in both coordinator and clinical corpsman positions were exclusively male, the division of labor might have seemed based on gender stereotyping.

As it turned out, management and technical opportunities for nurses generally continued to increase over the following years, rather than otherwise. And for at least some nurses, moving away from technical procedures and administrative detail would indeed prove a liberating process, freeing them to concentrate on optimizing their patients' mental and emotional as well as physical outcomes.

"The Focal Point for Patient Care"

No one ever doubted that nurses had a central position among all the employees from various departments who cared for the patients of Clinic physicians. Just as Barney Crile had acknowledged the crucial roles of Emma Barr and Lou Adams in making it possible for his father to perform so many thyroidectomies in the 1920s; just as in the 1940s the Administrative Board had realized that without enough nurses to keep open enough beds the whole Cleveland Clinic structure would crumble; so administrators in the 1960s knew that nurses played a key part in the institution.

"This department provides the focal point for patient care," declared James Harding. "So many aspects of the Foundation revolve around this department that the functions of nursing have tremendous impact." In 1970, the Clinic hoped to cut nurse recruitment expenses by relying more on its own employees and less on outside contractors like public relations agencies: "However, the economic impact of Nursing on the Foundation is so great, we must let nothing interfere with the professionalism of recruitment."[121]

Isabelle Muller spoke for her own department: "In order for the Medical Staff of the Cleveland Clinic Hospital to continue its present service, and in view of the planned expansion of that service, it is necessary that the Nursing Department maintain an adequate nursing staff which will provide nursing care commensurate in quality and dedication to that of the Foundation physicians."[122]

But the importance of nursing could not be calculated on a balance sheet or listed on a personnel roster. "The Nursing Department is the one that the patient looks to for whatever happens to them,"observed Mr. Harding. "Even though the actual work is done by other departments, the report of failure is directed by the patient to nursing."[123] Ultimately, as Sophia Larsen had pointed-ed out, the nurse was responsible to the patient.

The Convalescent Unit

The history of the Cleveland Clinic Hospital's Convalescent Unit illustrates just how crucial nurses were to patient care. In 1957, at "the suggestion of Dr. [Barney] Crile and others," the Hospital had opened its Convalescent Unit on 5 Central "utilizing no nurses. If this works, and it must, it could set the pattern for future expansion." The unit admitted convalescent patients, who had no need for "professional nursing care," but still had to be hospitalized "for

IN THE 1960s
At the beginning of the decade, the Hospital appointed its first chaplain. A Family Lounge opened for families of patients in surgery and Constant Care. In 1962, Room 768 of the pediatric unit was opened as a constant care room for pediatric cardiac catheterization patients. In 1964, cardiac arrest carts were placed on each Hospital floor. In 1965, more than 60 percent of the Hospital's patients came from outside the area. The number of open-heart cases cared for in Surgical Intensive Care rose from 323 to 406. The average length of stay for psychiatric patients was 26 days. The Operating Room purchased three fiberoptic lights, for the chest and ENT services. Deemed "unsatisfactory," they were all returned to the manufacturer the following year. Administrators planned to close the larger Hospital wards in 1967 because insurers favored semi-private accommodations. As of 1968, an average of 47 laboratory tests were performed on each Hospital patient. Scrubs, now worn by the growing staff of intensive care unit personnel, were "a noticeable item" in the Laundry Department's production by 1969. Hospital-supplied white uniforms were changed over from all-cotton to synthetic blends. Nurses received a starting salary of $650 a month, with a $150 differential for shifts or intensive care.

one reason or another." The idea was not entirely unprecedented. Convalescent Clinic patients had sometimes been housed in nearby buildings like the Bolton Square Hotel. During the Second World War, when the Clinic Hospital could not find enough nurses to keep all of its beds open, the Administrative Board had considered reopening the closed second floor for patients who needed minimal or no nursing, such as patients recovering from some types of eye surgery.[124]

In the "more relaxed atmosphere" of the new Convalescent Unit (soon moved to the 28 beds "of our best physical facilities on 5 South") patients were to take their own medications as per doctors' orders, bathe, and otherwise care for themselves, and be permitted "to move about as in their own homes."[125] The unit did not have registered nurse staffing, but a practical nurse worked the evening shift and took temperatures and pulses. In the daytime, a ward secretary handled clerical and receptionist duties, and an aide made beds. Another aide provided solo coverage on the 11 p.m. to 7 a.m. shift.

Apparently the self-medication policy was less than successful, because only a year later, Mabel Selfe listed as one of her goals around-the-clock R.N. staffing of the unit. Since Hospital policy did not at this time permit practical nurses to give medications, only R.N.s would do. The goal of registered nurse staffing could not be immediately met, partly because at the same time the Hospital was opening more constant care beds, and additional nurses were channeled in that direction.

In 1964, when the unit reopened in its third home (18 beds on 8 South), it had the following staff: on days, an R.N., an aide, and a ward secretary; evenings, a practical nurse and an aide; nights, a lone practical nurse. Even that was not enough. In 1970 Ruth Elmenthaler, the Assistant Director of Nursing for Patient Care, pointed out some of the problems with the convalescent divisions (of which there were now two). Most of the patients were cardiac cases, either cardiac catheterization, or pre- or postoperative. "Many third day post-operative cardiac patients present problems resulting from complex doctor's orders and a need for close observation (a high frequency of triple pages occur on these divisions)." When the R.N. came on duty in the morning she had to try and receive the shift report from the night L.P.N. and give early morning medications to preoperative patients at the same time. "The practical nurses are placed in a position of responsibility beyond their preparations; physicians...seem to ...expect performance similar to that of an experienced RN. Feelings run high amongst the LPN group; it has been impossible to find an individual to be oriented to 6 West." Miss Muller and Mr. Harding both agreed that putting this kind of burden on the practical nurses simply was not workable, nor was it fair. "Our hospital has no patients who can be cared for without [registered] nurse staffing."[126]

National and International Reputation

The importance that nursing personnel had in the patient's mind and the quality of nursing care that patients received would be reflected in the institution's public image. Mabel Selfe had said that she hoped to "promote better Public Relations by improving our Nursing Care."[127] The Cleveland Clinic was regaining the high profile it had enjoyed in the days of the founders, when Dr. George Crile's fame had attracted patients from all over the country and even the world. In 1956 the Clinic Hospital was the third largest in Cleveland, but had one of the busiest operating rooms in the country — not surprising, since its census showed a two to one ratio of surgical to medical patients.

In 1957, Sophia Larsen prepared a graph that showed a sharp increase in the number of operations after 1954. "This may be significant in that many of our surgeons enjoy national and international reputations because of constantly improved techniques," commented Mr. Harding. But, he added, "Bigness must never be a substitute for quality of care! This is the never-ending struggle our hospital faces as we expand to keep step with medical progress. The patient must be 'number one' always or voluntary hospitals will lose their reason for existence."[128]

Over the following years, surgeons certainly felt that the quality of the Operating Room Department was not measured by number of procedures alone. In 1966, Dr. Hoerr and the physician staff's Surgical Committee expressed the opinion that "Mrs. Martha Hoffman continues to run what is probably the smoothest department in the country."[129] The department continued to grow busier. On October 23, 1970, 79 patients underwent procedures in the Clinic Hospital operating suite, the record number to that date.

Due to the serious nature of many of the cases admitted, the average stay for Clinic Hospital patients was relatively long: approximately 10 days throughout most of the 1950s and 1960s. Patients and nursing staff had more of a chance to get to know each other. The Cresap, McCormick report had noted that although, statistically, the number of nursing hours per patient-day seemed low on the general medical-surgical nursing units, this was because housekeeping, dietary, messenger, and other functions, which in many hospitals were performed by nursing personnel, were handled at least in part by other departments at the Clinic Hospital. Nursing hours represented direct patient care.

In the Constant Care Units, statistics clearly showed that patients received intensive nursing care. In 1963, 1,652 patients, making up 10 percent of the Hospital's admissions, were cared for in these units. Each patient received 12 to 14 hours of nursing care per day, "or more than one nurse for every two patients - a phenomenal ratio....To our knowledge, few other hospitals in the world are giving equal care in this area."[130]

At this time, a Constant Care Unit in the Clinic Hospital required about seven to nine times the number of registered nurses needed to staff a general unit of the same size. But even this "phenomenal ratio" might not be enough for some of the critically ill patients admitted to the Hospital. "Our hospital must provide the most intensive nursing care possible, even on a one nurse to one patient ratio in some of the new medical discoveries. Costs in this area will skyrocket..., but balanced against the patient care required, it is a must here."[131]

Expanding Programs in Education

The Continuing Education office had the mission of assisting Cleveland Clinic nurses to "carry out our complicated pattern of care." By 1969, it offered both management training and clinical skills courses to nurses. "Monthly programs are conducted in each area of nursing skills, such as cardiovascular surgery, orthopedics, etc. Our hospital is unlike most, and nurses must be trained in skills needed to cope with the unusually complex medical and surgical patients who are admitted by our nationally known medical staff."

THE PRIVATE UNIT
The Cleveland Clinic Hospital had always set aside areas for the accommodation of private patients. In the original Hospital building, there were private rooms on every floor, plus suites with private baths and extra rooms on the third through sixth floors. Extra beds placed in rooms on the fifth and sixth floors during WWII concentrated private care on the third and fourth floors; eventually, nursing unit 4 West became the Hospital's "private" medical-surgical unit. For many years, beginning in 1966, Margaret Finefrock (center photograph on cover) managed the Private Unit as head nurse. The unit's patients included many people who had come from other parts of the U.S. and abroad, drawn to Cleveland by the national and international reputation of the Clinic's medical staff. Clinic physicians themselves often stayed on the unit when hospitalized. Miss Finefrock's management helped ensure that the unit's reputation matched that of the institution.

Decentralized in-service programs were offered to nursing personnel on the intensive care units.[132]

In 1969, the Department of Nursing entered into an affiliation with Cuyahoga Community College to provide clinical experience to students in its two-year associate degree nursing program. The Clinic now had affiliations with institutions offering three different types of nursing education: the B.S.N. program at St. John College; the associate degree at Cuyahoga Community College; and the Jane Addams School of Practical Nursing.

By offering tuition assistance, the Cleveland Clinic encouraged its employees to work toward degrees at area schools. A career ladder program paid for courses leading to R.N. licensure for practical nurses and other employees in Nursing, the Operating Room, and Central Service. Central Service Supervisor Eleanor Reilly took particular pride in the employees in her department who were working toward degrees, often mentioning them in her annual reports. Ken Wilson, R.N., appointed Assistant Supervisor of Central Service in 1970, was a notable example. Mr. Wilson was first employed at the Hospital as an orderly in the Operating Room in 1958, where he worked until breaking his ankle while playing baseball with the Clinic's team in 1965, according to the *Cleveland Clinic Newsletter.*

> Ken had a break in more ways than one, however, because in the six weeks he spent convalescing he got to know himself....He came back to temporary duties as a clerk in Central Service in October, 1965 and by December had proved his value in that department and was asked to stay, healed ankle and all.

> In September, 1966, Ken kept the promise he had made to himself during his convalescence — he enrolled at Cuyahoga Community College as a part-time student.[133]

After obtaining a government grant, he became a full-time student, and then received a scholarship, but remained a full-time employee as well. He graduated with an associate degree in nursing in 1970.

Although the Cleveland Clinic did not have a nursing school, it did start a school for nurse anesthetists in the winter of 1968-69. Since 1950 the Foundation had paid for nurses to receive training in anesthesia at other institutions, as part of its effort to obtain qualified nurse anesthetists. In that year Stella Taylor, R.N., enrolled in the Mayo Clinic's two-year program; in 1951, Mary Feran, R.N., the Recovery Room Supervisor, entered the one-year course at Western Reserve University. Both nurses returned to the staff of the Anesthesiology Department in 1952, which at that time consisted of 10 nurse anesthetists, 2 staff physicians (including Dr. Hale, the director), and 4 fellows. In the same year, Marietta DelCorso Portzer, C.R.N.A., who would be instrumental in founding the Clinic's own school, joined the staff.

From the Cleveland Clinic's point of view, "Paying a small stipend appears to be the best way to encourage nurses to study anesthesia and return to us. In this way, we...have a staff familiar with the hospital."[134] By 1964, the Anesthesiology Department had 18 nurse anesthetists on its staff, with 3 nurses attending anesthesia school.

The Clinic's own School of Nurse Anesthesia was instituted as a two-year certificate program. It was founded by Mrs. Portzer, Audrey Spence, C.R.N.A.,

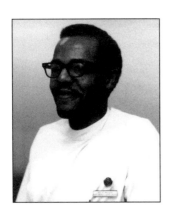

KEN WILSON
Mr. Wilson began his career at the Cleveland Clinic in 1958, as an orderly in the Operating Room. Within 12 years he had become a registered nurse, after graduation from Cuyahoga Community College with an A.D. degree, and had climbed the career ladder to the position of Assistant Supervisor of Central Service. In 1973, after Eleanor Reilly was promoted to Director, Mr. Wilson became Supervisor and LuVerna Eiland Assistant Supervisor of Central Service. The accomplishments of the department were, in Miss Reilly's words, a result of the "joint effort" of this team.

and Carl Wasmuth, M.D., Chairman of the Department of Anesthesi-ology from 1967 to 1969, a president of the American Society of Anesthesiologists, and, as Chairman of the Board of Governors, the Foundation's chief executive officer from 1969 to 1976. As of January 1969 the program had its first 9 students enrolled; a year later there were 17 students. The first class graduated in December 1970. "It was fitting that Dr. Wasmuth spoke to the graduates, since it was he who started this school, in answer to our former chronic shortage of these professionals, even though it meant incurring possible dis-pleasure of the anesthesiology profession."[135] The Clinic hired most of the first graduates.

From Births to Bypasses

By this time, the Clinic Hospital was admitting a large number of cardiovascular patients. For example, in 1965 the Surgical Constant Care Unit cared for 406 open-heart cases alone. In 1967 special care became more specialized, when the opening of the Cardiovascular Unit in effect departmentalized the Surgical Constant Care Unit. The new self-contained unit employed personnel from both the Nursing Department and the Operating Room. This concept treated the sur-gical procedure and the postoperative period as points along a patient care continuum in a single clinical area.

In a sequence that reflected demographic trends and the birth of Medicare, the Cardiovascular Unit replaced the defunct obstetrics unit on the Hospital's sixth floor. The Clinic had started its obstetrics unit too late, just before the baby boom began to abate. The number of deliveries in the unit peaked at 821 in 1960, and thereafter declined, to 732 in 1965, the last full year of service. Had the Hospital not begun admitting patients from the nearby Florence Crit-tenton Home (a home for unmarried mothers) in 1959 after the latter eliminat-ed its own medical facilities, the decrease would have been even more noticeable. Births to patients from the Crittenton Home rose from 15 to 20 percent of the total between 1963 and 1965. The 100-and-some annual deliv-eries added by the contract with the home did not fill all of the unit's empty beds, however. In 1964 "carefully screened 'clean' gynecology cases" were admitted to the unit, bringing the occupancy rate close to 80 percent.[136] The Clinic closed its obstetrics unit in 1966. A side effect of this was that the Gyne-cology Department lost its fellows. Subsequently, in the outpatient Clinic, an L.P.N. (under the tutelage of the department's chairman, Dr. James S. Krieger) began taking patients' full written histories, a task not customarily part of Clinic nursing duties at this time.

The unit's closing probably did nothing to damage the Clinic's growing national and international reputation. Many community hospitals had obstetric units. A world-class cardiovascular unit was a far more valuable asset for a tertiary referral center. The *Cleveland Clinic Newsletter* described the new facility shortly after its opening:

> The new unit is thought to be the only one in the United States that has combined the Surgical Suite of three Operating Rooms with a 39-bed post operative facility. It is staffed by a team of surgeons, anesthesiologists,

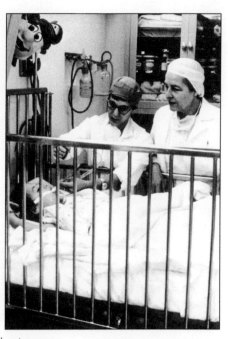

A CONSTANT PRESENCE
Throughout its history, the Cleveland Clinic employed nurse anesthetists, giving advanced nurse practitioners a presence at the institution from the begin-ning. In 1969, Marietta DelCorso Portzer, C.R.N.A. (at left in photo-graph), Audrey Spence, C.R.N.A., and Dr. Carl Wasmuth, Chairman of the Board of Governors, founded the Clinic's School of Nurse Anesthesia.

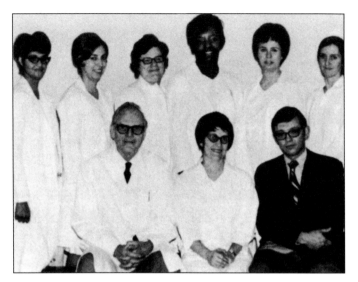

nurses, technicians and other specialist personnel all specifically trained in some phase of surgical and post-surgical care of the cardiac patient.

The patient is placed under anesthesia and intubated first in the Induction Room....The patient then goes to the Operating Room. From there he goes directly across the hall or next door to the large Intensive Care Division. This has 15 beds. It has its own full nursing desk. Nurses are in constant attendance in the room, besides modern controls at each bedside to monitor changes in pulse or blood pressure. Oxygen, suction and four electrical outlets for special equipment are at the head of each bed.

**SCHOOL OF
NURSE ANESTHESIA**

The Cleveland Clinic School of Nurse Anesthesia was a two-year certificate program for graduate nurses. The first class graduated at the end of 1970. In this photograph, Dr. J. Kenneth Potter, Chairman of the Division of Anesthesiology, Mrs. Portzer, and Hospital Assistant Administrator James Zucker are seated in the front row. Standing behind them are the graduates: (left to right) Marie Busby, Ruth Horning, Rosemary Wettach, Elizabeth Gates, Eileen Schefft, Jan Klinke, and Jessie Keith.

From Intensive Care, the recovering patient goes around the corner to the Intermediate Care section. When his condition warrants, he goes to the minimal care area. This is the concept of progressive patient care.[137]

The article went on to note that the "Clinic group probably does more heart surgery for acquired heart disease than any other institution"— usually 7 or 8 operations a day and, with the new unit, up to 10.[138] Clinic surgeons and cardiologists were by now renowned as leaders in the treatment of coronary artery disease, and patients came from great distances to undergo bypass and other operations in the Clinic's Cardiovascular Unit.

On September 4, 1968, the unit's surgical team performed Ohio's first successful heart transplant; the second quickly followed, on December 16.

A Faster Pace

The opening of the Cardiovascular Unit gave other clinical services more opportunity to use the Surgical Intensive Care Unit (SICU), and also made some reorganization of nursing services necessary: "As a result of the transfer of patients to 6 South, the number of nurses left in the Surgical Intensive Care unit was also diminished." Therefore, it was decided to combine under one head nurse the staffs of the SICU and the Recovery Room, "for better utilization of personnel and [to] provide continuity of care." The Recovery Room was remodeled, incorporating a new staging area where patients would receive preoperative medications. The In and Out Room was renamed the Ambulatory Care Room.[139]

The Medical Intensive Care Unit (MICU) also benefited from the wave of hospital remodeling, moving to a 13-bed unit on 3 East in 1968, which included three beds that could be separated from the main area by sliding glass doors, for peritoneal dialysis patients "and for patients who need quiet surroundings." The new facilities were said to have improved staff morale "immeasurably." Another bright spot for the ICUs was the excellent performance of the licensed practical nurses assigned to both the Cardiovascular and Surgical Intensive Care Units to supplement the stretched-too-thin R.N. staffing.[140]

In 1969, staffing dropped to such a low level in the SICU during the summer that the administration decided to offer a $150 per month "bonus," or differential, to R.N.s, and $112.50 to L.P.N.s working in intensive care units: "While this created a temporary 'tempest in a teapot,' it subsided, since we also gave a similar bonus for working evenings or nights on the medical-surgical division." Also, "individualized" orientation programs for the intensive care units seemed to increase nursing staff satisfaction.[141]

For these or other reasons, the situation changed rapidly. By the end of 1969, the SICU/Recovery Room was again well-staffed, although with "young and not experienced" nurses.[142] At the beginning of 1971, all intensive care units were for the first time fully staffed, and now with experienced nurses. There was actually a waiting list for nurses wishing to transfer to the ICUs. Unfortunately, concentrating experienced nurses in the intensive care units left a higher proportion of inexperienced nurses on the other units.

On the Cardiovascular Unit, nearly half — 820 of 1,504 in 1969 — of the patients were open-heart cases. The mortality rate was 5 percent in that year. The census (882 in 1969) on the SICU was divided more or less evenly into neurosurgical, vascular, and "other" patients. The MICU cared for 2,667 patients in 1969: 370 for peritoneal dialysis, 260 for cardiac problems, and the rest for a variety of diagnoses including diabetic acidosis, respiratory disease, gastrointestinal bleeding, and drug intoxication. In 1971, cardiac medical patients received their own unit when the Hospital opened its fourth intensive care area, the four-bed Coronary Care Unit, on 4 East.

The physical and mental demands of the job could take their toll on nurses. One nurse described her first day in the Cardiovascular Unit as frightening: "I had never experienced patients like that with so many tubes and machines to watch." Greater numbers of severely ill patients put pressure on employees throughout the institution, not only those in the intensive care units: "Every department experiences greater activity when sicker patients occupy our beds." As a tertiary care center, the Clinic cared for a great number of very sick patients. Everyone recognized that "the fast pace" could cause "tensions that many nurses find overwhelming." And the pace showed no signs of slackening.[143]

The innovations of the 1950s and 1960s had not been a sudden revolution; they had gone step by step. In 1950 the Nursing Department had considered employing "colored aides"; in the following years African-Americans actually were hired as aides, and then as L.P.N.s, and R.N.s, as well. By the early 1970s African-American nurses had been able to attain positions at the head nurse and supervisory levels. In 1954 the first class of student nurses from St. John College spent a few weeks visiting the pediatrics unit as observers. This soon grew into a full-fledged affiliation, with students observing and working in all areas of nursing; the Clinic affiliated with a practical nurse school in 1965, and with an associate degree program in 1969. Meanwhile, Hospital administration continued to entertain the possibility of opening its own nursing school. In 1957 the hospital tried, unsuccessfully, to separate medical and surgical patients onto separate floors; in the same year it opened a constant care unit staffed by private duty nurses. Gradually, some general medical-surgical nursing units did become specialized, first for the care of dermatology patients, and next for urology and gastroenterology patients. At the same time, several different intensive care units developed out of the original constant care area, including two units — Cardiovascular Intensive Care and Coronary Care — devoted to cardiac patients.

As hospital construction added beds, year by year, and medical specialization gradually but steadily added new medical and surgical services, the Cleveland Clinic hired more nursing personnel to care for more patients. The Hospital Nursing Department, Clinic Nursing, and the Operating Room Department all grew in size. These nursing areas also evolved, expanding the diversity of their personnel and changing the way that they did their work.

The changes of the 1950s and 1960s were not a brand-new beginning, like the founding of the Clinic in 1921; nor were they an improvised response to a near-impossible situation, as had been the case during the desperately short-staffed years of the Second World War. They were primarily managed changes — reasoned, sober responses developed after problems had been identified and solutions suggested. In the remaining decades of the twentieth century, change itself became both problem and solution.

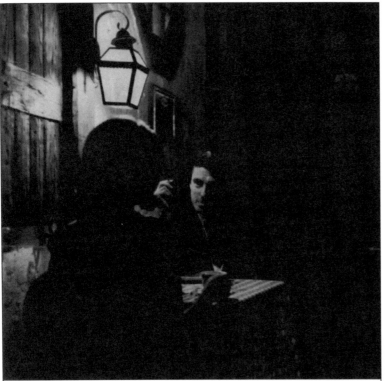

Do you flip for escargot, veal parmesan and wine after an evening of Debussy?

(OR A HOT DOG AND MUSTARD AT THE OLD BALL GAME)

Nursing at the Cleveland Clinic Hospital blends together the finest things from two fine worlds . . . on duty, challenging work alongside the very best medical talent . . . off duty, the world you wish to make in a city noted for an abundance of good things. You're a hop, skip and jump away from your favorite diversion while satisfying your appetite for professional growth and achievement. Clip the coupon and put yourself in the picture. Bon appetite!

The Cleveland Clinic Hospital
2050 East 93rd Street, Cleveland, Ohio 44106

TO: Director of Nursing — The Cleveland Clinic Hospital
2050 East 93rd Street, Cleveland, Ohio 44106

PUT ME IN THE PICTURE!

Please send me your new brochure.

Name

Address

City

State _____ Zip

☐ I am a registered nurse
☐ I am a student nurse. I will graduate

(date)

AJN 4 68

PUT YOURSELF IN THIS PICTURE
In 1968, the Department of Nursing hired a full-time recruitment director and, with assistance from public relations firm Edward Howard & Co., mounted an ambitious recruitment drive, complete with new convention displays, films, brochures, and advertisements. This ad, placed in national nursing journals, invited nurses to put themselves "in the picture."

5

Changing to Manage

*Change itself is not new, but it is the pace of change
which dramatically affects all of us....To succeed in change,
you do not need to like it. You must anticipate it,
understand it, immerse yourself in it, and move on.*

— Sharon Coulter, Chairman of the
Division of Nursing, during Nurses' Week, 1993

Cleveland and the Clinic Foundation

In the 1960s, the governing boards of The Cleveland Clinic Foundation had
a decision to make as they pondered new construction: "whether or not to
abandon the inner city location of the Clinic and move the entire operation
into or even beyond the eastern suburbs of Cleveland."[1]

The years between 1966 and 1980 have been called a period of "loss of confidence" for the city of Cleveland: "Cleveland was an aging city where nothing
seemed to go right, where even the river caught fire." This period began with
the Hough riots and culminated in 1978, when Cleveland became the first
major U.S. city to default since the Great Depression. The financial crisis came
about partly because of the city's loss of jobs and population in the preceding
decades. Cleveland had gone from the nation's sixth-largest city in 1940 to its
eighteenth-largest by 1980. Whole blocks of deteriorating buildings had been
first abandoned, and then demolished. Businesses left for the suburbs; manufacturing plants moved to the Sun Belt or even overseas.[2]

Amid this urban flight, the Cleveland Clinic ultimately stayed where it was.
It did set up a satellite in the Sun Belt when Cleveland Clinic Florida opened in
1988. Its International Center and contacts and affiliations with health care
organizations as far away as Istanbul, Turkey, gave it a presence overseas. But
the main campus remained where it had always been, inside the city limits of
Cleveland, and, in fact, grew substantially over the period. This growth had its
critics; they declared that the Clinic was contributing to neighborhood deteri-
oration by acquiring and razing houses and business blocks to make room for
its own expansion. An east-side businessman put up billboards denouncing
the Cleveland Clinic on this account. The overall effect of the Clinic's expansion, however, was positive. It provided additional jobs for people in the
neighborhood, the city, and the metropolitan area.

During the 1990s, civic boosters and some outside observers began to hail
Cleveland as a "comeback city," based on the completion of the much publicized Gateway sports complex and the Rock and Roll Hall of Fame. Neighborhood renewal projects also gave hope for the future. The continued presence
of major health care institutions like the Cleveland Clinic had helped the city
through the difficult years and gave additional grounds for optimism.

The growing importance of health care in Cleveland's economy in the second half of the twentieth century reflected its growing importance in the

nation's economy. Between 1960 and 1975, the number of beds in Cuyahoga County's general medical-surgical and maternity hospitals grew 30 percent, from 6,636 to 9,666. The average cost per patient day in Cleveland hospitals rose tenfold, from $28.40 in 1957 to $268 in 1980. Meanwhile, the relative importance of manufacturing in the city's economy had declined. In 1950, 42 percent of employed Clevelanders worked in manufacturing; by 1980, more than 70 percent had service jobs.[3]

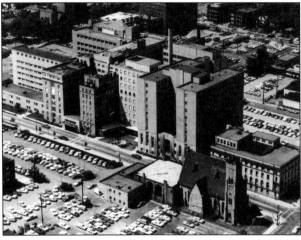

THE CLEVELAND CLINIC, 1968

Poised for another round of expansion in the 1970s and 1980s, the Cleveland Clinic stayed in the inner city rather than moving to the suburbs. Decisions to acquire and build on surrounding property were sometimes controversial, but represented a commitment to the future of the community. By the mid-1990s, the campus shown in this photograph would be ringed by newly constructed buildings and parking garages, and The Cleveland Clinic Foundation would be Cuyahoga County's largest non-government employer.

Health care jobs generally did not pay as well as manufacturing jobs. They did not necessarily replace manufacturing jobs, since a majority of health care workers were women, while most factory workers were men. Health care jobs, however, had one great advantage — they could not be exported. People from northeastern Ohio would not go to the Sun Belt, much less overseas, for medical care when they could get "world-class" care at Cleveland hospitals and outpatient clinics. On the contrary, Cleveland's medical centers — and the Cleveland Clinic in particular — attracted patients from beyond the metropolitan area. The Clinic's reputation for excellence in areas like cardiovascular care brought patients to Cleveland from around the world.

The continually escalating amount of money spent on health care resulted in pressures from third-party payors, most notably the U.S. government, for hospitals, physicians and other health care providers to control costs. The Cleveland Clinic, like most providers, underwent a period of belt-tightening in the 1980s. Everywhere, cost containment had significant effects on individual programs, which might be cut, and individual employees, who might lose their jobs. On a larger scale, some hospitals closed and others merged. But overall, health care maintained its important role in the national and local economies.

By the 1980s the Cleveland Clinic Hospital was the area's largest hospital. The Cleveland Clinic Foundation was one of greater Cleveland's largest employers, outranking most manufacturers. By far the greatest number of Clinic employees worked in nursing: as registered and practical nurses, as nursing assistants, and as unit and administrative secretaries.

Woman's Profession

A factor less measurable than economic trends (although in some ways linked to them) also had great importance for the nursing profession at this time — the women's movement, which was in a sense reborn during the social ferment of the 1960s. Books like Betty Friedan's *The Feminine Mystique* (1963) and Kate Millett's *Sexual Politics* (1969) helped create the ideological foundations for feminist activism. Demands for greater political equity and equal opportunity in the workplace followed. In 1971 the Supreme Court, in a landmark decision on gender discrimination in hiring, declared that employers could not refuse to hire women with preschool children unless the same standard was applied to men. In 1972 the Senate passed the Equal Rights Amendment and sent it on to the states for ratification. It was quickly approved by a majority of states but ultimately failed to obtain ratification by the 38 states necessary for it to become law. Nonetheless, progress in the workplace continued. Women gained admission to more occupations and higher positions, although their wages continued to lag behind those of men, and some analysts believed that a "glass ceiling" barred the advance of women beyond a certain level in the corporate world.

Although nursing was becoming less strictly a "women's profession" as more men entered the field, female nurses still greatly outnumbered male nurses, and nursing was influenced by the women's movement. Nurses increasingly began to examine their place in the health care system, and in some cases to demand greater autonomy in the practice of their profession. The number of advanced practice nurses (A.P.N.s), including certified registered nurse anesthetists (C.R.N.A.s), clinical nurse specialists (C.N.S.s), nurse practitioners (N.P.s) and certified nurse-midwives (C.N.M.s), grew. An article published in the *Yale Law Review* in 1992, which drew a great deal of attention, suggested that using A.P.N.s to provide more of the nation's primary health care could both improve quality and decrease cost.

Decentralization...

As the 1970s opened, most of the Cleveland Clinic's nurses worked in the Hospital Department of Nursing, as had been the case since 1924. They were represented by the head of the department, who since the mid-1960s had held the title of Hospital Assistant Administrator/Director of Nursing Services. That position was abolished in 1971, as part of a general reorganization of the Clinic's administrative structure.

In September 1971, James Harding resigned as Hospital Administrator. The Cleveland Clinic's Board of Governors appointed a committee "to study the administrative needs of the hospital and to recommend changes which would

be consistent with the overall administrative scheme of the Foundation." The new organizational chart grouped hospital departments within two divisions, Management Services and Patient Care Services, the latter initially headed by James Zucker. Made up of the Nursing Department and other departments "involved in direct patient contact," the Division of Patient Care Services had more than 1,100 employees.[4]

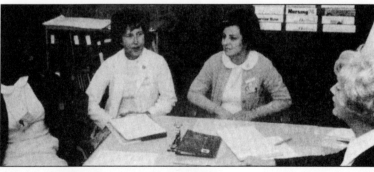

Hospital Nursing administration was decentralized: "The new organization places the authority and responsibility for nursing care of patients under seven Directors of Clinical Nursing; the old positions of Director of Nursing and Assistant Director of Nursing-Patient Care having been eliminated."[5]

The seven Directors of Clinical Nursing (also known as Nursing Directors, Clinical Directors, or Area Directors) administered the seven clinical areas into which Hospital Nursing had been divided on the basis of geography and clinical specialty. Doris Martin, R.N., was in charge of Area I, which included the Nursing Office, Psychiatry on 7 West, and the Emergency Room. Area II, headed by Sue Shoptaw, R.N., consisted of Intensive Care — Surgical Intensive Care/Recovery Room/Ambulatory Care Room, Medical Intensive Care,

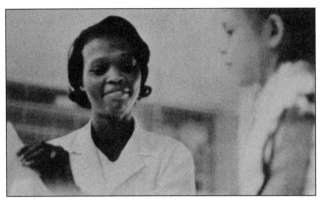

ALMA DAVIS
Ms. Davis, who had been head nurse of the Cleveland Clinic's pioneering Hemodialysis Unit since the 1960s, was appointed Clinical Director for the sixth floor nursing area, which included Hemodialysis. She also oversaw the Clinic Inn units: Dermatology, Intermediate Nursing Care, and two units for overnight cardiac catheterization patients. (The Inn was a hotel for patient families and other visitors, but also housed nursing units.) After recentralization, Ms. Davis served as Administrative Director for Medical Nursing and Director of Nursing Operations.

Coronary Intensive Care, and Cardiovascular Intensive Care — as well as the Cardiovascular Intermediate Care Unit on 6 North. Patricia Skerritt, R.N., oversaw Area III — 3 East, 3 North, and 3 West. Area IV was headed by Barbara Schmidt, R.N., and consisted of 4 West (Private Medical-Surgical), 4 North (Gastrointestinal/ Medical-Surgical), and 4 East(Hematology/ Oncology). Barbara Wisintainer's Area V was units 5 North, 5 West, and 5 East. Alma Davis, R.N., the Hospital's first African-American Director of Nursing, was in charge of Area VI, which included sixth floor Hemodialysis, the general Medical-Surgical unit 6 West, and four units housed in the Clinic Inn: Intermediate Nursing Care 4A, Dermatology 4B, and Cardiac Catheterization 3A and 3B. Area VII, headed by Margaret Verbic, R.N., M.S.N., consisted of 8 West (Orthopaedic), 7 East (Pediatric), 7 North (Renal Hypertension), and 7 U (Adolescent Pediatric).

Decentralization under clinical supervisors had been a recommendation of the Cresap report in 1965, and the actual abolition of the Director of Nursing position was a logical, if extreme, extension of the decentralizing principle. It also followed a trend within the organizational structure of Cleveland Clinic Hospital: the disappearance of the nurse from the highest levels of management. The Hospital's first superintendent had been a nurse, Abbie Porter, who had reported directly to the Cleveland Clinic's physician administrators. A Foundation-wide superintendent and general secretary had then been interposed between her and the Administrative Board; and finally, when she retired, a lay administrator, James Harding, was hired to head the Clinic Hospital. Now, the positions of Hospital Administrator and Associate Administrator/Director of Nursing both no longer existed.

By 1974, Gilbert Cook had been appointed Director of the Division of Patient Care Services. The division's department heads reported to one of two associate directors or the assistant director. The Hospital directors of clinical nursing, along with the supervisor of Clinic Nursing, the directors of Nurse Recruitment and Staff Development, the nurse epidemiologist, and the departmental assistants all reported to Associate Director Richard D. Thomas. In effect, Mr. Thomas served as a lay administrator of nursing services. (However, Mr. Cook also interacted directly with the nursing areas and departments, since nursing was by far the largest component of the Division of Patient Care.) The Operating Room remained separate from other nursing areas, reporting to a different associate director; Central Service reported to the assistant director.

...and New Connections

Hospital Nursing was now being led by a committee of nursing directors. Eventually, the drawbacks of this system came to outweigh its advantages. But in the meantime, the reorganization of the early 1970s had benefits. The Hospital Nursing directors and the Supervisor of Clinic Nursing, Corinne Hofstetter, all now reported to the same administrator within the Division of Patient Care Services. This meant that the common mission of Hospital and Clinic nurses — providing nursing care to patients — was finally recognized in the institution's organizational structure. However, Hospital and Clinic Nursing did remain separate; they were not merged into a single department, as had been suggested back in 1945.

At this time, the 84 full-time and 2 part-time Clinic Nursing personnel included R.N.s, L.P.N.s, nursing assistants, electrocardiography (EKG) and other technicians, and an enterostomal therapy instructor. The department had nearly doubled since 1962, when it had 48 employees. Besides the increased number of nurses, Clinic Nursing acquired responsibility for a number of "stray" departments over the years — mostly new areas staffed by technicians, like EKG, electroencephalography (EEG) and pulmonary function. These areas often started out staffed by one or two individuals and eventually grew into large independent departments with their own directors. But during their early years they were administered by Clinic Nursing. The supervisor of Clinic Nursing interviewed and hired new staff members, who were trained on the job by the senior technicians.

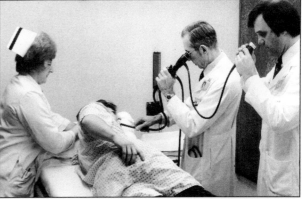

By this time the institution's rules had been changed so that Hospital nurses could transfer to work in the outpatient Clinic. Nurses now could move in either direction on the former one-way street, but it was more common for nurses to transfer from Hospital to Clinic. (Occasionally, nurses did transfer back again to the Hospital from the Clinic, declaring that they missed the Hospital patients.) Many Clinic nurses, and also Operating Room nurses, were initially attracted to these areas by the schedule, which had no evening, night, or weekend hours. One nurse referred to the Operating Room as "the only place that I can work and be guaranteed steady days and weekends off."[6]

The relatively small number of Clinic and Operating Room positions, compared to the large number of Hospital nursing personnel, ensured that there could be no mass exodus from the Hospital Nursing Department to the other areas. In 1974 the total complement of Hospital nursing personnel was 1,226, including 483 registered nurses, 454 licensed practical nurses, and 132 nursing assistants. The 148-member staff of the Operating Room included 63 R.N.s, 3 L.P.N.s, 38 O.R. technicians, and 16 nursing assistants. There were now 120 people in Clinic Nursing, including 38 R.N.s and 25 L.P.N.s.

In other ways, too, the "wall" between Hospital and Clinic was coming down. For instance, when deaths occurred in the outpatient area, Hospital personnel, usually including one of the nursing supervisors, would come over to help, for instance by bringing the necessary forms. When Ms. Hofstetter compiled a procedure manual for Clinic Nursing, she requested and received input from Hospital nurses. When individuals transferred between the two areas, the Clinic Nursing supervisor and the Hospital Nursing directors exchanged information on their past work performance. In 1972, Ms. Hofstetter reported that "The Nursing Education Staff Development department has invited the Clinic Nursing personnel to attend the in-service programs which is building a better rapport between Hospital and Clinic Nursing personnel."[7]

IRENE SPADA
Ms. Spada, a graduate of Spencer Hospital in Meadville, Pennsylvania, first worked at the Cleveland Clinic during the 1940s. Like many nurses, she stayed home when her children were small, but returned to work as a Clinic nurse in 1965, in the Gastroenterology Department. She is shown here assisting in an endoscopic procedure with Dr. Benjamin Sullivan and Dr. Richard Farmer (right) in the mid-1970s. The development of flexible scopes made more outpatient procedures possible, extending the practice of Clinic nurses.

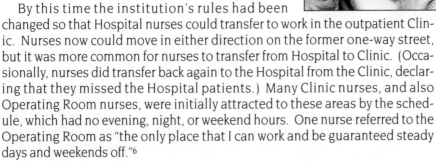

More Flexibility

In addition to bringing the separate departments of nursing closer together, another noticeably positive effect of the new organization was a change in atmosphere within Hospital Nursing. One of the aims of decentralization had been to make nursing administration more accessible, more flexible. At least in the beginning, this seemed to work. The nursing directors shared hospital-wide duties like weekend administrative coverage, reviewing departmental policies (for instance on vacation and sick time), and evaluating present practices and potential innovations (for example, instituting the unit dose system for medications). Where possible, however, managerial responsibility was delegated to head nurses, and staff involvement encouraged, as the Cresap report had recommended. One head nurse remarked on the difference this made:

> In the past year there has been a noticeable change in the structure of the nursing department. There is a less rigid attitude and positive changes are much easier to implement. There is more flexibility in supervision and I am more involved in decisions and responsibility. I think that most of the staff feels more involved because of the changes and are willing to accept additional responsibility and accountability.[8]

Area V Director Ms. Wisintainer observed the same effect on her nursing units.

> More effective utilization and involvement of personnel. Changing role of Head Nurse—"away from the desk," to increased direct patient contact, closer supervision of nursing staff with more frequent counseling and informal evaluation. These intangible changes are resulting in a generally improved staff morale, (a more relaxed working environment and improved communications both vertically and horizontally) as well as a more skilled and interested nursing staff thereby establishing a foundation for our goal of promoting and maintaining the highest possible standards of nursing care.[9]

Unfortunately, changes in management style could not solve all problems, as Ms. Schmidt's reports from Area IV indicated. She made rounds with physicians "to maintain open communications and good working relationships"; she encouraged units to hold team conferences. She hoped to hold management mini-workshops for her assistant head nurses, to encourage her L.P.N.s to become qualified to give medications, and to encourage all of her nurses to expand their skills.[10]

However, Ms. Schmidt's three units presented a mixed picture in 1972. She felt that morale had generally improved since the year before, and the quality of her staff had improved. But this was offset by the increased number of acutely ill patients admitted to the units. "The patient census on 4 North changed significantly from GI Medicine, General Surgery and Colo-rectal surgical patients to almost total Colorectal surgical patients. 4 East gained more Hematology and Medical Oncology patients as well as mixed Med-Surg patients after Dermatology moved to facilities in the Clinic Inn." She described the increased work load and the other conditions on her units:

> (1) More patients on bedrest and requiring total care (2) Heavy IV therapy and medications (3) Increased patient treatments such as N/G tubes, CVPs, dressings, I & Os, blood pressure and temperatures, chest physio

and respiratory care, etc. (4) More staff needed to care for the same number of patients. (Example: 5 years ago it was routine to have 8-10 patients daily as an LPN—today on 4 North an LPN may be totally tied up for an entire day with 1-5 patients.) (Example: on 4N and 4E 2 years ago, it was possible to function and meet the patient care demands with 2 nurses on 3-11 and 1 nurse on 11-7. Now, 3 nurses are needed on 3-11 every night and 2 nurses are needed on 11-7.)

Along with the increased work load and sicker patients, there are also increased pressures in dealing with physicians, who are demanding more and more service from the nurses. Also increased are related problems involving other departments. As medications increase, problems with pharmacy increase; as diets are changed daily for most patients, dietary problems increase....Obtaining staff is not so much a problem as retaining staff. 4 East and 4 West do not have people leave because they don't like the environment or the type of patients, but this is a continuing problem for 4 North....Because of the constant demands on the staff, and the types of patients on this floor, the young LPNs and RNs are ready for a transfer soon after they start working there. The Head Nurse is faced with an inexperienced staff and is constantly having to orient new people which leaves her little time....she is frustrated with not being able to make any gains in improving the floor or in meeting the needs of her staff....

Morale is always a problem on 4 East because of the terminal illnesses of their patients with cancers, leukemias, etc. The personnel do exceptionally well at keeping each other from becoming depressed. There is always the problem for young nurses of becoming too emotionally attached to these patients and their families.

For both 4 North and 4 East, the working environment does nothing to contribute to improved morale. There are crowded nurses' stations and physician charting areas. 4 East has no lounge facilities. 4 North uses the Central Exam room, which was painted in the old OR green, |and| is barren of anything aesthetically pleasing. Four North has burst the seams of its nursing station since the installation of the computer. The secretaries and charge nurse have virtually no place to work except on top of the computer terminal.

Ms. Schmidt closed by saying that 4 West was stable and there were no major problems on 4 East, but that stabilizing the staff on 4 North would be "an uphill battle."[11]

In Area VII, Ms. Verbic observed a different problem. She noted that the orthopaedic unit 8 West also had a high turnover rate. However, in contrast to the situation on 4 North, these nurses transferred — often to intensive care units — not because they were overworked or depressed, but because they were bored.

When Ms. Martin retired in 1973, her area was divided up among the remaining directors. Two more areas were divided when two more directors (Ms. Schmidt in 1975 and Ms. Wisintainer in 1976) left and were not replaced. Meanwhile, Area II, the Intensive Care Units and Recovery Room, was becoming increasingly separated from the other Hospital Nursing areas.

The other large departments within the Division of Patient Care Services headed by nurses — Clinic Nursing, the Operating Room, and Central Service — remained relatively stable, in administrative terms, during the 1970s.

IN THE 1970s

In 1970, tape recorders were placed on all Hospital nursing units for change-of-shift reporting. Spanish-language information sheets were written for cardiac surgery patients. A laminar air flow unit was installed in Operating Room 10. In 1972, visitors' passes were abolished. The costumed character "Gerry Germ" led a 1973 campaign to promote infection control. Pediatric nurses now wore colored uniforms, and no caps. In 1975 a Catheter Care Team was started. Official policy allowed Hospital nursing personnel to wear pantsuit uniforms as of 1976. In 1977, the SICU received stationary EKG monitors for every bed space. Nurses noticed that infusion pumps had "caught on" throughout the Hospital. CICU personnel received a reminder: "No hemostats on TV antennas." In 1979, the purchase price of a suction machine was $185; the Hospital had 64 machines. Statistics showed 31,555 Clinic patient registrations, 30,558 Hospital admissions, and 24,904 surgical procedures during the year. The Cleveland Heights Light of Yoga Society conducted a stress reduction seminar for Cleveland Clinic head nurses.

Corinne Hofstetter continued as Supervisor of Clinic Nursing, and Eleanor Reilly as Director of Central Service. Ms. Reilly also temporarily took charge of the Operating Room in 1973 and 1974, when no supervisor was appointed immediately to succeed Martha Hoffman. Irene Werley was then named Operating Room Director, and Ms. Reilly was again able to devote all of her attention to Central Service, which she continued to direct as of 1995.

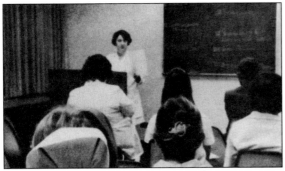

HEAD NURSES'
MEETING, 1977
With decentralization, Hospital head nurses became more involved in management. Each month, they met together as the Head Nurse Committee to discuss matters of common interest. An elected chairman — in this photograph, Maria Zickuhr of the Recovery Room — presided at meetings and served as a liaison with the nursing directors. In turn, head nurses held monthly meetings with their own unit staffs.

The Head Nurse Committee

In the autumn of 1972, the nursing directors instituted monthly meetings for Hospital unit head nurses. At their first meeting, the group, which became known as the Head Nurse Committee, "expressed a desire for informality at meetings and freedom for expression from any member present."[12] (Head nurses also served on other Foundation committees at this time: Physician-Nurse Liaison, Records and Statistics, Hospital Procedure, and Computer.)

Administrators of the Division of Patient Care Services looked at the Head Nurse Committee as a conduit through which they could channel directives and information to nurses at the unit level. Head nurses, on the other hand, saw the meetings as a forum in which they could discuss their concerns and offer nursing input into decisions that affected them. At first, they directly refuted the notion that they could speak for the division's administrators: "Head Nurses view themselves primarily as nurses, not as management and are devoted in their own minds to patient care rather than managerial functions."[13]

At this time, head nurses often took patient assignments as a matter of course, and were counted in the staffing numbers. They did not do budgets for their units and did not select or hire new staff members; the central nursing office handled these matters. Head nurses prepared time sheets, but nursing directors and supervisors could make changes.

In 1975 the Head Nurse Committee members drew up a list of 14 proposals which they presented to Mr. Cook for consideration. They focused on expanding the head nurses' authority to include: approving vacations, leaves of absence, and overtime; interviewing new nurses; and evaluating staff. They also requested office space and file cabinets. Patient care, not management, was still the first love of many head nurses. But they had realized that if they were to be accountable for the care given on their units, they needed more managerial tools and more independent authority to use them.

The Head Nurse Committee gave head nurses the opportunity to share information on matters of common interest, promoting communication among the different areas created by decentralization. For instance, Committee members discussed the use of verbal orders, a perennial bone of contention among nurses, residents, and staff physicians; expressed concern about the untidy appearance of nursing personnel; and pointed out the need for clinical instructors on the units. They received reports on new patient care supplies and equipment, like disposable tracheostomy care sets ("cheaper than our present clean method"), and isolation carts prepared by Central Service.[14]

In 1978 the large Head Nurse Committee was dissolved and replaced by the Head Nurse Executive Board. The new group, which reviewed policy, was made up of a head nurse representative and an alternate from each of the four nursing areas. It could call special meetings of all head nurses when necessary. Head nurses would continue to meet together at quarterly seminars, and separate meetings for head nurses within each area would continue to be held, but for the time being, there was no forum in which all head nurses could meet together on a regular basis to discuss policy.

The Delivery of Nursing Care

In 1971, when decentralization became the organizing principle for Hospital Nursing, nurses at the unit level were still struggling to implement team nursing. For instance, the psychiatry unit started a "better team nursing program," with "permanent team leaders" in 1972. "Team conferences were encouraged but certainly have not appeared with any regularity" in Area VII. The "Experiment in Nursing" on 3 East was the most thorough approach to team nursing, and in fact went a step beyond it. The entire unit was built from the ground up

> to develop new concepts in the delivery of nursing care. The idea is to get the nurse away from paper work enabling her to devote more time to the patients. The unit will have teams of 16-17 patients with both medical and surgical problems. The Team Leaders, RNs, will coordinate patient care. Practical Nurses following sufficient instruction will administer medications. One of the major tasks of the experiment is evaluation. Ideas are needed regarding methods for assessing the quality of care.[15]

The area directors selected Betty Bartel, R.N., B.S.N., of Staff Development as the coordinator of the new unit, a position designed to replace the traditional head nurse role. Two administrative service coordinators were assigned as unit managers, to work with her in the operation of the unit. Housekeeping was requested to take more responsibility in cleaning and related work on 3 East. The goal of all this was to provide "patient centered care" which recognized the patient

> as a unique individual within a family unit and social setting....our nurses would feel accountable primarily to the patients, and not primarily to the physicians and hospital administrators....This type of nursing care would mean making nursing decisions about patient care which are written down and used by other nursing personnel so that continuity of nursing care could be maintained from shift to shift, day to day.

The nursing coordinator did not take on the "traditional" role of the head nurse as charge nurse on the day shift. She occasionally worked as a team leader or even as a team member: "sometimes because of staffing, sometimes to give an example: sometimes for teaching purposes, and sometimes for the sake of [unit] morale." She was responsible for planning, coordinating, and assessing patient care on a 24-hour basis, scheduling staffing time for nursing personnel, evaluating employee performance, and working with the unit manager to coordinate all unit activities. Finally, the job description included orientation, in-service, staff development, and the creation of patient and family teaching programs.[16]

All R.N.s on the unit took turns performing team leader duties. The most difficult aspect of this was assuming responsibility for the team members as well as the patients. "These Team Leaders are attentive to detail; they make

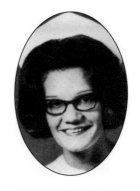

ELIZABETH BARTEL
Beginning in 1972, nursing unit 3 East was the site for an "experiment in nursing," which featured team nursing, and management by a nursing coordinator rather than a head nurse. Since the unit, staffed by personnel from all over the Hospital, was organized according to new concepts, "even the most basic of procedures" involved decision-making. As the unit's first coordinator, Ms. Bartel led unit staff members in this process. In her career at the Cleveland Clinic Hospital, she also held positions in Staff Development, nursing supervision, and the Private Medical-Surgical Unit.

rounds with doctors; they get their questions answered; they respond to their patient's needs with the concern that a charge nurse must have."[17] L.P.N.s often served as medication nurses on the teams, and handled this new responsibility "with apparent ease." Overall, team members were working well together. The unit managers were also working well with the nursing coordinator: "The 3 East project would not be possible without the help of these two men." The unit's two "exceptionally competent" secretaries reported to the unit managers.

As might be expected in the trial of a new concept, problems arose. For instance, patients admitted to the unit were supposed to stay there throughout the remainder of their hospitalization. This did not happen and was one of the great disappointments of the "experiment," since it interrupted continuity of care. A key objective of the project had been to eliminate "the impersonal characteristics which can result from specialization of services."[18] Yet, despite the problems, Ms. Bartel felt that even as she was writing her report, the unit had begun to jell.

As the 1970s progressed, team nursing became more securely established as the Cleveland Clinic Hospital's standard model for nursing care delivery.

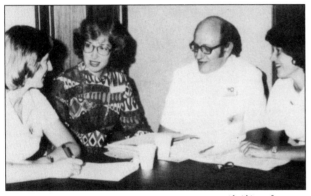

PLANNING PRIMARY NURSING, 1977

In 1977, primary nursing was piloted on two Cleveland Clinic Hospital units. Here, members of the Primary Nursing Care Planning Committee — Hospital registered nurses Michele Magdinec (left), Richard Calvin (center right), and Susan Cancian (right) — meet with consultant Karen Ciske. Mr. Calvin, neurosciences supervisor, chaired the 18-member committee, which also included L.P.N. representatives.

However, at the same time, a new model — primary nursing — was gaining popularity nationwide. Team nursing had been an improvement on the functional system, making nurses responsible for their own groups of patients within the unit, rather than for unit-wide tasks like passing medications. But with separate teams of six or seven people on three shifts, each caring for 17 or 18 patients, and with assignments sometimes changed daily, the link between nurse and patient was not as strong as it could have been. Primary nursing aimed to restore that link, by assigning around-the-clock responsibility for a patient's care throughout the hospital stay to a "primary nurse," assisted by an associate nurse or nurses. Primary nurses, who planned and evaluated their patients' care, assumed increased responsibility. The goal was increased continuity of care for patients.

In the summer of 1977, a pilot project to study the primary nursing care model was set up at the Cleveland Clinic Hospital on 5 North and 5 West, under the department's Primary Nursing Care Planning Committee. "For the study, a 'primary' nurse and an associate nurse will be in charge of the same four to six patients from the day of admission through discharge." Committee member Richard Calvin, R.N., explained the reason for the proposed change: "We hope to increase the feeling of 'my nurse and my patient,' something both nurses and patients often feel is lacking."[19]

Changing Roles

Changes in the nursing care delivery model meant that the roles of workers on the units changed. The move away from functional nursing required the R.N. to assume the role of team leader. Some of the R.N.'s functional tasks, such as passing medications, had to be assumed by L.P.N.s, as was done on the experimental unit.

A considerable amount of attention was given to preparing the Cleveland Clinic's L.P.N.s for these additional duties. As of 1971, the practice of hiring by waiver ended. All newly hired practical nurses had to be graduates of accredited schools. The Continuing Education office stated that in 1971 it hoped to "teach Pharmacology, Administration of Medications and Charge responsibilities to carefully selected groups of licensed practical nurses who are assigned to nursing divisions where these additional skills and knowledge are needed."[20] (L.P.N.s had already taken on charge duties in the convalescent units.) In 1972, staff development instructor Elaine Dvorak, R.N., developed and taught a pharmacology course for L.P.N.s. After completing the course (or an equivalency exam) and two weeks of clinical experience, L.P.N.s were certified to give medications at the Cleveland Clinic. They were encouraged, although not required, to apply for national certification as well.

The course was offered to L.P.N.s working in both inpatient and outpatient settings, and Ms. Hofstetter in the Clinic and Ms. Shoptaw in Area II cited positive results: "This past year six Clinic LPNs were able to attend the Drug Course for Practical Nurses provided by the Foundation. Their new knowledge plus satisfaction of completing the course and new self-esteem was worth the time and effort of planning and providing replacements during their 60 hours of class." "Miss Shoptaw reports that LPNs giving medications are taking pride in themselves and their work." As the course developed, it placed additional emphasis on not only "technical skill in pouring and passing medications," but also on knowledge about dosages, effects, and side effects of medications. "This increased knowledge is useful in assessing the patients' condition and understanding certain signs thereby enabling the LPN to carry out more meaningful patient care even if she is not actively engaged in dispensing medicines all the time."[21]

Eventually, the Hospital Nursing administration began to consider requiring all L.P.N.s to be able to administer medications. Some L.P.N.s did not wish to do so, and Ms. Hofstetter kept it optional rather than mandatory for Clinic L.P.N.s. Hospital Nursing administrators also worried that "good bedside LPNs" might leave if giving meds were made a requirement.[22] In the end, a senior L.P.N. position was created in 1975 for L.P.N.s with additional qualifications, including the ability to give medications. In 1983, L.P.N.s who could not administer medications were put in a separate job classification.

Nursing administrators had hoped that the Pharmacy Department's unit dose system, piloted in the early 1970s on some nursing units, would eventually be extended throughout the entire Hospital as a permanent measure. With medications prepared in the Pharmacy, nursing unit personnel would only have to pass them, not pour them, and a considerable amount of nursing time would be saved. The Nursing and Pharmacy directors strongly supported the unit dose system, but it was dropped after a few years.

In 1976, Staff Development began offering a 60-hour "Psychology of Human Behavior" course for L.P.N.s, which emphasized understanding and working with patients. L.P.N.s received credit from the National Association of Practical Nurse Education for the course.

An example of someone able to push the envelope of the traditional L.P.N. role was Susan Richards, L.P.N. She worked in the Clinic's Department of Gynecology for more than 30 years beginning in 1964, holding the positions of

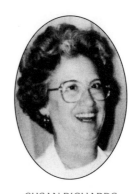

SUSAN RICHARDS
Ms. Richards, a licensed practical nurse, had a long and outstanding career in Clinic Nursing, as staff nurse for Dr. James Krieger, Chairman of the Department of Gynecology. She was also Coordinator of the Clinic's Reproductive Center. In this position, she worked with infertility patients; her first such patient, who became pregnant and had a son, continued to keep in touch with Ms. Richards over the years.

staff nurse and Coordinator of the Reproductive Center. She took patient histories, researched and developed a form to be used for sexual assault victims "so everything would be done for these patients," worked with infertility patients, and helped to set up a donor sperm program, for which she also produced patient education materials.[23]

Over the years, the role of the nursing assistants had changed as well. Originally, they had cared more for the patient's physical surroundings than for the patient. By 1970, the assistants were not only helping patients with the activities of daily living, but were also taking TPRs and changing dressings — tasks only a few decades back considered key duties of the registered nurse. The "Senior Ward Aide Training Course" prepared by Jacqueline Heed in 1966 covered apical pulse, blood pressure, irrigations, enemas, colostomy and ileostomy care, clean dressings, application of heat, surgical skin preps, isolation, traction and suspension, and review of the cardiac arrest procedure. As team nursing was established at the Clinic Hospital, nursing assistants were included, and teams always had one or two assistants assigned to them. Their role in direct patient care was acknowledged in 1977 by a new title, Patient Care Assistant.

One nurse gave this description of the way the division of labor worked in the 1970s: "Head nurses did patients the same as everyone; L.P.N.s did everything R.N.s did except orders; aides did everything L.P.N.s did except meds."[24]

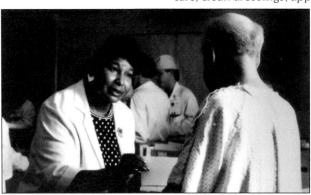

AT THE DESK
The Nursing Department's secretarial staff worked in two major areas. As part of the central Nursing Office staff, administrative secretaries and clerical workers provided necessary support within the nursing management area. Unit secretaries worked on the units, either in permanent assignments or as floats.

By the 1980s, they were present on all three shifts, doing everything from answering visitors' questions to organizing patient records to helping nurses learn how to use computers. Here, secretary Irene Echols of the Peripheral Vascular Unit assists a patient on G80 (circa 1988).

The Unit Secretary

Although not involved in direct patient care, the unit secretary was an important member of the nursing unit staff. She was often the first person visitors met. She made calls and took calls from physicians, families, laboratories, and other units. She transcribed orders, filled out requisitions, and scheduled tests. By 1972 unit secretaries covered two shifts, seven days a week. They were trained by a staff development instructor and reported to the nursing directors. More than 40 unit secretaries worked on the day shift alone. Nursing and Patient Care Division administrators decided that since there were now so many, they needed their own spokesperson/teacher/leader. Karen Bourquin, who had "demonstrated ability and...leadership capabilities," was chosen as the "Secretarial Team Leader."[25]

In 1975, unit secretaries were transferred out of Nursing and into their own department, headed by Ms. Bourquin as Supervisor. She would now be responsible for evaluation, assignment, and payroll, and would report to the Assistant Director for Patient Care. The new department had 116 employees. Under Ms. Bourquin's direction, staff members began developing a unit secretary handbook. As of 1976, unit secretaries worked in 42 locations throughout the Hospital, including all inpatient units, and were "heavily relied upon by nursing" to handle the clerical duties of the units.[26]

Eventually, it was decided that unit secretaries, as an integral part of nursing unit staffs, should rejoin the decentralized Nursing Department. As part of the general process in which head nurses were assuming increased responsibility for personnel matters on their units, secretaries assigned permanently to nursing units would report to head nurses. Float secretaries would report to Ms. Bourquin, who remained responsible for orientation and in-service for all unit secretaries.

New Positions for Nurses

During the 1970s, more Cleveland Clinic nurses began to work outside the traditional settings of nursing unit, Clinic department, or operating room. A new job category developed: the nurse clinician, also known as the departmental assistant. Departmental assistants worked for medical departments, and were not bound to a particular care setting. A surgeon's nurse clinician might scrub with him in the operating room, round with him in the Hospital, and assist with his ambulatory patients in the Clinic.

In 1973, the head nurse on the gastrointestinal medical-surgical unit 4 North was hired as the nurse clinician for the Department of General Surgery. In her new position, she made rounds on all general surgical patients:

> "She is seeing them pre-op and post-op; talking, listening to the patients and their families. She is teaching patients and staff and rendering some discharge consultation. She has permission to write verbal orders concerning such things as ambulation, removal of Foley catheter, etc. She will see that these orders are countersigned by the residents. Miss Hall has been instructed to bring nursing care problems and complaints to the Clinical Directors of the areas."[27]

The role of the departmental assistant at first developed informally. Medical departments hired assistants on an individual basis. Often, a nurse already working at the Hospital or Clinic was hand-picked by a physician to become his assistant. In late 1974 was it decided that the position should have a job description. In 1977, the Departmental Assistants Committee, composed of physicians and administrators, listed duties typically performed by departmental assistants: taking histories; performing physical examinations; making decisions regarding data gathering and management and treatment of patients; ordering standard lab tests; identifying normal and abnormal findings on examinations and tests; handling emergency situations; and counseling and instructing patients regarding common problems. Departmental assistant chemotherapy nurses administered drugs in both ambulatory and inpatient settings beginning in the mid-1970s.

Some difficulties had to be overcome in establishing this new position. For example, departmental assistants, under the clinical direction of medical departments, at first had no one to whom to report administratively. The Clinic Nursing supervisor ended up with the responsibility. It was important to have someone in nursing do this, since administrators in other areas might not be aware of the importance of requirements such as nursing license renewal. Despite the difficulties, the departmental assistant position grew in importance during the 1970s and in subsequent years.

Nurse anesthetists (known as C.R.N.A.s after the institution of certification in 1945) had been the Foundation's first advanced practice nurses in the 1920s. As the place of A.P.N.s in the health care system grew nationwide during the last quarter of the twentieth century, the variety of advanced practice roles at the Cleveland Clinic also grew. The Clinic hired a nurse practitioner,

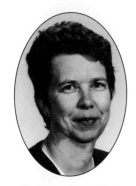

KAREN BOURQUIN
Ms. Bourquin played a major part in developing the unit secretary role at the Cleveland Clinic Hospital. She came to the Clinic as a hostess/secretary in the Obstetrics Department in 1964, and later worked as a unit secretary on Hospital units including the 6 North Cardiovascular Unit. Ms. Bourquin was promoted to Secretarial Team Leader, and then Unit Secretary Supervisor, during the 1970s. Her responsibilities included scheduling, orienting, and evaluating the growing number of Hospital unit secretaries, and also revising forms used on the units.

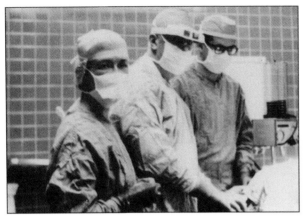

ALEXA McCUBBIN
During the 1970s, increasing attention to infection control led to the creation of nurse epidemiology positions at the Cleveland Clinic. Janet Serkey was appointed the institution's first nurse epidemiologist in 1972. Ms. McCubbin was the first nurse epidemiologist in the Operating Room, holding the position from 1977 to 1988. A native of Germany, her career in the Cleveland Clinic Hospital's Operating Room Department began in 1958. After two years in general surgery, she transferred to the eye service, where she was head nurse for fifteen years. At the same time, she also served as a staff nurse in neurosurgery. The photo above shows Ms. McCubbin (left) with Dr. Roscoe J. Kennedy, (center), head of the Ophthalmology Department, in the operating room in the 1960s.

"the first of many," to work in the Primary Care Department (the employee health service) in 1975.[28]

By 1982, the Department of Nursing had hired its own clinical nurse specialists: Chris Platt, R.N., M.S.N., to serve as a resource to all nursing units in the area of endocrinology (especially diabetes), and Gayle Whitman, R.N., M.S.N., as a specialist in cardio-thoracic nursing. Nursing administrators explained how the role of the C.N.S. within Nursing differed from that of the departmental assistant. The C.N.S. reported to Nursing and acted as a liaison with physicians; departmental assistants reported to physicians and liaised with Nursing.

When the Cleveland Clinic reinstituted an obstetric service in 1995, the new Birthing Services Department included certified nurse-midwives, under the direction of Cindy Cover, R.N., C.N.M. The Cleveland Clinic now had nurses working in all four advanced practice areas.

Other roles added to the traditional nursing structure during the 1970s and 1980s included the nurse epidemiologist and the quality assurance nurse. Janet Serkey, R.N., B.A., who had been a head nurse on 4 East, became the Hospital's first nurse epidemiologist in 1972. By 1982 both she and Emily Smith, R.N., were working in Infection Control. Alexa McCubbin, R.N., formerly in charge of the eye service in the Operating Room, became the Operating Room's first nurse epidemiologist in 1977. P. Mardeen Atkins, R.N., M.P.A., in charge of nursing quality assurance, had worked on the development of the nursing audit at the Clinic Hospital beginning in 1973. In 1981, she took on responsibility for building a quality assurance program when the Nursing Department's Audit Committee was succeeded by the new Quality Assurance Committee.

Reality Shock

In the 1960s, Hospital and Nursing administrators were already expressing concern about the "fast pace" and the "pressure" on Cleveland Clinic Hospital nurses. New graduates were considered particularly vulnerable to the stressful working conditions on the units, since more of them were coming from associate or baccalaureate programs, where they did not have the advantage of immersion in the daily work of patient care that diploma graduates did. One nurse who came to the Cleveland Clinic during the early 1970s remembered that by the third day of her orientation, she was working on the floor. By the end of the first week, she had been given an assignment and was doing it.

At least some veteran nurses had doubts about associate degree (A.D.) graduates, in particular, being ready to take on the responsibilities of the registered nurse without additional preparation. The Clinic Hospital began hiring associate degree nurses in significant numbers in the late 1960s, after local community colleges began offering A.D. nursing degree programs. These nurses were given a longer orientation program, and barred from charge nurse duties until they had at least six months' experience. Several early A.D. graduates went on to distinguished careers at the Cleveland Clinic, but in the early years some received "the impression that this type of nurse is [considered] inferior."[29] By 1972, however, the official policies differentiating A.D. nurses from other nurses in terms of orientation, salary, and charge duties had been changed.

For instance, all new nurses now received the same three-week orientation, since it seemed that all new graduates, not only A.D. graduates, might need extra help. Intensive care unit nurses received two additional weeks of orientation. As specialized units became the rule, rather than the exception, the need for more orientation on the individual units became evident. In 1976 nursing directors expressed the wish that staff development instructors could spend more time with new employees on the floors, since staffing levels were too low for unit nurses to do so.

Late that year, the Clinic Hospital instituted a mandatory internship for all new graduate nurses. "This program is designed to shorten and smooth the adjustment period from the role of student to the role of professional nurse."[30] The graduates worked as interns for four months (later shortened to three months) before beginning the three-month probation period required of every new employee. In another move to give new nurses on-the-job support and instruction, head nurses were permitted to create the clinical instructor position. These instructors, appointed at the assistant head nurse level, would be part of the nursing unit staff, present on a full-time basis and thoroughly familiar with the unit. Working with Staff Development, they would orient new employees, conduct unit in-service programs, and participate in patient care.

In 1980, orientation was expanded to 16 weeks, and a preceptor program was started in which experienced staff nurses served as mentors to new graduates on their units. In addition, Nursing Education incorporated "reality shock" sessions into orientation. "All graduate nurses who had no prior hospital job experience were eligible to attend the five sessions. They were thereby able to share experiences with other new graduates....ways to deal with erroneous and/or inadequate perceptions and problems were discussed." Initially, the response was good, as evidenced by the reaction of veteran nursing unit personnel: "They too wanted to attend Reality Shock classes." The program also gave nursing administrators insight into the difficulties experienced by newly employed nurses, at a point before those difficulties led to resignation.[31]

Since the 1950s, the Nursing Department's educational programs had had a dual purpose. Although the more obvious goal was preparing nursing personnel to perform patient care according to the standards of the institution, educational programs also served to recruit and retain nurses. Affiliation programs, for instance, helped to attract nurses to the staff, and benefits like tuition aid helped to keep them. By 1980, Cleveland Clinic nursing administrators were giving increased attention to the orientation period and the first year of work, as a crucial time for a nurse's career. This was when she bonded to her profession and to the institution that employed her. If she had a bad experience, she might leave nursing altogether. "Reality shock" and the presence of unit-based instructors would help ease nurses over the difficult transition from school to workplace, and help retain them on the staff.

PSYCHIATRIC/MENTAL HEALTH NURSING
In 1961, the Cleveland Clinic Hospital opened its first psychiatric nursing unit. By the 1980s, there were four psychiatric/mental health units located in the P Building (formerly the Clinic Inn): adult psychiatry, P77; adolescent psychiatry, P78; chemical dependency, P47; and pain management, P58. Care planning involved multiple disciplines and also the patients. In 1988, registered nurse Peg Palmer (below), clinical instructor on unit P77, participated in implementing a new, comprehensive format for documenting multidisciplinary care.

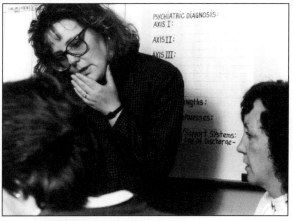

The Nursing Audit and Documentation

Clinic Hospital nurses whose careers spanned the 1970s and 1980s remarked on the great increase in documentation of nursing care over the period. The keeping of notes had had a place in professional nursing since the days of Florence Nightingale. The observations of the nurse, who was "always there," would ideally be recorded, to aid in the patient's care. But in practice, documentation, or "charting," was often sketchy at best — TPRs and intakes and outputs — or non-existent at worst. In 1955, at the request of the physicians on the Hospital Committee, the Cleveland Clinic Hospital nursing units began charting medications, as "an aid to the physician, even though it does take more nursing time."[32]

By the last quarter of the twentieth century outside entities such as government agencies, insurers, and accrediting bodies, notably the Joint Commission for the Accreditation of Healthcare Organizations (JCAHO), were the great motivators of paperwork. JCAHO representatives found nursing care plans to be inadequate during their accreditation visit to the Clinic Hospital in 1971. In 1972, administrators, nurses, and physicians were still evaluating care plans, debating how nurses' notes (which were also said to "need improvement") fit into the patient record, and determining how nursing documentation could be used in discharge planning.[33] No separate form for nurses' notes existed at this point, but it was suggested that they could be written on the patient progress sheet. In July 1973, nurses' notes were made mandatory throughout the Hospital.

In the same month the new Nursing Audit Committee had its first meeting. The committee stressed that neither documentation nor audits were ends in themselves. The goal of the audit was to evaluate nursing care in order to maintain or improve its quality. Emphasis was to be "not on the technical performance of tasks but on professional judgement and skills." The audit would evaluate quality of care "through appraisal of nursing process as it is reflected in the patient care record" of discharged patients. The nursing audit — and therefore quality of care — depended on the existence of complete information in the patient's chart.[34]

Documentation and audits tied together a number of concerns and trends within nursing and health care current at the national level. Professionalism, accreditation, and finance were all involved. Nursing leaders emphasized the exercise of nursing judgment and the application of the nursing process — patient assessment, determination of the nursing diagnosis, and planning, implementing, and evaluating nursing care — as the basis of a professional approach to nursing. Accreditors began to judge nursing care accordingly. Third-party payors were checking patient records, including nursing records, and sometimes refusing to reimburse hospitals for portions of patient stays that were not recorded properly.

Clinic Hospital nursing administrators found that putting new documentation policies into practice was not easy. In the first place, even though nurses might in theory support the idea of keeping better records, they might in practice find it difficult to take time to do so. Also, nursing directors observed, "nurse's notes are being written but not the problem oriented type of notes. It was felt that the nursing staff are still afraid of the 'nursing diagnosis' and are

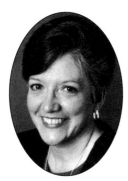

MARDEEN ATKINS
In 1973, Mardi Atkins, a staff nurse and team leader on nursing unit 3 East, became a member of the new Nursing Audit Committee. She went on to lead work on the nursing audit and the nursing quality assurance program. As Manager of Nursing Quality Management, Ms. Atkins also had an important role in helping the Division of Nursing prepare for JCAHO surveys. In the 1990s, the division shifted its focus from quality assurance to the broader concept of quality improvement. "The healthcare quality arena has moved from simply assuring quality care to continuously assessing and identifying new opportunities to improve the quality of care," Ms. Atkins wrote in the September 1993 issue of *Cleveland Clinic Nurse*.

getting this confused with medical diagnosis."[35] Although all nursing personnel involved in patient care could write nursing notes, R.N.s had to cosign
notes written by L.P.N.s and nursing assistants. The forms for nursing documentation were continually being added to and revised. For example, in 1978,
new care plans and assessment sheets were developed following an audit on
documentation itself.

A Critical Point

In the late 1970s the recurring cycle of nurse shortage at the Clinic Hospital
had reached a critical point. Understaffing and overwork made for low morale.
As the Division of Patient Care Services struggled to recruit and retain nurses,
it became evident that the problem would require a radical solution.

In 1975 the nursing directors had argued against a proposed staff reduction, pointing out that Nursing was already under its budgeted number of
positions. In 1976, they noted an urgent need for experienced nurses on the
Hospital's off-shifts. In 1977, they declared that staffing levels were critically
low: several units had only one R.N. scheduled for the evening shift on weekends; supervisors sometimes had to pass meds; and not enough employees
were available to work overtime.

Nurse Recruitment obtained permission to hire up to 250 nurses, and in the
following months the Hospital also turned to temporary agencies to supplement its staff. In 1978 the nursing directors called upon Staff Development,
Recruitment, Clinic Nursing, and the Operating Room for help, asking if they
could spare any nurses for temporary assignment to the units. But in February
1979, staffing was still "critical in all areas."[36] Nurses finally suggested that
some Clinic Hospital beds be closed. As had been the case in the 1940s, this
notion was resisted. This time, one of the reasons was fear that it would be
difficult to reopen closed beds in the tightly regulated health care environment of the 1970s.

Reunification

Many nurses felt that the administration had not taken seriously the warn-
ings about critical staff shortages during the 1970s. By 1980, administrators
began taking stronger action to resolve nursing concerns.

Some changes in the administration itself had occurred. In 1977, a request
from head nurses for a nursing representative on the Foundation's Policy and
Procedure Committee had been denied. Nursing would continue to be represented indirectly by the Director of the Division of Patient Care Services. But
in 1978, the Division of Patient Care Services was absorbed into the Division of
Operations. In the same year, Nursing lost its ex officio representation on the
Cleveland Clinic's Hospital Committee when the committee was decreased in
size and all ex officio members were dropped.

Overall, the decentralized Nursing Department seemed to have drifted yet
further away from the center of power, but its course was about to change. Not
only the low levels of staffing and morale, but also the way that the Nursing
"area" concept had worked out in practice over the years, made it evident that
a new departmental structure was needed. The area directors stated the case
succinctly: "Nurses wish greater involvement in high level decisions that
affect them."[37]

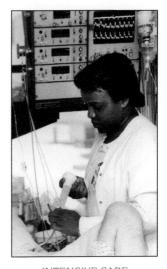

INTENSIVE CARE
The Hospital's early constant care
rooms (see pp. 159 and 167)
appeared simple and bare compared to the intensive care units of
later years. The gastric tube and
cardiac monitor visible in this
photograph were only a small part
of the equipment used by intensive care unit personnel like registered nurse Sarah Jordan (above).
In 1977, the Hospital had seven
intensive care units, including
three cardiac units, out of a total
of 35 nursing units; by 1984, the
Hospital had 180 cardiac beds
and 93 ICU beds. Stepdown units
accommodated patients who did
not need intensive care but were
not yet ready for transfer to a
regular nursing unit.

Long before this, the number of areas headed by the directors had leveled out at four. The logic of the original structure had been lost by this time, as directors had left and nursing units had been moved from one floor of the Hospital to another. Of the first directors, Ms. Verbic and Ms. Davis had remained; Norma Clifford, R.N., promoted from nursing supervisor, had joined them in 1977. The fourth director's position was vacant at the beginning of 1980.

The continued expansion of the Hospital during these years also contributed to increasing the responsibilities of all of the directors. As their areas had grown, and the administrative duties connected with nursing had grown even more, the nursing directors' roles had become more removed from the original clinical supervisor ideal. Another problem was that although the directors met together to review and approve policies, these same policies might be administered very differently in the different areas, creating disunity. The advantages of decentralization had dwindled along the way, making the disadvantages appear greater in contrast.

A subcommittee on nursing structure, composed of Ms. Clifford, Ms. Davis, Dr. John Eversman, Chief Operating Officer of the Cleveland Clinic, and James Lees, Director of Operations, made two recommendations at the beginning of 1980. First, fill the fourth nursing director position as quickly as possible; and second, create a new position to represent Nursing at the administrative level and conduct a nationwide search to fill it.

Ms. Clifford and Ms. Davis also served on a subcommittee on nurse retention. This group also recommended a nurse representative in administration, "i.e., an R.N. in charge of nursing to report directly to the Chief of Operations." In addition, it recommended more involvement of staff nurses in policy planning, expansion of in-service education, enhanced communication between Nursing and the medical staff, development of an "objective" acuity classification system, better coordination among offices involved in hiring nursing personnel, and competitive salaries and benefits.[38]

To improve communication between physicians and nurses, the Clinic's Professional Liaison Committee was re-established immediately. A pilot study to create a patient classification system took place in 1981. In the spring of 1980, salaries were raised. A registered nurse now started at $8.16/hour, one of the highest rates in the city, and an L.P.N. at $6.16. The search for a nursing administrator also got underway in 1980.

The search process took time. Meanwhile, the four area directors, now including Catherine Baur, R.N., who was hired in 1980, were meeting together on a regular basis with Mr. Lees, the directors of Nursing Education and Nurse Recruitment, and Operating Room Director Irene Werley. This group constituted an administrative committee for Hospital Nursing. Even before anyone was hired to fill the new administrative post, the pendulum had begun its swing back toward centralization, and toward Nursing's participation at the top level of management.

The Nursing Education staff members had long since found it impossible to function under the decentralized structure as a group of instructors, without a head, responsible to a group of nursing directors. In 1974, Ken Whidden, R.N., had been appointed Director of Nursing Education. During this period, the increasing employment of men in the Nursing Department included appointments to nursing management positions. Mr. Whidden and Robert Brent, R.N., Director of Nurse Recruitment since 1977, both served on the new administrative committee.

A New Hierarchy

Late in the summer of 1981, Sharon L. Danielsen, R.N., M.S.N., assumed the new position of Associate Director of Operations/Nursing. After 10 years of decentralization, the Cleveland Clinic Hospital Department of Nursing again had a single director at its head. The unified department included the four areas headed by the directors of clinical nursing, and also Nursing Education, Nurse Recruitment, and the Operating Room, which rejoined Nursing after more than 30 years as a separate department.

During the next few years, the Nursing Department's administrative structure was completely revamped. The numbered areas were replaced with a clinically-oriented scheme, which seemed more appropriate for a highly specialized tertiary care center. The aim was to promote clinical excellence by creating an administrative organization based on nursing specialties.

With the Associate Director of Operations/Nursing at the apex of the structure, the Nursing Department was divided into medical and surgical areas headed by clinical directors. These areas were in turn divided into "clusters." Each cluster was headed by a department chair, and each nursing unit was assigned to one of the clusters. Medical Nursing had four clusters, with nursing units initially organized as follows: General Medicine - 5E and 7N (both Medical-Surgical), 5U (Precautionary Care), 6N (General Medical), 4W (Private Medical-Surgical), 4E/U (Hematology/Oncology), Medical Intensive Care Unit, and the Emergency Room; Pediatrics - 7E, and 7U (Adolescent); Psychiatry - 7B, and 7A (Adolescent); and, Renal Dialysis - 8U (Peritoneal), 8U/6D (Hemodialysis), and 8W (Hypertension/Research). Five clusters made up Surgical Nursing: General Surgery - 3W, 3N, and 3E (all Gastrointestinal Medical-Surgical and General Surgical), 4N (Ophthalmology/Otolaryngology/Plastic), 4B (Dermatology/Plastic), 6W (Peripheral Vascular/Endocrinology), Pediatric/Surgical Intensive Care Unit, Post-Anesthesia Recovery Unit, and Outpatient Surgery Unit; Genitourinary/Gynecology - 5Q and 5S; Neurosciences - 5W, 5N, and Neurosurgical Intensive Care Unit; Orthopaedics - 6S and 6Q; and, Cardiothoracic - 8S and 8Q (Cardiology/Pulmonary), 7W (Cardiology), 7S and 7Q (Cardiovascular), Coronary Intensive Care Unit, and Cardiovascular Intensive Care Unit.

As of 1983, Medical Nursing was directed by Carol Thompson, R.N., and Surgical Nursing by Linda J. Lewicki, R.N., M.S.N. Operational areas were added, with Ms. Clifford now serving as Director of Strategic Planning for Nursing, and Ms. Davis as Director of Nursing Operations. The department's executive committee, which became known as the Nursing Administrative Group, was chaired by Ms. Danielsen and had responsibility for decision-making in major policy, practice, and administrative areas. In addition to Ms. Danielsen, Ms. Clifford, Ms. Davis, Ms. Lewicki, and Ms. Thompson, the group included Ms. Werley, Operating Room Director; Shirley Moore, R.N., M.S., Director of Nursing Education; Mr. Brent, Director of Nurse Recruitment; and Timothy Gibbons, in the staff position of Ms. Danielsen's Administrative Assistant. Barbara Flewellyn, R.N., M.S.N., later joined the group in the new position of Director of Program Development.

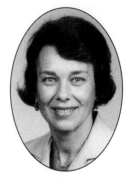

SHARON L. DANIELSEN
Appointed Associate Director of Operations/Nursing in 1981, Ms. Danielsen led the process of forging a new identity for the Cleveland Clinic's reunified Department of Nursing. She had previously held positions as director of a community hospital in Wisconsin, and Assistant Professor in the University of Minnesota School of Public Health, in a program that prepared nursing administrators. At the Cleveland Clinic Hospital, Ms. Danielsen implemented a nursing structure based on clinical specialties, with department heads responsible for clinical "clusters" of nursing units like pediatrics or orthopaedics. In 1983, testifying before an Ohio Legislature committee, she cited the need for greater educational opportunities for nurses, in view of the "knowledge explosion" in health care. At the same time, she noted, "the necessary responses to technological advances cannot overshadow the cornerstone of nursing practice — care and comfort. The nurse... is the constant resource to patients and families."

By the end of 1984 this structure was simplified into four divisions, three of them clinical: Surgical Nursing; Medical Nursing, now headed by Francine Wojton, R.N., M.S.N.; Operating Room and Treatment Areas, headed by Isabelle Boland, R.N., M.S.N.; and Nursing Resources under Ms. Moore. Nursing Resources had four components: Nursing Education, Nursing Human Resources (which included Nurse Recruitment), Nursing Information Systems, and Nursing Physical Resources. Ms. Boland had administrative responsibility for the Post-Anesthesia Recovery Unit, the Outpatient Surgery Unit, the Emergency Room, the Intravenous Therapy Team, and Infection Control, as well as the Operating Room. The Nursing Administrative Group was now made up of Ms. Danielsen and the four division heads, plus Sandra S. Shumway, R.N., M.S.N., who joined the administrative team in 1984 in a staff capacity as Director of Program Development, and Amy Caslow, the department's fiscal coordinator.

The Nursing Operations Group

During the department's reorganization, it was decided to terminate the Head Nurse Executive Board and return to a format in which the entire head nurse group met together. By this time, the head nurse's role as a manager was unquestioned. But the assignment of nurses within the department, the Hospital, and the entire Cleveland Clinic had become more complex. Individuals in nursing positions other than head nurse were also serving at the middle management level. If the new head nurse meetings were to provide a forum in which nursing administrators could meet with all management personnel within the department, the administrative group had to decide exactly who should attend.

The Nursing Operations Group, formed in 1982, finally included nursing administrators, supervisors, and head nurses from the nursing units and the Operating Room, clinical nurse specialists, infection control nurses, and the quality assurance nurse. The group received information, made decisions, and formed subcommittees and task forces to investigate specific issues.

The Nursing Operations Group was particularly important during 1982 and 1983, when the department's new direction was being charted. It began by investigating and discussing some major issues, like the new departmental structure, and the way in which various care delivery models were used on nursing units. The group and its subcommittees then settled in to fine-tuning the Nursing Department's activities in specific areas.

In 1983 the Nursing Operations Group discussed the issue of divisional status for the Department of Nursing. Within the Cleveland Clinic Foundation, divisions were the largest units of organization, and departments were included within divisions. (For instance, the Department of Orthopaedics was part of the Division of Surgery.) Besides its clinical divisions — Medicine, Surgery, Anesthesiology, and Radiology — the Foundation had divisions of Laboratory Medicine, Research, Education, and Operations. The division heads met as the Management Operations Group. This group was responsible for overseeing the day-to-day management of the Cleveland Clinic, and reported to the physician Board of Governors, the institution's policy-making body.

Although Ms. Danielsen, as Associate Director of Operations/Nursing, attended Management Operations Group meetings, she was not a divisional

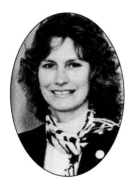

ISABELLE BOLAND
The new nursing organization had four internal divisions — Nursing Resources, Surgical Nursing, Medical Nursing, and Operating Room and Treatment Areas. Each division included several departments or areas. Ms. Boland, hired in 1983 as Director of Nursing Resources, was appointed head of Operating Room and Treatment Areas in 1984. Besides the Operating Room and Outpatient Surgery Unit, she had responsibility for the Post-Anesthesia Recovery Unit, the Emergency Room, the IV Team, and Nursing Infection Control, with a total of 319 nursing personnel who cared for an average of 430 patients daily. She was also instrumental in starting a departmental publication, *Memo to Nursing Staff*. Ms. Boland served as Associate Director of Nursing from 1986 to 1988.

chairperson; she reported to the chairman of the Division of Operations. The Nursing Operations Group unanimously supported seeking divisional status for Nursing. Ms. Danielsen presented the proposal to the Board of Governors, but it was not approved at that time.

Departmental Mission

By early 1983, the Department of Nursing had identified four departmental missions: "to provide the patients with professional nursing care"; "to provide all levels of nursing personnel with opportunities for on-going education"; "to contribute to the body of nursing knowledge"; and "to be a resource to the nursing community at-large." The first three of these corresponded to the Cleveland Clinic's historic three-part mission — "better care of the sick, investigation of their problems, and further education of those who serve" — as interpreted by nurse administrators of the 1980s. The fourth departmental mission added a role for nurses in keeping with the Cleveland Clinic's status as a state-of-the-art medical center.[39]

Throughout the history of The Cleveland Clinic Foundation, nursing personnel had always concentrated on "better care of the sick." Education supported that goal, but education itself was not of primary concern, as it was in nursing schools. As for research, nurses often assisted physicians, but had no organized framework in which they could carry out nursing research. During the 1980s, and after, the Department of Nursing continued to emphasize the first mission, providing high-quality nursing care to patients. Under the new administration, specific objectives related to this mission included both restructuring and professionalization.

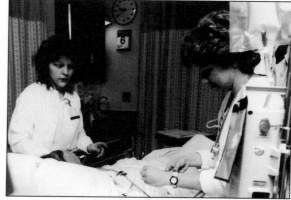

Restructuring meant the implementation of the new departmental organization with its clinical clusters and Department of Nursing Resources, and also a change in the nursing care delivery system. Professionalization meant increasing the proportion of registered nurses in the department, and increasing the use of professional tools such as standards of care, nursing assessments, nursing diagnoses, and care plans to rationalize care delivery.

Although the Nursing Department now included the Operating Room, as well as Nurse Recruitment and Nursing Education, substantial differences in the work setting meant that the Operating Room would contribute to the departmental mission in somewhat different ways. The ever-increasing amount of expensive and sensitive equipment used in the operating suite meant that organization of the physical environment and attention to cost containment were key objectives, although the Operating Room, too, proposed to contribute to professionalization by delegating non-nursing tasks to ancillary personnel, and by developing nursing care standards.

"Patients are Smart"

As part of the "new structure," Ms. Danielsen wanted to see an overall shift toward the primary nursing model of care delivery, stating that "nursing care should be given by an R.N. and every patient should know his/her nurse." A

PATIENT CARE
The primary mission of the Department of Nursing had always been patient care. In the 1920s, registered nurses, assisted by a small number of orderlies and "ward maids," gave all direct care. They monitored patients through sight and touch, recorded TPRs and I & Os, and gave medications and supportive care. By the last quarter of the century, nurses were using cardiac monitors and infusion pumps, administering CPR and chemotherapy, and caring for patient populations that included organ transplant recipients and AIDS victims. But the goal of helping patients to attain optimum health remained the same.

survey conducted in 1982 by the Nursing Operations Group's Patient Care Delivery Task Force indicated that although some units designated primary nurses for patients, team nursing still remained the predominant assignment system on Cleveland Clinic Hospital nursing units. When the survey asked, "Can patients identify a single nurse who perhaps knows the most about their care?", the answers ranged from "Rarely" to "Not always" to "Yes, patients are smart."[40]

In answer to the question, "Describe your present mode of nursing care delivery," 10 of the Hospital's 35 nursing units said they used the team method. Eight used a modified team approach. Eight more used modified primary nursing. Three units were, theoretically, primary nursing units, but were not well-enough staffed to operate fully on the primary model. Six units listed their delivery model as "total patient care," in which an individual nurse would handle all care for an individual patient on a given day.

> This model was largely seen in the ICUs in which the bedside nurse performed all care, administered meds, took off own orders etc. It was not viewed as a primary model since assignments may not be consistent. Some of these divisions practiced a modified primary model since their more acute or long term patients had a designated primary nurse. No division felt their model was totally a primary nursing model at this time.[41]

Four units had daily patient care conferences; 11 had conferences "rarely"; one unit defined conferences broadly, stating that it had them "during the day, at breaks, and at the desk, whenever the nurses discuss the patients." Patients who figured most frequently as the subjects of conferences were long-term, difficult patients. More often than not, colleagues from other departments, such as Physical Therapy, Social Service, and Dietary, participated. Most units (25) had charge nurses; most units (25) had team leaders. Team leaders and charge nurses made most of the nursing rounds, at intervals and in ways which varied from unit to unit: hourly; two or three times a shift; with M.D.s; to check patients and IVs; and, "spontaneously, whenever Head Nurse 'grabs' somebody."[42]

More R.N.s

In 1974, L.P.N.s and nursing assistants had together outnumbered R.N.s on the Hospital Nursing Department staff. By 1986, this had changed. Of the department's 2,072 employees, 1,097 were R.N.s. Had all 2,345 budgeted positions been filled, 1,426, or fully 60 percent, of the department's employees would have been registered nurses.

This new staffing balance was the result of a conscious policy decision within the department to provide more care by R.N.s for Clinic Hospital patients and to emphasize the primary nursing care model. Team nursing allowed a relatively few R.N.s, as team leaders, to manage the care of a relatively large number of patients by depending on auxiliary staff to provide much of the direct care. In the early 1980s, L.P.N.s were also serving as team leaders on some units. If registered nurses were to handle more direct care, and to spend more time planning and evaluating the care of individual patients, more R.N.s would be needed.

The Surgical Nursing division evaluated the L.P.N. and Patient Care Assistant roles. It was concluded that "patient needs and educational background affirmed the L.P.N.'s appropriate role as one of support for R.N. work," and that assistants should have their "technical skills [used] in a more appropriate support function." In 1986 the Department of Nursing changed the Patient Care Assistant title to Nursing Unit Assistant (N.U.A.), underscoring the position's revised role: "The department clarified the work of registered nurse and NUA staff....The RN was identified as responsible for the provision of direct care. The NUA provides support to the RN and to the unit."[43]

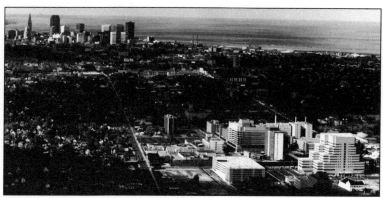

At the same time as the nursing administration was trying to increase the proportion of R.N.s on the staff, the Hospital itself was expanding, adding new beds and units. Numerically, the number of R.N.s working in the Hospital Department of Nursing (not including the Operating Room) rose from 559 in 1980 to 918 in 1986. This 64 percent increase resulted from an intensive recruitment and retention effort. It was an especially impressive accomplishment, noted Ms. Boland in 1986, "given the significant shortage that exists locally, statewide and nationally for nurses, especially those prepared for critical care."[44] However, the Nursing Department's need for more R.N.s seemed nearly insatiable; 329 R.N. positions remained open at the end of 1986.

The attrition rate had dropped somewhat in the early 1980s, following efforts to improve both salaries and morale. As of mid-1981, R.N. salaries ranged from a $9.20/hour start rate to an $11.79 maximum, with a standard job rate of $10.70. Mr. Brent had cited a steady decline in attrition, from 38 percent in 1979, to 25 percent in 1982. Nonetheless, Nurse Recruitment had to attract hundreds of R.N.s each year. Advertisements in professional journals and in local newspapers supplemented person-to-person recruitment, which included campus visits, convention booths, and open houses. Attempts were made to hire nurses from other countries, "especially from the Philippines."[45] Recruitment brochures were painstakingly constructed to feature nurses from various educational and ethnic backgrounds, as well as both genders, working in the various specialized areas of nursing at the Cleveland Clinic.

In 1986, the Department of Nursing hired 87 nursing students to work on the units as undergraduate nursing assistants: "This program provided an opportunity for nursing students to learn about nursing opportunities at The Cleveland Clinic Foundation."[46] Although this differed from affiliation programs, in which students from designated schools came to receive formal clinical instruction to fulfill their curriculum requirements, it had similar value as a recruitment device.

A New Look

The changes of the 1970s and 1980s had given nursing organization at the Cleveland Clinic a new look. The Clinic's campus was also taking on a new look, with the remodeling of old buildings and the construction of new ones, culminating in the mid-1980s. The pyramid-shaped "A" Building (officially named the Crile Building in 1992) opened in the autumn of 1985 as the new home of the institution's outpatient area. Clinic Nursing, now often referred to as Ambulatory Nursing, was headquartered there.

The new "G" wing of the Clinic Hospital was completed at almost the same time. Nursing units began moving in during January 1986. The old system of naming nursing units by a number indicating a floor and a letter designating a location on that floor — for instance, 5S (South) or 7Q — was revised. Now unit names began with a letter indicating the unit's building, followed by a number with the first digit indicating the unit's floor. For instance, G80 (the first nursing unit to move into the new area) and G81 were both located on the eighth floor of the new Hospital wing.[47]

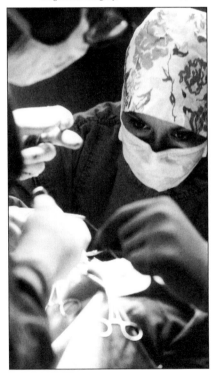

SCRUBBING
This photograph shows registered nurse Linda Hopkins of the ENT service in the role of scrub nurse, with operating surgeon Dr. Howard Levine of the Department of Otolaryngology. In the 1980s, Cleveland Clinic Operating Room nurses were assigned to 10 surgical specialty services, as well as general surgery.

Change upon change also took place in nursing practice, which significantly affected the daily working lives of nursing personnel in caring for their patients. Organization and practice of nursing at the Cleveland Clinic did not evolve independently of each other. For instance, nurse administrators played a key role in encouraging and sometimes requiring innovation in nursing practice. On the other hand, new medical technologies and associated changes in nursing practice could affect the Nursing Department's organizational structure. For example, the increased use of ventilators and sophisticated monitoring equipment resulted in a greater proportion of intensive care and telemetry nursing units.

Looking back, many nurses pinpointed the mid-1970s as the time when practice changes began to snowball. Trends at the national and international level in medicine and nursing had a great impact on practice over the next 20 years. New materials, some of them developed for or by the space program, made possible the development of new techniques and instruments, like flexible scopes. New drugs, like cyclosporine, expanded treatment options. The role of research in nursing grew. Nursing specialty organizations and nursing specialty certification programs were proliferating. For example, the American Association of Critical-Care Nurses (AACN) was founded in 1969, the Oncology Nursing Society (ONS) in 1975, and the Society of Otorhinolaryngology and Head and Neck Nurses (SOHN) in 1976. During the 1980s, the first certification exams were held in specialties including post-anesthesia, oncology, nephrology, and orthopaedic nursing.

As a tertiary care center with an international reputation, the Cleveland Clinic handled patients with severe or unusual illnesses in the ambulatory departments, operating rooms, and Hospital units on a daily basis. It was important for Cleveland Clinic nurses to stay at the forefront of knowledge in their fields, incorporating innovations into the everyday routine of patient care and assisting in advancing nursing practice.

Operating Room Nursing

Operating room nurses experienced a great deal of change in administrative organization and in nursing practice between the 1970s and 1990s. They also saw some changes in their work area. Existing balconies were removed from the operating rooms in the 1970s. In the 1980s, remodeling transformed the suite's old layout, with its single large setup room and central scrub room. In the new layout, a number of smaller rooms located between the various operating rooms provided more convenient areas for preparation and cleanup, and made it easier to maintain sterile conditions.

The most important feature of the Operating Room's administrative structure was the assignment of nurses to specialized surgical services. With minor revisions, this system remained in place. As a rule, Operating Room nurses filled in as necessary on other services besides their own. For a short time, however, the idea of having a service staffed only by its own nurses, with no substitutes from other areas, was tried out. This plan took full advantage of nurses' specialized expertise, but was also prohibitively expensive.

Throughout this period, the assignment areas for Operating Room nurses stayed basically the same as in this 1984 listing: General, Cardiothoracic, Colorectal, Otolaryngology, Eye, Genitourinary, Gynecology, Neurosurgery, Orthopaedic, Plastic, and Vascular services. Some specialties were at times grouped together with another area, like Gynecology with General Surgery. Asked what was distinctive about working at the Cleveland Clinic, Operating Room nurses most often cited the highly specialized nature of their practice, along with the opportunity to work with renowned surgeons who performed rare operations on an almost daily basis.

One unsettling aspect of Operating Room nursing during this period was frequent turnover in the director's position. The position changed hands six times between 1983 and 1991. Different directors implemented different management structures within the Operating Room: "Every time there was a new head, management positions were changed and people had to reapply for their jobs." The situation created tension and turmoil, making it difficult for everyone in the department. Most agreed that Betty Bush, R.N., B.S.N., who assumed leadership in 1991, had a "very calming effect" on Operating Room personnel.[48]

Administrative change was only the tip of the iceberg. Operating room nurses active from the 1960s through the 1980s and 1990s pointed out the numerous challenges they had confronted: "sophisticated technology, complicated sterilization technique, budget planning, documentation, personnel management, evaluation of products etc." They referred in particular to the sheer amount and variety of equipment and instrumentation used in the operating room as "the hard part about OR nursing now."[49]

Advances in endoscopy, microsurgery, synthetic implants, and heart-lung equipment, along with the introduction of new technologies like lasers, meant that operating room nurses had responsibility for ordering, storing, and maintaining a dazzling array of complicated, delicate, and expensive items. They had to know how to use this equipment, and, upon occasion, to be able to instruct surgeons in its use.

Nurses agreed that most of the new technology represented genuine advances. "In my way of thinking, probably the greatest innovative thing that has been devised [is] fiberoptics," declared a nurse, remembering when bronchoscopies had been performed using rigid scopes and light carriers with "little tiny bulbs" that worked outside the patient but seemed to go out every time they were inserted into a patient's throat.[50]

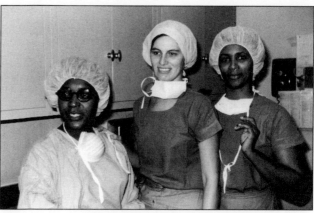

IN THE O.R.
So that surgeons could concentrate on surgery, nurses coordinated everything that went on in the operating room, from before the patient's arrival, through the operation, and on to cleanup and preparation for the next procedure. Operating Room nurses like (left to right) Josephine Smith, Linda Solar, and Betty Williamson could look forward to substantial changes in their practice between the late 1960s, when this photograph was taken, and the 1990s. The variety, fragility, and sheer amount of equipment used in the various surgical specialties added to the complexity of their work.

The availability and fragility of the new equipment ended, for the most part, the old "do-it-yourself" days. (Some nurses found that they missed the challenge to their ingenuity.) Also, with the huge increase in the use of disposables, operating room nurses often simply threw away supplies they formerly would have cleaned. Disposable plastic syringes replaced glass syringes and reusable needles, and paper masks, drapes, and gowns replaced green linen. "Now they throw practically the whole room away!" exclaimed one nurse.[51] More technicians were added to handle those items that still needed to be cleaned. Personnel in new positions, like laser technicians, assumed some of the responsibility for new technologies.

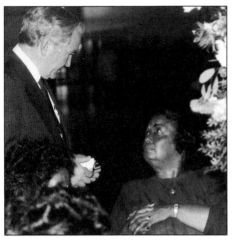

ANN REE GRAY
The Cleveland Clinic's 25 Year Club was instituted to honor employees with a quarter century of service. Ms. Gray, who joined the club in 1984, is seen here at the Club's 1985 dinner with Dr. William S. Kiser, Chairman of the Board of Governors. A licensed practical nurse, she worked in the Cleveland Clinic Operating Room as a technician (O.R.T.) for many years.

The new division of labor still left the operating room nurse in charge of everything that happened in her room. As long as the patient was there, at least one nurse stayed to keep watch. "The nurses are so important in the OR as advocates of the patient. Technicians, like surgeons, are focused, and properly so, on their own particular part of what is going on. If there is no nurse, no one is responsible for the overall welfare of the patient." The circulating nurse, in particular, managed the flow of work in her room. However, most nurses agreed that scrubbing was "more fun." If at least two R.N.s worked on a case, they could decide between themselves who would scrub and who would circulate. Like the days of improvised equipment, the days of circulating two or more rooms were mostly over. "Now, you just don't even think of it."[52]

By the 1980s and 1990s operating room nurses were more likely to call surgeons by their first names. They spent more time on paperwork. With increasing awareness of risks like acquired immunodeficiency syndrome and hepatitis, they had to take more precautions against infection. "You handled sponges with your bare hands in the old days....Now it's rubber gloves and plastic bags to put everything in."[53] Eye protection and laser masks were mandatory, since the plume from laser surgery could carry a virus.

Other aspects of operating room nursing remained the same. For instance, the nurse had to be able to organize her work. "There's a lot of things that have to start all at once, and you have to be able to figure out, do I take care of the patient now, do I start my sterile supplies now, do I get this equipment, what's first, what's the most important....[You have] to prioritize your list in about two minutes flat." Shorter cases with faster turnover meant more cleaning up and setting up, more paperwork, more time settling patients into the room. Contrary to what an outsider might have assumed, most operating room nurses considered short cases more difficult than procedures lasting many hours. But for short cases or long ones, said nurses, "if you're in good control of your room and know what's going on, [and have] what you'll need...you can relax and have a good day, because you have organized yourself well."[54]

The Post-Anesthesia Care Unit

The evolution of the old "Recovery Room" into the Post-Anesthesia Care Unit (PACU) at the Cleveland Clinic Hospital reflected the development of post-anesthesia care into a recognized nursing specialty nationwide. Maria Zickuhr, R.N., B.S., head nurse from 1973 to 1993, and her successor Deborah

Atsberger, R.N., B.S.N., were charter members of the American Society of Post Anesthesia Nurses (ASPAN), founded in 1980.

During the 1970s, the Clinic Hospital's Recovery Room was administered within Nursing as part of Area II, the ICU area, remaining under the medical direction of the Division of Anesthesia. In 1978, after the appointment of Azmy Boutros, M.D., as Division Chairman, the Recovery Room's hours were extended so that it was open around the clock, five days a week. This decreased the need to send patients who needed close observation for a short time to an intensive care unit. After an overnight stay in the post-anesthesia unit they could go immediately to a regular nursing floor. Also at this time, the name of the unit was changed to Post-Anesthesia Recovery Unit (PARU).

After the reorganization of the Department of Nursing in the early 1980s, the PARU was initially administered as part of Surgical Nursing, but in 1984 became part of the Operating Room and Treatment Areas division of the Nursing Department, as did the Outpatient Surgery Unit (OPSU) and the new To Come In (TCI) Unit. The name was eventually changed to Post-Anesthesia Care Unit.

Meanwhile, the growth and development of the unit continued. In 1970, the Recovery Room had 10 beds and a tiny full-time nursing staff supplemented by floats. In the following decade, bed space expanded to 25. In 1986, the Post-Anesthesia Care Unit moved to a 47-bed facility made up of four smaller nursing units, each under the direction of an assistant head nurse. The new PACU included a separate 5-bed pediatric unit. In 1987 Post-Anesthesia Care took on responsibility for the TCI Center, and in 1989 the Pre-Care area was added. By the early 1990s, the PACU had 57 beds and a staff of 70.

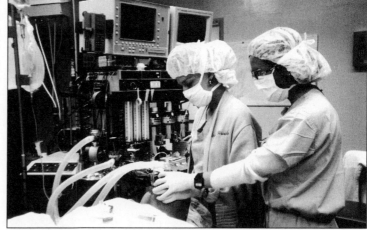

Knowledge of anesthesia agents and side effects, and skill in airway management and respiratory care remained the cornerstones of post-anesthesia nursing, but new responsibilities, like monitoring venous and arterial pressures with invasive lines, had added complexity to post-anesthesia practice. In 1983, a post-anesthesia nursing career ladder was developed and put into practice at the Cleveland Clinic. It identified four levels, from Beginner to Advanced Post-Anesthesia nurse, with knowledge and clinical competency requirements for each. In 1986, the unit implemented an innovative Post-Anesthesia Care Record based on the use of the nursing process and nursing diagnoses in the post-anesthesia setting. The record included space for nurses to note both expected and actual outcomes.

Perioperative Nursing

At the Cleveland Clinic, as elsewhere, efforts by third-party payors and others to control costs by decreasing hospital stays, along with encouragement from nursing specialty organizations like the Association of Operating Room Nurses (AORN) and ASPAN, helped to create expanded roles for both

CONTRAST
AND CONTINUITY
The sophisticated anesthesia and monitoring equipment used by nurse anesthetists in the late 20th century contrasted with the very basic setup of earlier years (see p. 30). Nurse anesthetists continued to practice at the Cleveland Clinic, and to teach the next generation of anesthetists at the Clinic's School of Nurse Anesthesia (above). In 1989, through affiliation with the Frances Payne Bolton School of Nursing at Case Western Reserve University, the Clinic's existing two-year certificate program became a 28-month M.S.N. degree program.

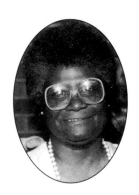

NURSING UNIT ASSISTANTS
The Cleveland Clinic Hospital began employing nurses' aides during WWII. Although administrators complained of high turnover among the first group, they were soon praising the "excellent aides" trained in the following years. The nurses' aide position developed into the nursing unit assistant (N.U.A.) role, filled by both women and men. A number of the N.U.A.s hired in the 1960s were still with the Cleveland Clinic in the 1980s and 1990s, among them Mary Ann Parker (above), who joined the 25 Year Club in 1988. She spent her many years of service caring for patients on G81 and its predecessor units, where mostly ENT and, later, pulmonary patients were admitted.

operating room and post-anesthesia nurses. The AORN promoted use of the term "perioperative nurse," rather than "operating room nurse," to convey "the concept that the nursing care of the patient having surgery should extend prior to and beyond the doors to the surgical pavilion."[55] At the Clinic, operating room nurses had always met and greeted patients as they arrived in the operating suite, but this greeting now included a presurgical interview to verify the patient's identity and surgeon, the existence of any allergies, and other significant information. Attempts were also made to enable operating room nurses to visit inpatients on the day before surgery.

The number of patients admitted on the day of surgery increased as lengths of stay decreased. Nursing personnel in the To Come In Center provided gowns, medication, and instruction to these patients in preparation for surgery. They assessed and interviewed patients. They also provided reassurance and emotional support to patients and families alike. "Aware that the TCI experience appears to the patient to be a highly technical, task-oriented and rushed 'production-line-like-process,' we try to create a warm, cheerful and accepting atmosphere. We begin by greeting each patient with a smile."[56] When the TCI Center was transferred from the Outpatient Surgical Unit to the PACU in 1987, post-anesthesia nurses took on these preoperative duties.

Nurses also gave patients the information they needed to prepare themselves for surgery. The Divisions of Nursing and Anesthesia had collaborated to set up a preadmission process in 1985, adding a facet to perioperative nursing at the Cleveland Clinic. Nurses in the Anesthesia Clearance area in the A Building did preoperative assessments, gave instructions, answered questions, and helped patients cope with anxiety.

In 1988 a new, separate Outpatient Surgery Center opened in the M61-63 area. It included a reception area, preoperative staging area, five operating suites, and adult and pediatric post-anesthesia units. Here, the expanding roles of operating room nurses and post-anesthesia nurses intersected most visibly. The Outpatient Surgery nurses were oriented to the post-anesthesia care specialty. They rotated "through the pre- and postoperative area, PACU areas and the preadmit area at A38 and O.R."[57]

At the same time, the new PreCare preoperative holding area opened for Hospital inpatients. (It was also occasionally used for TCI and OPSU patients.) "In the past, patients awaiting surgery were placed in a small induction room and occasionally in the hallways." In the greater privacy and quiet of the PreCare area, nurses assessed patients, completed preoperative medications, placed or checked IV access, and also answered questions and offered "reassurance and emotional support...and warm blankets." An operating room nurse coming to PreCare to escort a patient to the operating room had the chance to meet family members and check the patient's status with PreCare nurses.[58]

Complexities of Care

One of the areas for which the Cleveland Clinic was well known was the treatment of renal disease. The Clinic, and its Department of Artificial Organs, had been a pioneer in the field of hemodialysis since the 1950s. Decades later, some of the challenges of providing nursing care to people with end-stage renal disease and other severe kidney problems remained the same, but patients, nurses, and all members of the health care team faced new complexities as well.

By the mid-1980s, care of the dialysis patient was well-established at the Cleveland Clinic. Following admission, the nurse assessed the patient. Weight and vital signs were recorded. The dialyzer was prepared, the inflow and outflow lines connected to the patient, and the blood pump turned on. Assessment of the patient continued throughout dialysis. The blood in the dialyzer was then re-transfused to the patient, another assessment made, and any necessary medications given.

In addition to being knowledgeable about the highly techni-cal procedure itself, nursing personnel had to be aware of emotional and social factors. "Virtually no other procedure of long-term care requires individuals to be as dependent....There are varied behavioral manifestations to the overwhelming stress and forced dependency," noted nurses who worked on the dialy-sis unit, M82. "For much of our patient population, the disease is chronic necessitating frequent hospital admissions. This represents a big change in lifestyle" for the patient and family. One of the nurse's most important roles was to provide educa-tion and information, helping patients comply with treatment regimens and enabling them to participate in their own care.[59]

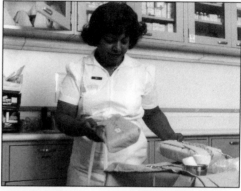

AMBULATORY SURGERY
Trends in medical technology and financing encouraged outpatient surgery. At the Cleveland Clinic, this included operations in the Hospital's Outpatient Surgery Unit, and also in the Crile Building outpatient areas, so that some Ambulatory Nursing staff mem-bers were involved in operating room work. In this photograph, Ambulatory Nursing patient care assistant Beverly Henderson restocks supplies in the Plastic Surgery Department's Crile Building operating suite.

The care of the dialysis patient had been, from the beginning, a collabora-tive effort at the Cleveland Clinic. In the 1980s and 1990s, dialysis technicians, social workers, and dietitians continued to work alongside physicians and nurses in caring for dialysis patients and patients with other nephrologic dis-orders. In 1986, nurses and social workers on the nursing unit H80 began meeting weekly to identify patients in need of social services, facilitate dis-charge planning, and improve communication. A renal dietitian was available for patient consultation and teaching on the units of the nephrology/urology cluster, H80, H81, and M82.

Also in 1986, extracorporeal shock wave lithotripsy, a new treatment for patients with renal calculi (kidney stones) was introduced at the Cleveland Clinic. The patient was immersed into warm water, which transmitted shock waves that pulverized the stones. New nursing care procedures were intro-duced as well. Nursing personnel had to make sure that patients took in enough fluids after the procedure to keep the urinary tract healthy; to strain urine to save calculi fragments for analysis; and to watch for signs of hemor-rhage. Patient education, both before lithotripsy and before discharge from the hospital, was an integral part of the nursing care of these patients.

Organ Transplantation in the 1980s

Some patients with end-stage renal disease underwent kidney transplanta-tion. The first renal transplant surgery performed at the Cleveland Clinic was done in 1963. All major organ transplant procedures were high-profile treat-ments that offered great hope but involved great difficulties for patients and caregivers alike. The medical hurdles to be cleared were daunting: tissue typ-ing and matching of donors and recipients, a long and complex operation, the possibility of rejection, the risk of infection. Beyond these life-and-death con-cerns, caregivers and patients had to face many strategic, ethical, social, and emotional challenges. Nurses worked with patients from screening to surgery through hospital stay, and on to home care and periodic checkups that might continue throughout a lifetime.

Pediatric patients represented a special challenge. For example, patient teaching had to be tailored to meet the needs of children. The nursing staff on H80 did this by giving their young renal transplant patients a "jobs list" to be completed each day, with the help of the primary caregiver. "The list included daily recording of...creatinine level, blood pressure, temperature, weight, intake and output, ambulation, and use of the incentive spirometer. Also included on the list for our school-age patients are daily routines such as bathing and brushing teeth."[60]

The development of a powerful anti-rejection drug, cyclosporine, gave new impetus to organ transplantation during the early 1980s. At the Cleveland Clinic, surgeons had made headlines by performing Ohio's first heart transplants in 1968. Disappointing outcomes overall later led to the abandonment of heart transplants at the Clinic until 1984. The first liver transplant at the Clinic was also performed in 1984.

However, cyclosporine, an immunosuppressive agent, increased the risk of infection. The first transplant patients, recalled one nurse, "spent much of their time alone" because of the strict isolation precautions considered necessary.[61] Nurses were responsible for monitoring patients for signs of both rejection and infection, as well as administering prophylactic antibiotics under doctors' orders.

During the mid-1980s, anti-rejection therapy was "a rapidly expanding field."[62] High-dose steroids were being administered to transplant patients, and monoclonal antibody therapy also showed promise. At the Cleveland Clinic, a monoclonal antibody, administered as an IV push medication, was used to treat renal transplant patients beginning in 1986. Helped by cardiac nurses, nurses on unit H80 developed guidelines and a self-instructional learning packet to prepare nurses to give the medication. Since the incidence of reaction — including fever, chills, vomiting, diarrhea, pulmonary edema, tachycardia, and hypotension — was highest during the first three once-a-day doses, those were administered by physicians. Nurses gave the remaining doses for the duration of the 10 to 14 days of therapy.

During the liver transplant program's first year, recipients included two adolescent patients. In 1986, a 19-month-old girl named Carla was the first young child to undergo the procedure at the Cleveland Clinic. Carla had been born with biliary atresia, and a transplant was "her only hope of survival."[63]

Pediatric and other nurses had been preparing to care for young liver transplant patients from the moment the program began. They communicated with other institutions, visited the Pittsburgh Children's Hospital, and prepared an educational presentation for co-workers on the care of pediatric transplant patients.

During the weeks-long wait for a suitable donor, little Carla and her mother stayed at the Clinic's Transition Care Unit. Nurses from the Pediatric/Surgical Intensive Care Unit (P/SICU) and pediatric unit M73 worked with mother and child to prepare them for the transplant and the hospital stay. After an eight-hour operation on August 27, 1986, Carla went to the P/SICU, where she remained for two months. She was then transferred to M73, where she stayed for another month. During this time

> Carla's mother needed to learn post-transplant care regimens, medication administration, techniques to promote Carla's development both

physically and emotionally and tube feeding procedures, since Carla had feeding difficulties. A notebook was developed by the nursing staff to organize the written instructions, home records of vital signs, weights and medications.

Nursing, Social Services, Clinicare, Nutrition Services, Occupational Therapy, Physical Therapy and the Administrative Coordinator worked hand-in-hand to assure that the parents had the needed medical supplies and thorough instructions to care for their daughter at home.

Caring for Carla and her family took a great deal of work and planning, but the results were well worth it. When discharge day finally arrived, three months from the day of transplant, we sent home a happy, well-adjusted child and a mother who felt confident and competent in her child's care.[64]

The child's family and nurses were still in touch a year later. "Carla's mother still calls her primary and associate nurses, requesting advice and seeking suggestions on home care. Sometimes she calls just to let us know how Carla is doing. Staff look forward to family visits and share the parents' joy in watching her grow into a beautiful little girl."[65]

Cardiac Nursing in the 1980s

By the time the reborn heart transplant program had its second birthday in August of 1986, members of the cardiac transplant team were encouraged by the percentage of successful transplants as well as the "excellent" quality of life enjoyed by heart recipients. Members of the transplant team who met weekly to plan patient care included nurses, social workers, physical therapists, and dietitians. The nurses were "intensely involved" in educating and supporting the patient and family, as well as in providing physical care.[66]

Heart transplant recipients were an important but small part of the patient population cared for by cardiac nurses. Patients with many types of heart disease came to be treated by Cleveland Clinic cardiologists and cardiac surgeons. As in other specialties, economic and other factors were resulting in a greater proportion of severely ill patients on cardiac nursing units.

For example, the patient with alteration in cardiac output who requires cardiac monitoring is now being treated and discharged from the cardiac nursing floor rather than the intensive care unit.

....Telemetry/cardiac monitoring and patient education begin from the moment the patient arrives on the unit....

....Our goal is the prevention of life-threatening situations and the education of patients and families in lifestyle modification.

Nurses needed to be well-versed in "EKG interpretation, cardiovascular physical assessment, disease pathology, and the integration of laboratory results into the nursing data base."[67]

On a routine basis, nurses on the cardiac telemetry units were caring for patients with pacemakers and other surgically implanted devices, as well as patients on ventilators and IV medications. One nurse, noting that ventricular tachycardia (V-Tach) no longer necessarily called for a "triple," illustrated how the extraordinary had become the commonplace: a patient with V-Tach might, as a matter of course, be defibrillated or interrupted for assessment during a game of checkers or a walk down the hall. Even more extraordinary, electrophysiology testing involved "an attempt...to reproduce |in order to treat| the dysrhythmia which may have previously resulted in syncope or sudden death." During pre-procedural patient teaching, the nurse had the challenge of explaining this while trying not to frighten the patient.[68]

Another innovation of the 1980s was the external pacemaker, for use in emergencies when there was no time to insert a pacing wire. It could also be used for patients who needed only intermittent pacing, or for patients who could not undergo invasive procedures. Since it was a new medical practice, nurses had to assess patients frequently and develop appropriate nursing strategies and interventions to reduce the considerable discomfort that the external pacemaker caused.

Nurses also helped to develop new technologies. Nurses in the Cardiothoracic Intensive Care Unit (CTICU), along with cardiac perfusionists, collaborated with Delos M. Cosgrove, M.D., Chairman of the Department of Thoracic

Cardiac Nursing from Catheterization to Rehabilitation

Several key events in the history of cardiac nursing at the Cleveland Clinic occurred in the 1950s. In 1951 Sophia Larsen organized the Operating Room into specialized nursing services, creating a "Chest" service for heart and lung surgery. In 1952, Vae Lucile Van Derwyst began her career at the Clinic as nurse in the one-year-old Pediatric Cardiology Department; by the end of the decade, she was serving as the first nurse in the new Cardiac Catheterization Laboratory. Specialized nursing care for Clinic Hospital cardiac patients began with the opening of the Constant Care Unit's "Heart Room" in 1957.

In 1967, a unit for cardiovascular surgery patients opened on the Hospital's sixth floor, with its own operating suite, intensive care unit, and stepdown unit. Nurses from the second-floor operating pavilion and the Surgical Intensive Care Unit transferred to the new Cardiovascular Unit; Virginia Myers Meserko served as its first head nurse. Cleveland's first, and the world's 40th, heart transplant was performed in the unit in 1968. The surgical team included six nurses.

In 1972, registered nurse Emily Wagstaff assisted Dr. Floyd Loop in establishing the Cleveland Clinic Cardiovascular Information Registry, the first of its kind in the world. It quickly grew to include information on tens of thousands of patients.

In 1985, the Clinic introduced a new program devoted to health recovery and wellness for cardiac patients. The Cardiac Health Improvement and Rehabilitation Program (CHIRP) included regis-

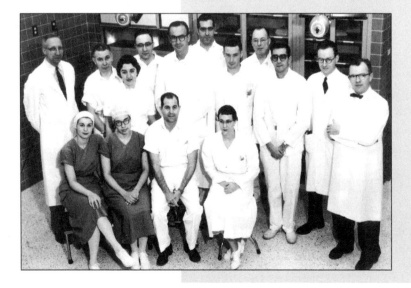

Cardiac team, 1956, including: (left to right) nurses Donna Adamcin and Betty Lou Gary; Rose Litturi (standing); and nurse anesthetist Del Portzer (seated at right)

and Cardiovascular Surgery, to develop a cardiotomy autotransfusion system. Autotransfusion, using the patient's own blood for transfusion, had several advantages over conventional transfusion. It decreased risk of disease transmission or transfusion reaction and reduced demands upon the blood bank. It also could be offered to patients whose religious teachings forbade them to receive donated blood. During cardiac surgery patients often lost a great deal of blood, but existing technologies to recover and use this blood were "both expensive and plagued with complications."[69]

The new system, which was more economical and efficient, used

> a reservoir from the cardiopulmonary bypass circuitry as the post operative chest tube drainage system. The conversion is made intraoperatively by the perfusionist with the assistance of the cardiac operating room nursing staff.

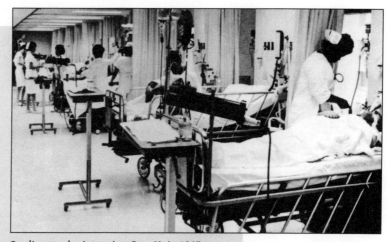

Cardiovascular Intensive Care Unit, 1967

CHIRP activity and education coordinators, Ben Meola (center) and Betsy Stovsky (right), with a patient, 1987

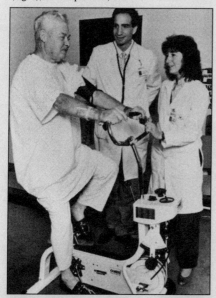

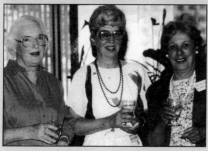

Lucile Van Derwyst (left) and Emily Wagstaff (right) with lab technician Betty Root, 1987

tered nurse activity and education coordinators.

Within the Division of Nursing, a Department of Cardiac Nursing was created in 1987. Its director, Gayle Whitman, had served as head nurse of a cardiac unit and one of the first clinical nurse specialists in the Hospital Nursing Department. A contributor to numerous nursing texts and journals, she was subsequently named a Fellow of the American Academy of Nursing.

By the 1990s, the Cleveland Clinic Hospital had 12 medical and surgical cardiac nursing units. In the Clinic and the Hospital, nurses cared for cardiac patients from all over the world.

> Upon admission to the CTICU, negative suction is applied as well as an infusion pump with tubing. Any blood drained from the mediastinal or pleural chest tubes is returned hourly to the patient via the infusion pump as the patient's condition permits, up to 12 hours post op....After that time, the cardiotomy serves as a drainage collection system until the chest tubes are discontinued.[70]

In 1989, cardiovascular intensive care nurses collected data for a multi-site clinical trial of the sodium nitroprusside titrator, a closed loop infusion pump that made it possible to control a patient's blood pressure automatically. The titrator had also been designed under the direction of Dr. Cosgrove with the assistance of the nursing staff.

Writing about "Cardiac Interventional Nursing," a Clinic Hospital nurse highlighted the differences between caring for patients with coronary artery disease in the 1960s and the late 1980s. During the earlier period, nursing care consisted mainly of "close observation, assessment of vital signs and palpating the pulse for arrhythmias." In those days, "there was no talk of 'stopping' a heart attack!" A quarter of a century later, physicians tried "to identify high-risk patients as early as possible and intervene before myocardial damage occurs."

> This approach to care has resulted in new avenues for nursing practice.
>
> The nurse's role frequently begins with identifying possible candidates for intervention. When a patient experiences angina, the nurse must not only attempt to relieve pain by conventional methods, but must also assist the physician in diagnosing the event by obtaining stat EKGs and communicating changes in the patient's condition. Once an acute cardiac event is confirmed, it is the nurse's responsibility to act swiftly in preparing the patient for a cardiac catheterization and possible intervention. Concurrently, the nurse must maintain a calm, reassuring environment and continue to relieve the angina with intravenous vasoactive drips and analgesics as ordered by the physician.

After intervention by the cardiologist

> the patient may return to the interventional stepdown unit. It is the RN's responsibility to monitor the patient for possible complications and intervene. Nursing care of the post PTCA atherectomy patient includes careful and frequent arterial monitoring....If a decreased cardiac output or altered tissue perfusion does occur, the RN must act quickly to prevent a MI [myocardial infarction].
>
> Patients are usually stable by the following morning....Prior to discharge, patients are given strict diet instructions and reminded of the importance of medical compliance and physician follow-up....
>
> While care of the cardiac patient is now more of a challenge, it is also rewarding. Our unit [G91] is a blend of an ICU and telemetry floor. Although special skills are required to nurse the patient through an unstable sixteen hours after intervention, the reward is seeing the patient return home to his normal lifestyle within three days.[71]

Getting the cardiac patient back to his normal lifestyle was also the goal of the Cardiac Health Improvement and Rehabilitation Program (CHIRP), an interdisciplinary effort directed by a physician and supervised by nurses in the roles of education and activity coordinators. Patients had their endurance monitored during exercise in the program's activity center or on the nursing units, and received individualized activity programs to follow at home. During

CHIRP rounds, members of several disciplines met to set goals for patients and discuss their progress. The CHIRP education coordinator also conducted a patient education group for cardiac nurses. All of these activities aimed toward promoting and maintaining optimum health for the cardiac patient.

• Overall, nursing services for cardiac patients, both medical and surgical, continued to expand. In May 1986 the Cardiovascular Intensive Care Unit, which by this time had a staff of over one hundred nurses, subdivided into four smaller units. On the cardiothoracic unit G90, a stepdown area was developed to care for angioplasty patients. It grew so quickly in size and patient diversity that it was soon decentralized to form a separate unit.

Oncology Nursing in the 1980s

Oncology nursing came into its own as a specialty in the 1970s. The founding of the Oncology Nursing Society in 1974 was a key event. At the Cleveland Clinic, an Oncology Nurse Task Force was founded in 1976 to fill the need for "an informal support group for nurses caring for patients with cancer."[72] In the following years, the task force brought together nurses working in a growing variety of settings and roles, including medical departments, Hospital nursing units, radiation therapy, the Chemotherapy Team, and the Clinic's Cancer Center.

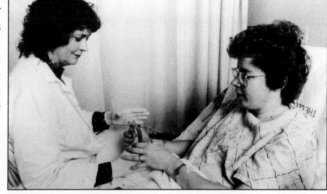

When the Cancer Center was established in 1985, "nursing was acknowledged as a key area for development in order to integrate new concepts of care along with established forms of practice. Specific areas were identified that required a nurse functioning at an advanced level of practice."[73] Cancer Center nurses worked closely with physicians and other disciplines. They were involved in research and program development, cancer prevention and detection, therapy and follow-up care, and patient education. They coordinated care given in inpatient, outpatient, and community settings.

While the treatments available to cancer patients had expanded, and remission rates in patients with some types of cancer, like leukemia, were encouraging, they also produced significant side effects and after effects. Highly skilled and supportive nursing personnel were needed to manage these effects, as well as to administer some of the treatments. Nurses worked together to develop nursing care protocols and care plans to meet new situations and ongoing problems in the care of cancer patients.

On G91, a hematology/oncology unit in the mid-1980s, nurses investigated various mouth-care treatments in order to develop a mouth-care protocol for cancer patients. "Oral care is one of the cornerstones of oncology nursing practice," pointed out one of the nurses involved in the project.[74] Head-and-neck radiation and especially chemotherapy, received by many Clinic cancer patients, damaged the oral mucosa and led to the development of stomatitis, or inflammation of the mouth. This painful condition, which sometimes had to be relieved with narcotic drugs, might make it impossible for the patient to eat or drink, necessitating the use of enteral nutrition.

THE NURSE CLINICIAN Some nurses, including a number of specialists in oncology nursing, worked as nurse clinicians in medical departments. Registered nurse Ina Hardesty (shown here with a patient) joined the Department of General Surgery after working in Hospital Nursing on unit 3 East. Her many years of work with breast cancer patients, and her "caring attitude and extra effort" in ministering to their emotional needs earned her The Cleveland Clinic Foundation's Emma Barr Award for Clinical Excellence in 1991.

However, nurses could offer some hope: "If patients are given proper mouth care before stomatitis develops, its severity may be decreased or its occurrence prevented."[75] Perceiving their ability to promote the health and comfort of these patients, the G91 nurses proceeded to draw up protocols for the care of two groups of cancer patients, those receiving high-dose chemotherapy (including many bone marrow transplant and leukemia patients) and those receiving other treatments like radiation or conventional-dose chemotherapy.

Guidelines for mouth care included instructions for cleaning the teeth and using specific mouthwashes and anti-fungal treatments. Regular assessment of the patient's mouth completed the protocol. Development of the protocol combined a scientific approach to problem-solving with a humane approach to patient care: "We feel our patients will benefit from our identification of the nursing care problem, our studies of products and the resolution of the problem."[76]

A potentially fatal complication of chemotherapy was infection, which accounted for many of the deaths among leukemia patients. Good oral care was one weapon nursing personnel used to help protect patients against infection. Since patients with low platelet counts also had to guard against bleeding, ordinary items used in personal care, like toothbrushes and razors, had to be avoided.

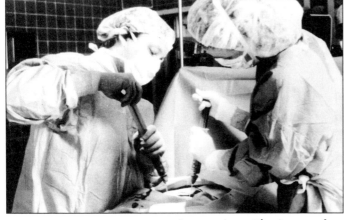

Nurses continually assessed patients for signs of bleeding, and for other signs that all was not well. "There is great pressure to assess carefully and constantly for subtle changes. These assessments must occur while the nurse is administering antibiotics and blood products and performing all the other technical tasks involved in the care of the patient."[77]

Not all patients receiving chemotherapy were on oncology units. A check of the census reports in the mid-1980s revealed that on an average day 20 to 30 such patients were being cared for on other units. The number of treatments given on an outpatient basis was also increasing. The issue of safe handling of the cytotoxic agents used in chemotherapy was addressed by a Foundation-wide policy in 1986, and oncology nurses participated in drafting a procedure to be used by Department of Nursing personnel. As the role of the staff nurse expanded to include the administration of chemotherapy, the nurses of the chemotherapy team, expert in the field, served as a resource.

Other responsibilities of chemotherapy nurses included performing bone marrow aspirations and biopsies for diagnostic purposes and working with physicians who were conducting research. "Our institution is involved in many Phase I/II research protocols which require time-consuming involvement on the part of the chemotherapy nursing staff. We must be flexible to meet the demands of physicians and their individual protocols. Each nurse is involved with one or more protocols."[78]

In addition to being knowledgeable about established cancer treatments, nurses caring for oncology patients had to keep up with new developments. New treatments often had serious side effects, which appropriate nursing

ONCOLOGY NURSING
Oncology nurses' responsibilities covered the whole spectrum of patient care, from research to teaching, from technical procedures to emotional support. Here, two nurse clinicians do a bone marrow aspiration and biopsy. The procedure involved a small incision under local anesthesia, and helped in diagnosing a patient's condition. By 1990, chemotherapy nurses were performing approximately 1,000 such procedures annually.

interventions could counter. Innovative treatments also held great promise. Nurses "witnessed tumor regression and remission in patients with aggressive disease which has been unresponsive to other therapies....The nurses on M70 and M71 share daily in the hopes and frustrations of our patients." In caring for patients receiving new treatments, nurses had the opportunity to help them by working to "develop creative strategies" to ease pain and discomfort.[79]

The Division of Nursing
of The Cleveland Clinic Foundation

While nurses were incorporating changes like these into their practices, administrative changes had continued to take place within Hospital Nursing. Reunification might have seemed to mark the end of the Nursing Department's troubles, but this was unfortunately not the case. The transitional years, during which entirely new departmental structures and philosophies were implemented, proved a difficult time for nursing personnel. In retrospect, it could be seen that the changes provided a basis for the future development of nursing at the Cleveland Clinic Hospital. However, it remained for new leadership to bring about that development.

Sharon Danielsen headed the Department of Nursing from 1981 to 1986. During this time, the decentralized nursing areas were once again consolidated under one administrator. After her tenure, Isabelle Boland, who had been handling the operational functions of the department since the beginning of 1986, took over as acting head while the Cleveland Clinic conducted a nationwide search for a new director of nursing. The search committee sought input from Nursing Department personnel, Ambulatory Nursing, physicians, and others. Sharon J. Coulter, R.N., M.N., M.B.A., was chosen for the position, and assumed her duties in May 1987. One of her first acts was to make another application to the Board of Governors for divisional status for nursing. This time the Board approved the request, affirming that the department now met the criteria for being designated a division. Her title became Chairman of the Division of Nursing.

The new division encompassed all areas of Cleveland Clinic nursing, including inpatient facilities, surgical services, and other treatment areas, except Ambulatory Nursing, still independent. (Nurses working in non-nursing departments, for example nurse anesthetists, also were not part of the division.) As of 1985, Ambulatory Nursing was headed by E. Mary Johnson, R.N., B.S.N., who had come to the Clinic as a staff nurse in 1974.

Nurses had never lost their historic importance in the work of The Cleveland Clinic Foundation. But, over the years, they had lost organizational ground since the time when Abbie Porter served as Hospital Superintendent. Finally, that ground had been recovered, as nursing was reunified into a department, and then, for the first time, became an independent division.

The name "Division of Nursing" disappeared again in 1993, when the Pharmacy Department was brought into the division, and the new grouping became known as the Division of Patient Care Operations. But the situation differed from that in the 1970s, when the Patient Care Services Division of which nursing was a part had included two layers of lay administration at the top. This time, the Chairman of Nursing, Ms. Coulter — now the Chairman of

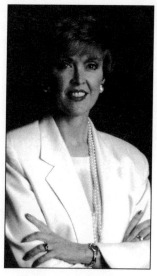

SHARON J. COULTER

A graduate of Research Medical Center (diploma), Avila College (B.S.N.), the University of Kansas (M.N.), and Rockhurst College (M.B.A.) in Kansas City, with a clinical background in critical care and oncology nursing, Sharon Coulter was appointed the Cleveland Clinic Hospital's Director of Nursing in 1987. Upon successful application for divisional status for Nursing in the same year, Ms. Coulter became Chairman of the Division of Nursing, and, in 1993, Chairman of the larger Division of Patient Care Operations. In 1990, she was named an Assistant Dean of Case Western Reserve University's B.S.N. program. Before coming to Cleveland, she had held vice president (Research Medical Center) and director of nursing (Trinity Lutheran Hospital) positions in Kansas City, and had also served for eleven years in the U.S. Air Force Reserve as a flight nurse, instructor, and training officer.

Patient Care Operations — headed the division. The incorporation of Nursing and Pharmacy into a single division was seen as a way of enhancing the professionalism of both. This arrangement allowed pharmacists and nurses to collaborate even more closely and take advantage of each others' expertise in preparing and delivering medications, administering them according to physicians' orders, and monitoring their use and effectiveness.

New Leadership, New Structure

With the arrival of a new administrative head in 1987, Nursing's table of organization was again modified. The division continued to be structured along clinical lines, maintaining a feature that had been key to "building an innovative, premier nursing organization" under Ms. Danielsen.[80] However, the unit/cluster/division/department structure was reduced to three levels, unit/department/division. Nursing Operations Managers (similar to nursing supervisors) and assistant head nurses remained part of the chain of command, handling administrative and managerial responsibilities on the off-shifts. With the elimination of a layer of management, Nursing Resources was broken down again into separate support departments.

By 1988, the Division of Nursing had six clinical departments and three support departments, each headed by a departmental director. The clinical directors were Mary Ann Brown, R.N., M.S.N. (Medical Nursing); Cathy M. Ceccio, R.N., M.S.N. (Neuro/Ortho/ENT Nursing); Angela Janik, R.N., M.S.N. (Critical Care Nursing); Ms. Lewicki (Surgical Nursing); Marian K. Shaughnessy, R.N., M.S.N. (Operating Room Nursing); and Ms. Whitman (Cardiac Nursing). The support department directors were Kathleen Lawson, R.N., M.B.A. (Physical and Environmental Resources); Deborah M. Nadzam, R.N., Ph.D. (Nursing Research); and, Elizabeth Vasquez, R.N., M.S.N. (Nursing Education).

The Nursing Administrative Group was renamed the Nursing Management Group (in 1989 its name changed again, to the Nursing Executive Council). Chaired by Ms. Coulter, it included the nine department directors and also two members in staff positions, Fiscal Coordinator Amy Caslow Maynard and Ms. Shumway, now Assistant to the Chairman.

An additional clinical director, Meri Beckham Armour, R.N., M.S.N., joined the group as director of a new clinical department, Oncology Nursing, in 1989. More modifications of the organizational chart were made during subsequent years. Ms. Armour eventually assumed responsibility for the combined area of Medical/Surgical Nursing, which included Oncology.

The support departments were again reorganized when the Center for Nursing was created in 1989. The Center, directed by Marlene Donnelly, R.N., M.B.A., included Nurse Recruitment and Retention, Nursing Education, Quality Management, Staffing and Scheduling, Nursing Operations Managers, and Information Systems. Nursing Research remained a separate department.

As of 1993, the Division of Nursing had six departments: Medical/Surgical Nursing, Critical Care Nursing, Cardiac Nursing, Surgical Services, the Center for Nursing, and Nursing Research.

Directorships of some departments also changed hands. While searches were being conducted for permanent directors, Jane Soposky, R.N., M.S.N., head nurse of P78, the adolescent psychiatric unit, and Madeline Soupios, R.N., head nurse of the P/SICU, served in 1991 as acting directors of Medical

Nursing and Critical Care Nursing, respectively. Jo Ann T. Birch, R.N., then became director of Medical Nursing; Deborah Peeler Charnley, R.N., M.N., was named director of Critical Care Nursing. Marcia Orsolits, R.N., Ph.D., directed Nursing Research from 1989 to 1991; Christine Wynd, R.N., Ph.D., then assumed the position. Lorraine Mion, R.N., Ph.D. became director of Nursing Research at the beginning of 1995. During the years between 1989 and 1994 the Operating Room, renamed Surgical Services, had four directors. Bernice Butler, R.N., served as acting director in 1989. Claudia Wormuth, R.N., was director for several months beginning in late 1989; Ms. Bush served in the position from 1991 to 1993. Lois Bock, R.N., who had served as acting director immediately before Ms. Bush's tenure, was appointed director of Surgical Services in 1993.

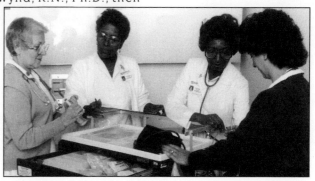

EMERGENCY CART
Cleveland Clinic ambulatory patients, as well as Hospital patients, often suffered from serious illnesses and sometimes needed on-the-spot emergency care or resuscitation. Here, registered nurse Betty Gurney and licensed practical nurses Colleen Elbert, Mae Grice, and Angelina Foliano of the Clinic's Nephrology and Hypertension Department review one of the emergency carts kept ready for use in the outpatient area.

Expense Reduction

The Cleveland Clinic Foundation administrators and nurses had never had the luxury of working with unlimited financial resources. The advent of Medicare's Diagnosis Related Group (DRG)-based prospective payment system in the mid-1980s represented neither a turning point nor a culmination of trends toward fiscal restraint in the health care industry, but it was a key event. The DRG system reimbursed hospitals for a patient's stay according to a formula based on the diagnosis. "Cost containment" had become a watchword in the late 1970s, and the attempt by public and private payors alike to find new ways of controlling health care expenses continued to intensify after DRGs went into effect. Health care, like other sectors of the service economy, was labor intensive. Salaries and benefits made up a substantial portion of the annual operating budget in hospitals. Since more hospital employees worked in nursing than in any other single area, it was difficult to cut hospital costs without cutting nursing costs.

The Cleveland Clinic Foundation implemented an expense reduction program in 1988. Although the Division of Nursing was not required specifically to reduce its number of positions, the limit placed on the division's overall expenses made it necessary for the new administrative team to reduce positions in some job categories. The Clinic-wide expense reduction and program review were merged with the division's own restructuring process.

In 1985, the Clinic Hospital had put in place a patient classification system, which categorized patient populations on the basis of acuity, that is, the severity of illness and the amount of care needed. The system was now to be used to help determine staffing levels. Differing patient acuities on the various units would affect the number of personnel in various job categories assigned to them. To provide the required flexibility, some unit-based positions were eliminated and the float pool of R.N.s and L.P.N.s was expanded. Patient classification systems were not perfect, but they were an improvement over traditional staffing methods, in which nursing personnel were assigned to a unit based on the number of beds, or the average patient census, without regard to the levels of nursing care needed by different kinds of patients.

The Nursing Unit

The Division of Nursing's goals had been identified in the early 1980s as patient care, education, research, and outreach. The new administration re-affirmed these four goals as the division's mission, but also redefined them, mostly through broadening. The first goal now became: "To provide patients and family or significant others with professional nursing care."[81] The change in wording took into account the connection between patient and family, as nurses already did in practice.

Most of the division's personnel cared for patients on the Hospital's 40 nursing units. Within the nursing unit itself, organization remained basically the same. Each unit had a head nurse and (in most cases) two assistant head nurses. In 1992 the title Nurse Manager came into general use in the Clinic Hospital, replacing the traditional title of Head Nurse. The following year, the title of the nurses who headed the nursing staffs of the various medical departments in the outpatient Clinic was changed from Ambulatory Nursing Coordinator to Nurse Manager, so that the same title referred to corresponding positions in the Division of Nursing and Ambulatory Nursing. Nurse Managers also headed the nine clinical services — Cardiac, Otolaryngology/Ophthalmology, General Surgery/Gynecology, Neurosurgery, Orthopaedic, Urology, Colorectal, Plastic, and Vascular — and the Outpatient Surgery Center and the Post-Anesthesia Care Unit within the Nursing Division's Department of Surgical Services.

By this time, many nursing units had 50 or even more employees. Some nurse managers, who headed two units, had more than 100 employees reporting to them. Little more than 10 years before, head nurses had expressed the collective sentiment that they were nurses, not managers. Now they were managers of nurses, or, more accurately, managers of nursing units. They interviewed candidates for job openings and evaluated all unit personnel; they did their units' budgets; they worked with other disciplines and departments; they gathered information to share with unit staff, and with patients and families.

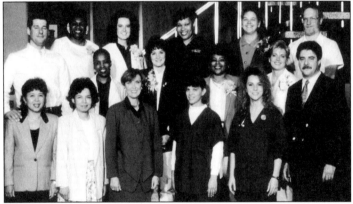

PATIENT CARE
TECHNICIANS
The Patient Care Technician (PCT) role was developed by cardiac head nurses in the late 1980s, and implemented in the Hospital's intensive care units beginning in 1992. The role combined technical and unit support activities. Here, Sharon Coulter (front row, third from left), congratulates the first graduating class of the division's PCT training program in 1992.

Responsible for all of the care that was given on their units, they themselves had relatively little time to participate in bedside nursing. "I am truly a clinician," said one head nurse; "I truly enjoy patient care." But she found that, as a nurse manager, she had a difficult adjustment to make: giving up a little of her clinical expertise in order to devote herself to managing her unit. "I had to accept the fact that my staff can work the floor better than I can, because things change so fast."[82]

Units were staffed by R.N.s, L.P.N.s, nursing unit assistants, and unit secretaries. In the early 1990s, the desired mix of R.N.s to other staff was set at four to one in the intensive care, pediatric, and bone marrow transplant units; at three to one in telemetry units, and at seven to three in all other units. Overall staffing levels were set partly on the basis of the acuity levels determined by the patient classification system. Before the role of the nursing unit assistant had been redefined in the early 1980s to emphasize support to the unit, rather than direct patient care, N.U.A.s had done many nursing procedures — for example, suctioning, tracheostomy care, tube feeding — that now again had to be done by R.N.s and L.P.N.s. R.N.s also had to handle more of the administration of intravenous therapy after a new state law put restrictions on its performance by L.P.N.s.

Another nursing unit role, the Patient Care Technician, was trialed during this period. First proposed by the head nurses of the division's Cardiac Nursing Department in the late 1980s, it was implemented in various intensive care units of the Hospital by 1992. The goal of the program was to "enhance patient care despite a declining supply of nurses....by freeing registered nurses" to concentrate on activities like patient assessment, care planning and patient education.[83] The patient care technician would work closely with the nurse and would be able to perform some of the technical tasks needed in the intensive care setting, as well as the unit support activities of a nursing unit assistant.

Documentation and Automation

In 1989, the blue "Nursing Documentation Record" binders became a familiar sight on the nursing units. Each binder collected together the numerous forms and documents that recorded the nursing care given to an individual patient. The JCAHO, in summing up the importance of the data kept by nurses, had declared: "Nursing documentation is the difference you make in the care the patient received."[84] Without this paper trail, the progress of the patient, and the performance and effectiveness of the nursing interventions, could not be tracked. Documentation and the division's quality assurance program went hand-in-hand. One facet of the quality assurance effort involved improving the rate of completion of several components of the nursing record. At the same time, the information contained in the nursing documentation made it possible to monitor quality of care. Documentation not only touched on issues of quality, but also continued to have a financial impact. Third party payors might refuse reimbursement if parts of the record were not completed properly, particularly those relating to medications and treatments.

Improvement of nursing documentation did not necessarily mean the cumulative addition of new forms — in 1991 new forms were added, but seven old forms were eliminated at the same time. The implementation of the Planning, Intervention, and Evaluation (PIE) charting system in 1991 and 1992 included as its centerpiece the "Nursing Progress Record." This documented the application of the nursing process to the care of the individual patient. Nurses assessed patients, and recorded nursing diagnoses and their resolution during the hospital stay on the associated "Problem List." At the end of 1994 the "Charting-By-Exception" system of documentation was introduced.

Automation also affected nursing practice and unit routine. Computers and printers began to appear at nursing stations in the 1970s, and over the years came to be used in a variety of ways, for instance, to communicate lab results. The patient classification system depended on the automated storage and tabulation of data. But the use of automation expanded in the 1990s. Beginning in 1994, the division's operating budget was placed on-line. On the units, three major areas were being automated: distribution of supplies, distribution of pharmaceuticals, and order entry.

Automated drug distribution was piloted first, with Pyxis medstations placed on three nursing units in 1991. During the next year medstations were installed on all units. Also in 1992, the unit dose system was reinstated on a trial basis on four nursing units. The coordinated work by the Pharmacy Department and the Nursing Division on these projects pointed the way toward the creation of the Division of Patient Care Operations in the following year. Pyxis stations for automated distribution of supplies were piloted and approved for use throughout the hospital in 1993. Both Pyxis systems were designed to save the time of nursing personnel by automating inventory control and the process of charging items to patients.

Although planning began in 1988, the PHAMIS order entry system did not go into effect until 1994. Through use of the system, nursing personnel could relay physicians' orders for services from support departments via personal computers installed in Clinic departments and on Hospital nursing units. To begin with, automated order entry covered laboratory tests and radiology exams, but eventually, physical and occupational therapy, EKG, transport, and other services were to be added. The automation of order entry was a milestone in the automation of the patient record and a step toward the elimination of some paper forms. Unit secretaries, who of all unit personnel generally had the most skill and experience in using computers, were the first group of Hospital Nursing employees trained to use the system, followed by staff nurses. In the Clinic as well, both clerical workers and nurses learned the system.

Always There

By the second half of the twentieth century, most people looked at nursing less as a calling and more as a job or a career, although one requiring special qualities of character or personality. Early in the century, some patients and families had expected private duty nurses to be on duty 24 hours a day. Nurses at many hospitals had worked 12-hour shifts six days a week, and a half day on Sundays. Over the years, the working week had been gradually reduced to the standard 40 hours.

But hospital nursing personnel still had to be, collectively, "always there": on duty 24 hours a day, seven days a week. Clinic Hospital nurses, like nurses at other hospitals, rated shift rotation and working weekends as major reasons for dissatisfaction. If more people could be placed on permanent evening, night, and weekend shifts, there would be more straight day shifts, with fewer weekends worked, for staff members who wanted or needed those hours.

The "Weekender Option Program," implemented in 1990, attempted to deal with one part of this dilemma. Part-time R.N.s and L.P.N.s could elect to work two 12-hour shifts during the weekend. By 1991 it was reported to the Nursing Executive Council that full-time staff in most areas were working one out of every three to six weekends, as opposed to every other weekend before the weekender option had been made available. As for shift rotation, a survey of Clinic Hospital nurses in 1989 indicated that increased shift differentials might encourage more individuals to work straight evenings or nights, so a shift incentive program was eventually instituted.

Nurses also gained more control over their work schedules when "self staffing" or "self scheduling" was developed as an option for nursing units. Defined as "the process by which staff nurses on a unit collectively decide and implement the monthly work schedule," it was piloted on nursing unit G71 in 1990.[85] Ambulatory nurses, too, gained more independence in setting their own hours, according to the needs of the work in their departments, when they were placed on a salaried rather than an hourly basis in 1991. When the Division of Nursing looked at self scheduling in that year, the director of Ambulatory Nursing served on the committee that studied the issue and drew up guidelines for general use.

Nursing Education

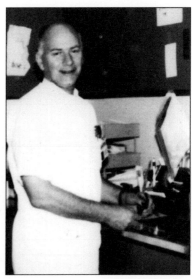

The division's second goal changed very little in wording from the early to the late 1980s: "To provide all Division of Nursing employees with opportunities for ongoing education, both personal and professional."[86] However, the responsibilities of the Nursing Education Department were continually expanding. In 1980, the Foundation had affiliations with one practical nurse program, at Jane Addams High School; one diploma program, at Huron Road Hospital; and two college programs, Ursuline College (successor to the St. John College program, offering a B.S. degree) and Cuyahoga Community College (A.D.). By the end of the decade, the division had affiliations with seven northeastern Ohio college or university-based programs alone: the Frances Payne Bolton School of Nursing at Case Western Reserve University, Cleveland State University, Cuyahoga Community College, Kent State University, Lakeland Community College, the University of Akron, and Ursuline College.

The Division of Nursing strengthened its ties with the Frances Payne Bolton School of Nursing in 1990 when the latter reinstituted its B.S.N. program. (An earlier baccalaureate program had been discontinued when school decided to offer the world's first Doctor of Nursing program in 1978.) The Cleveland Clinic Foundation, along with University Hospitals of Cleveland and Cleveland Metropolitan General Hospital, agreed to collaborate in the program and to provide tuition support and clinical experience to the students, who would in turn be committed to service at the sponsoring hospitals after graduation. Ms. Coulter was named an assistant dean at the school. The first class of "Bolton Scholars" sponsored by the Cleveland Clinic graduated in 1994.

The Nursing Education Department had responsibility for the Undergraduate Nursing Assistant (later called Nursing Associate) program, which brought nursing students to the Cleveland Clinic as summer employees. The department also was involved in the John Hay High School health careers and unit hostess projects, which combined education and community outreach by employing Cleveland high school students at the Cleveland Clinic.

Nursing Education also administered tuition assistance. The "internal incentives" program enhanced the skills of the current staff, and was also an attractive benefit. "External incentives," or scholarship grants, went to nursing students who would later join the Hospital's nursing staff.

Orientation, including the preceptor program, remained one of the most important functions of Nursing Education. The length of the orientation period was shortened and standardized according to the previous experience and the job assignment of the orientee. The unit-based clinical instructor program was changed in the late 1980s, so that instructors were assigned to the clinical nursing departments rather than the units.

KEN WHIDDEN
From 1974 to 1982, Mr. Whidden directed Nursing Education at the Cleveland Clinic Hospital. During this period, a new management course for nurses was offered, an internship program for new graduates created, orientation lengthened, and a preceptor program started. Mr. Whidden's nursing career at the Cleveland Clinic Hospital also included positions on the Private Medical-Surgical, Colorectal, and ENT nursing units. This photograph was taken in G81's stepdown unit, designed for postsurgical observation of patients having undergone head and neck procedures.

The preceptor program was maintained and strengthened. Now that each unit did not have its own clinical instructor, the role of the preceptor became even more important. By 1990, two hundred staff nurses were serving as preceptors for new nurses. The Nursing Education Department offered training and refresher courses for preceptors. An overwhelming majority of new nurses found their preceptors more helpful than anyone else during the orientation period. "The unit preceptor really made a difference," was a typical comment.[87] In 1990 the Performance-Based Development System (PBDS) became part of the division's orientation program. It was designed to assess the skills of new nurses and tailor their orientation accordingly.

For Nursing Division employees past the orientation level, the department coordinated numerous educational activities. State law, Cleveland Clinic policy, and the challenges of caring for a tertiary care facility's patients set ever-higher standards for nursing personnel, often with certification or other proof of proficiency required. The Nursing Education Department helped to make sure that Cleveland Clinic nurses were prepared. In 1993 its Continuing Education section offered 93 courses with 289 Continuing Education Unit (CEU) contact hours for R.N.s and L.P.N.s. The contact hours could be used toward the mandatory CEU requirement for licensure renewal. Cardiopulmonary resuscitation (CPR) certification was an employment requirement for Cleveland Clinic nurses, and Nursing Education provided CPR instruction at all levels.

Advancing Knowledge...

Meetings of nursing specialty organizations and other nursing and health care associations gave nurses a chance to discuss professional issues and share knowledge about basics and innovations in nursing practice and medical science. Of the hundreds of Cleveland Clinic personnel who attended national, regional, and local meetings each year, many presented papers, poster sessions, and workshops. Others served in their organizations as elected officers or committee members; in 1994, 13 individuals in the Division of Patient Care Operations were serving as officers of national organizations.

The sharing of knowledge at meetings and symposia took place both inside and outside the walls of the Cleveland Clinic. Inside, nurses conducted grand rounds, like a 1986 session held by the Neuroscience Nursing Department, which gave all Cleveland Clinic nurses the opportunity to learn about the functions and diseases of the cerebral cortex and related nursing diagnoses. Nursing personnel also exchanged information at meetings of journal clubs. The MICU Journal Club, established by the unit's night shift for all nursing staff members on the unit, chose a different article "pertinent to the patient population and practice of the MICU" for discussion each week.[88] Beyond its original intent of supporting a high level of nursing practice through exploration of the literature, the club also turned out to promote interdisciplinary communication: residents and respiratory therapists joined in the discussions.

As the number of meetings and conferences held by nursing and other health care organizations continued to grow during the 1980s, Cleveland Clinic nurses had increased opportunities to learn and to teach outside their home base. For instance, the 1986 American Nephrology Nurses' Association Symposium included three presentations by Cleveland Clinic nurses: "Dialyzing the AIDS Patient and Its Impact on Nursing Care" by Ernesto Jimenez, R.N., assistant head nurse on M82; "Is Cyclosporine Toxic to Nurses?" by Caroline Buszta, R.N., renal transplant coordinator; and "Adaptation to Pancreas/Renal Transplantation" by Kathleen Sweeny, R.N. The following year, Karen Ann Deluca, R.N., spoke on "CAVH/SCUF Nursing Implications in Implementation and Management," and Dolores Jackson-Bey, L.P.N., presented a poster on "Helping Patients Select the Most Appropriate Mode of Home Peritoneal Dialysis."[89]

June Romeo, R.N., M.A., clinical instructor on the NICU, collaborated with a physician to present a poster, "Adult Viral Encephalitis and Increased Intracranial Pressure: Patient Outcome," at the Academy of Neurology's national conference. The content was later submitted to the *Journal of Neurosurgery*. Four nurses from a variety of care settings — Mary Lynn Droughton, R.N., M.S.N., from the Cancer Center, Connie Miller, R.N., from G81, and Molly Dully, R.N., and Sandra Rustin, R.N., from the Operating Room — presented a poster, "Preoperative Patient/Family Assessment and Education: A Collaborative Nursing Practice Enhances the Road to Recovery," at the SOHN national congress. Betsy A. Kuhn, R.N., M.S.N., presented a workshop on "Clinical Strategies Which Facilitate a Child's Coping with Death" at a symposium of the Piedmont Oncology Association.

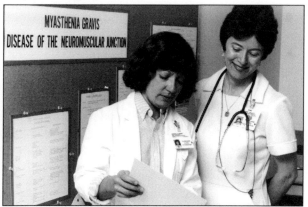

SHARING KNOWLEDGE
Angela Janik (left) directed the division's Department of Critical Care Nursing from 1987 to 1990. The department included the Hospital's Medical, Pediatric/Adult Surgical, and Neurology/Neurosurgery Intensive Care Units. Seen here with Suzanne Goertz (right), Ms. Janik designed this poster session on myasthenia gravis. By keeping up with advances in nursing practice, and sharing knowledge with colleagues both inside and outside the institution, nurses supported one of the Cleveland Clinic's three missions, "further education of those who serve."

Cleveland Clinic nurses continued to be active in giving presentations, and also in writing for publication, in the 1990s. For example, in 1993, Janet Serkey, T. Keys, M.D., R. Stewart, M.D., and D. Zabell, R.N., B.A., authored a presentation made at the international meeting of the Association for Practitioners in Infection Control. They reported on an investigation conducted by the Clinic's Infection Control Department, which indicated polyurethane dressings as a possible risk factor for infection among cardiovascular surgery patients. In both 1993 and 1994, cardiac nurses made several presentations at the American Heart Association's annual scientific sessions, often in collaboration with physicians and others. Topics included "Timing of Vasovagal Reactions Associated with Removal of Femoral Arterial Sheaths," by Kimberly Brown, R.N., B.S.N., Daniel Evans, Michelle Casedonte, R.N., Ellen Montague, R.N., and Gayle Whitman, and "Correlates of Costs of Coronary Bypass Surgery," by Nowa Omoigui, Ms. Brown, Dave Miller, Mark Hanson, John Sideras, Bruce Lytle, and Floyd Loop, M.D., Chairman of the Cleveland Clinic's Board of Governors.

In addition, nurses contributed their expertise through service on editorial boards or as reviewers for journal and books. Jean Cross, R.N., M.S.N., Josephine Dimengo, R.N., M.S.N., Linda Lewicki, Kathleen Tripepi-Bova, R.N., M.S.N., and Ms. Whitman were among the latter, reviewing current literature for the periodical AACN *Nursing Scan in Critical Care*.

In 1994, the Division of Patient Care Operations tallied 141 presentations and 91 publications to the credit of its staff members.

Articles, book chapters, and other publications written or edited by Cleveland Clinic nurses in the 1980s and 1990s covered a variety of subjects, using a variety of approaches. Many journal articles had as their subjects the specifics of patient care or nursing practice, often within a particular clinical area. For instance, P/SICU nurse Kathleen A. Singleton, R.N., collaborated on a case study article for *Critical Care Nurse* in 1985. Alexa McCubbin wrote about "The Role of the O.R. Department in Infection Control" for a 1986 issue of *Asepsis: The Infection Control Forum*. The journal *Dimensions of Critical Care Nursing* published the article "Cardiac Output: Iced versus Room Temperature Solution" by CCU head nurse Ms. Cross and clinical instructor Rita Vargo, R.N., M.S.N. Also in the Department of Cardiac Nursing, Lillie Hicks, R.N., and Ms. Whitman had an article on nursing care of the cardiac transplant patient published in the *Journal of Cardiovascular Nursing*. In a 1988 issue of *Heart & Lung*, CHIRP coordinator Betsy Stovsky, R.N., M.S.N., and clinical instructor Peggy Dragonette, R.N., wrote about communicating with intubated patients.

In the 1990s, articles appearing in the AACN journal *Clinical Issues in Critical Care Nursing* included "Surgical Alternatives for Patients with Heart Failure" by Ms. Vargo and Ms. Dimengo, and "Laser Angioplasty and Intracoronary Stents: Going Beyond the Balloon" by Nancy Albert, R.N., M.S.N. "Safe Handling of Cytotoxic Agents," by Shirley Gullo, R.N., M.S.N., first published in 1988, was scheduled to be reprinted in 1995 as a "landmark" article in the twentieth anniversary edition of *Oncology Nursing Forum*.

An increasing number of articles authored by Cleveland Clinic nurses focused on emotional and psychological factors involved in patient care, and on patient teaching and support by nurses. Ms. Droughton and Margaret Verbic wrote about "Body Image Reintegration after Head and Neck Cancer Surgery" in SOHN's journal. Cathy Ceccio of Neuro/Ortho/ENT nursing and Jan Horosz, R.N., of the PACU collaborated on an article appearing in RN, "Teaching the Elderly Amputee to Meet the World." "Recovering from Cancer: A Nursing Intervention Program Recognizing Survivorship" by Shawn Ulreich, R.N., B.S.N., and Joanne Gambosi, R.N., M.A., appeared in the *Oncology Nursing Forum*, as did Ms. Gullo's article "Props and Jokes Provide Patients with 'Healing Hugs.'" Melissa J. Gurley, R.N., M.S.N., examined the effect of visitation policies on patients, families, and nursing staff in her MEDSURG Nursing article "Determining ICU Visiting Hours."

Some nurses' writings dealt with the basics of disease pathologies or nursing care, appearing as textbook chapters, manuals, published standards, and the like. For example, Ms. Miller, head nurse of G81, collaborated with Howard Levine, M.D., on the second edition of the *Tracheostomy Care Manual*, designed to help "prepare patients and families for discharge and home care."[90] The book *Every Nurse's Guide to Cardiovascular Care* featured a chapter on vascular surgery by Carol Benedum, R.N., M.S.N., and one on cardiac surgery by Ms. Whitman.

Among Ms. Whitman's numerous other contributions to nursing texts were chapters on cardiac surgery and related topics in *The Recovery Room: A Critical Care Approach to Post Anesthesia Nursing*, *Critical Care Nursing: Body-Mind-Spirit*, and AACN's *Clinical Reference for Critical-Care Nursing*. Her chapter, "Shock," in the latter text explained, in modern terms, a physiologic state that Dr. George Crile, Sr., had studied in the early part of the century, and one that was important for the critical care nurse, "as the consistent presence at the patient's bedside," to understand.[91]

Members of the nursing Department of Surgical Services contributed modules to Medcom, Inc.'s *The Role of the Circulator Series*. Janine Stone, R.N., B.S.N., Doris Samstag, R.N., B.S.N., Laurie Canala, R.N., and Nancy Burkle, R.N.,M.S.N., authored Module 1, an "Overview of the Circulating Nurse's Activities," designed to acquaint the reader with "the basic competencies required to coordinate patient care in surgery" and the "duties and responsibilities of the circulating nurse."[92] Ms. Canala also wrote Module 21, "Surgical Counts." Patricia E. Chapek, R.N., B.A., co-authored Module 11 on "Potential Complications: The Malignant Hyperthermia Patient."

Deborah Atsberger, of the PACU, contributed "Interpreting Arterial Blood Gases" to the *Core Curriculum for Post-Anesthesia Nursing*, published by W. B. Saunders. She and Maria Zickuhr edited Saunders' *Pre- and Post-Anesthesia Nursing Knowledge Base and Clinical Competencies*. Rose Anne Berila, R.N., M.S.N., nurse manager on the adult psychiatric unit, wrote a chapter, "Dementia," for the book *Functional Performance in Older Adults* detailing the forms, causes, and symptoms of the condition, and management of patients with Alzheimer's disease and other dementias. Meri Beckham Armour's writings included *Standards of Care for Oncology Nursing Practice*, a 1991 publication of the Oncology Nursing Society. Dorothy Calabrese, R.N., M.S.N., and Mary Anne Matcham, R.N., wrote "Tumors of the Upper Tract" for the Saunders text, *Urological Nursing: Principles and Practice*. The chapter "Complications of Advanced Disease," written by Ruth Krech Fritskey, R.N., and C. Chernecky, R.N., appeared in both the first and second editions of *Cancer Nursing: A Comprehensive Textbook*.

Other publications by Cleveland Clinic nurses communicated the development of new procedures. For instance, Ms. Stone and Richard V. Dowden, M.D., wrote about "Breast Implant Endoscopy: Detecting Leaks in Silicone-Gel Breast Implants" in a 1994 issue of the AORN *Journal*. The article described the procedure, as developed by Dr. Dowden, and went on to detail the role of the perioperative nurse in pre-, intra-, and postoperative care of patients undergoing it.

Some chapters and articles focused on particular approaches to patient care being used at the Cleveland Clinic. Psychiatric nurse Kathleen Weiss, R.N., M.S.N., collaborated with five colleagues from other disciplines to produce the chapter "A Multidisciplinary Approach to the Treatment of Drug and Alcohol Addiction" for the textbook, *Comprehensive Handbook of Drug and Alcohol Addiction*. The authors provided an extensive review of the general dynamics of the team approach as applied to the treatment of chemical dependencies. They also described its practical application at the Clinic's Alcohol and Drug Recovery Center, where it allowed for "a degree of creativity" and fostered a "sense of personal specialness" among staff and patients alike.[93]

The commitment to case management at the Cleveland Clinic was evidenced by publication on the subject by nurses. The chapter "Case Management Model: Oncology" in *Outpatient Case Management: Strategies for a New Reality* was written by Eileen Groh-Smyth, R.N., M.S.N., Ms. Calabrese, and Ms. Droughton. Ms. Dimengo collaborated with Patrick McCarthy, M.D., Geoffrey J. Suszkowski, D.P.S., and Steven Nissen, M.D., in writing an article, "Cleveland Clinic Strategies: Five-Day Recovery Plan, Kaiser Affiliation, Regional Centers, and Satellite Clinics," describing the Clinic's approach to providing quality cardiac surgical care cost-effectively.

The Cleveland Clinic's patient satisfaction program, which approached patient care on the basis of the patient's own perceptions, was the subject of a chapter in *Improving Quality and Performance: Concepts, Programs, and Techniques*, published in 1994. "Patient Satisfaction: A CQI Pilot Project" by Sharon Coulter, Mardeen Atkins, Dawn Bailey, R.N., B.S.N., Mary Ellen Blatt, R.N., B.S.N.,

Lori Blashford, R.N., B.S.N., and Sandra Shumway reviewed the implementation and results of the pilot phase of the project.

...To Advance Practice

Many articles by Cleveland Clinic nurses communicated research results. Research articles and abstracts appeared not only in national journals, but also in institutional forums. In the fall 1987 issue of the Division of Nursing's quarterly publication *Essence of Nursing*, Nancy Burkle published an abstract of her pilot study on intraoperative hypothermia in the elderly. Subsequently, the division's biannual publication *Cleveland Clinic Nurse*, which first appeared in 1993, regularly featured abstracts of research studies carried out by Cleveland Clinic nurses. In the September 1993 issue, orthopaedic nurse Karen Mae Smith, R.N., in collaboration with Dr. Wynd of the Department of Nursing Research, published an abstract of her pilot study on postoperative urinary retention in patients undergoing total hip and total knee procedures. The pilot indicated that nurses might need to be especially aware of increased risk among older patients and patients "who received more fluids postoperatively," and pointed the way toward further research with direct application to nursing practice: "A thorough understanding of factors contributing to urinary retention will assist nurses in making appropriate assessments in designing interventions to prevent postoperative complications."[94]

Another abstract, published in May 1994, was authored by cardiac nurses: case managers Ms. Brown and Ms. Casedonte, staff nurses JoAnne Hughes-Morscher, M.S.N., R.N., and Ms. Montague, and Director Ms. Whitman, along with biostatistician Marion Piedmonte, M.A. Their study, based on a sample of 490 patients, looked at the incidence of "bleeding and vascular complications in [percutaneous] coronary interventional patients," and identified a "high-risk subset of patients." In this study, too, the connection of research and practice was made clear: "Specific assessment needs and monitoring activities can be tailored to this subset. Early identification of patients at risk may minimize complications and enhance discharge outcomes."[95]

Nursing Research

The third goal of nursing at the Cleveland Clinic, "To participate in nursing research thereby contributing to the body of nursing knowledge," had also changed very little in wording at the time the department became a division in 1987.[96] But nursing research was then in an embryonic stage at the Cleveland Clinic. The first step had been the original mission statement, identifying research as a nursing function, under Ms. Danielsen's leadership in the early 1980s.

No formal program of nursing research existed until 1984. In that year the process by which nursing research proposals would be approved within the Nursing Department and the Foundation was developed. In 1986 the Nursing Research Committee was established to "facilitat[e] nursing research activities at the Cleveland Clinic Foundation, in order to enhance the quality of nursing care and institute new approaches to patient care."[97] The Committee had responsibility for identifying priorities and initiating research, as well as reviewing proposals and making recommendations on them to the Foundation-wide Research Program Committee. Dr. Nadzam, the Director of Nursing Information Resources (and later of Nursing Research) chaired the committee.

The primacy of patient care was clearly stated in the Nursing Research Department's own statement of mission in 1991: "Nursing research at the Cleveland Clinic Foundation is defined as a systematic process of investigation involving problems relevant to nursing practice....Although the importance of nursing research aimed at extending theoretical nursing knowledge is recognized, emphasis is placed on applied research concerned with the delivery, organization and evaluation of nursing care." In 1993 one of the Division of Nursing's goals was to "increase the number of research projects related to quality patient care outcomes." In 1994 a nursing research utilization conference was sponsored by the Division of Nursing in connection with the regional Sigma Theta Tau convention, focusing on facilitating research into practice issues and incorporating the results into policy-making.[98]

The Nursing Education and Research Fund, established in 1993, provided monies for nurses to participate in "educational experiences" and to conduct studies "having scientific merit and significance for nursing practice at The Cleveland Clinic Foundation."[99] Appropriately, this fund was started with gifts from patients and families who wished to say "thank you" for the nursing care they had received at the Hospital. Additional contributions came from vendors, pharmaceutical companies, and nurses. A circle of support, with past recipients of patient care funding education and research, which would in turn benefit future patient care, was created through the fund.

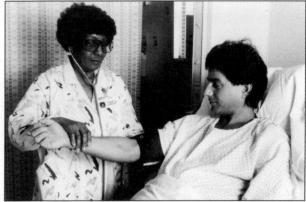

LICENSED PRACTICAL NURSING
In 1954 the Cleveland Clinic trained 7 of its own senior aides as the Hospital's first practical nurses. Nursing administrators soon began hiring large numbers of practical nursing school graduates for positions in the Clinic and the Hospital. Over the following decades, L.P.N.s assumed responsibility for an increasing variety of patient care duties, for instance, administering medications. In 1960, there were 80 practical nurses on the Hospital Nursing staff; by 1985, there were 270. Here, Alyce Pitts, a Hospital L.P.N. for 32 years, is shown taking vital signs and assessing a patient.

Skin Care: Integrating Research and Practice

Studies of pressure ulcers and skin care had immediate practical relevance to patient care, and led to a major initiative by the Division of Nursing. In 1989, physicians and a research nurse in the Department of Plastic Surgery had begun looking at the "incidence, prevalence, and etiology of pressure sores" in hospitalized patients.[100] It was clear that this was an area in which nurses had an important role. They could assess patients' vulnerability, intervene to prevent ulcers or at least lessen their severity, and evaluate the effectiveness and cost of different types of intervention. In the same year, the Department of Nursing Research became involved in relating research on pressure ulcers to nursing practice. Ongoing studies of skin care accompanied the development of an ongoing program aimed at preventing pressure ulcers in hospitalized patients. This resulted in the appointment of the Division's Skin Care Team, chaired by Betsy Kuhn, in 1990.

The program developed as a multidisciplinary effort: "The CCF approach to skin care is that pressure ulcer prevention is everyone's responsibility." The team itself included:

> staff nurses, nurse managers, and clinical instructors, as well as nurses from enterostomal therapy, nursing education, and infection control. The advisors to the Skin Care Team consist of representatives from these departments: plastic surgery, quality management, hospital pharmacy, musculoskeletal research, physical medicine and rehabilitation, and

hospital dietary. The functions of the Skin Care Team include planning and implementing strategies to decrease the prevalence of pressure ulcers, addressing cost issues related to various therapeutic bed equipment and skin care products, and acting as a resource for staff nurses in the prevention and treatment of pressure ulcers.[101]

Skin Care Team nurses made rounds on the units to check on the status and assist in the care of patients with pressure ulcers. Also helpful was a new section on skin condition in the patient chart, as Donna Behrendt, R.N., M.S.N., chairman of the Skin Care Task Force in 1991, noted: "If [skin] is breaking down, nurses have to plan for treating it. Two years ago you wouldn't have found anything about skin care anywhere on the charts."[102]

The prevention and treatment of pressure ulcers, although not as dramatic an intervention as something like CPR, could reduce patients' suffering significantly, as nurses knew well. Pressure sores could be very painful, difficult to treat once acquired, and even "associated with an increased mortality rate, especially among the elderly."[103] They could also be very expensive to treat.

Between 1990 and 1993 the prevalence of pressure ulcers among Clinic Hospital patients decreased from 7.0 to 5.4 percent. Other aspects of skin care, such as wound and stoma care, also received attention. The Skin Care Team's success temporarily threatened to become the project's downfall. Nursing unit staff members came to "rely heavily" on the team to identify patients at risk for pressure ulcers and to plan their care.[104] The large number of referrals made it difficult for the team to see all patients as promptly as they would have liked.

To solve these problems, late in 1993 the program recruited a nurse on each unit to serve as a Unit Based Skin Care Nurse. A unit's skin care nurse acted as "the primary resource person to assist the nursing staff in developing a patient's plan of care for the prevention and treatment of pressure ulcers and to evaluate the effectiveness of that plan," leading to earlier intervention and, it was hoped, a further decrease in the prevalence of pressure ulcers.[105] The units' skin care nurses also liaised with the team, which continued to coordinate skin care efforts overall, and whose members were available to consult on difficult cases. Skin care protocols were posted on bulletin boards on each unit. By the end of the first year of this phase, the incidence of hospital-acquired pressure sores had dropped from 0.15 to 0.07 per 100 patient days, the lowest rate ever recorded at the Clinic Hospital.

Meanwhile, the U.S. Agency for Health Care Policy and Research had published its clinical practice guideline, *Pressure Ulcers in Adults: Prediction and Prevention*, in 1992. Division of Nursing and medical staff members had contributed to its development, with the Cleveland Clinic serving as a pilot review site. Within the division, research on pressure ulcers continued. In 1994, a prospective study on pressure ulcer development among cardiovascular surgical patients involved three nursing departments, Surgical Services, Cardiac Nursing, and Nursing Research. The highest prevalence of pressure ulcers at the Cleveland Clinic Hospital occurred among its large population of cardiovascular surgical patients. By examining characteristics of patients who developed pressure ulcers, the investigators hoped to determine which patients were at greatest risk so that prevention programs could be accurately targeted.

Focusing on Outcomes

The Department of Nursing Research had two goals: advancing nursing practice through the "systematic examination of nursing practices and delivery-of-care models"; and advancing the professional development of nursing personnel. By 1995, the Department of Nursing Research had refined its goal of advancing practice to focus specifically on patient, nursing, and institutional outcomes: that is, "to examine how and what nurses practice as it relates to patient care outcomes, cost and systems of care."[106] At a time when concerns about the high cost of health care threatened to dominate debate on the subject, nurses could contribute to patients' well-being by finding ways to provide care of equal or better quality while holding down costs.

Director of Nursing Research Lorraine Mion stated that research could be generated at any point in the "knowledge/policy/practice" cycle that governed the actual giving of nursing care.[107] As of the beginning of 1995, examples of nurse-initiated research recently completed, under way, or proposed, stemming from issues in all three areas, could be identified. Gaps in the area of knowledge about patient population characteristics and responses to illnesses were being addressed by the study on pressure ulcers in cardiac patients, as well as studies on self-extubation and weaning from ventilators.

Through the division's quality management program, it was discovered that risk factors for self-extubation, which might include patient characteristics, medical practices, and nursing practices (such as the use of analgesics or physical restraints), were unknown. A multidisciplinary investigation was undertaken by Ms. Atkins from Quality Management, Dr. Mion, Walter Mendelson, M.D., from Neurology, Robert Palmer, M.D., from Geriatrics, Thomas Franko, R.Ph., and bioethicist Jacquelyn Slomka, R.N., Ph.D.

A study being done on the Respiratory Care Unit (ResCUnit) looked at factors influencing successful weaning from ventilation, which might include respiratory, nutritional, metabolic, and psychological elements. Ventilator dependence was a major obstacle to stepping patients down to less-intensive nursing care. Weaning could be very difficult, however, for patients with chronic respiratory diseases. Finding out which factors interfered with weaning would enable nurses to devise practices to help patients become independent of ventilators.

Nursing research also examined the influence of both external and internal policy on patient care. For instance, in recent years, JCAHO and U.S. Food and Drug Administration standards regarding physical restraint and sedation had become more restrictive. The departments of Nursing Research, Geriatric Medicine, and Bioethics undertook a study that looked at patient characteristics and patient outcomes (use of restraints, use of sedation, falls, pressure ulcers, disruption of therapy, and satisfaction) to determine which types of non-restraint strategies would be most effective for which groups of patients. The investigators hoped that a study of this nature in the acute care setting could provide a model for the entire nation, since most information had previously come from the long-term care field.

Another study of patient outcomes examined an internal policy, the use of case management as a nursing care delivery system, by looking at two types of case management models and their effects on specific patient outcomes in

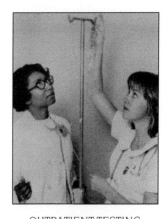

OUTPATIENT TESTING
Many Clinic patients came for diagnostic testing upon referral of their primary physicians. Ambulatory Nursing staff members played an important part in the testing procedure, preparing patients, setting up equipment, helping to administer tests, and, in the case of some advanced practice nurses, interpreting results. Licensed practical nurse Mae Grice (left) and registered nurse Chris Acker (right) of the Clinic's Nephrology and Hypertension Department are seen here preparing an intravenous solution for use in a test.

the areas of disease symptoms, knowledge, and self-management. With the Cleveland Clinic serving as a leader in implementing case management in the acute care setting, this study also had national and even international importance.

Research on urinary retention in orthopaedic patients continued, and was related to internal practice policy. Nurses believed that the use of IV infusions containing morphine as a patient-controlled analgesic medication under current policy increased the incidence of urinary retention. The study "revealed that it was not the type of narcotic, per se, but the length of narcotic usage, that influenced urinary retention. As a result of this study an assessment tool for risk of urinary retention was developed. Nursing interventions focus on pain management, especially non-narcotic strategies after 24 hours."[108]

Recent research on issues arising out of practice included a study comparing types of IV dressings, and studies relating to the nursing care of cancer patients. Clinical nurse specialists Kathy Tripepi-Bova, Kathleen Daum Woods, R.N., and Michelle Loach, R.N., from the Cardiac, Medical/Surgical, and Critical Care Nursing Departments, respectively, studied the use of peripheral IV catheter dressings to see whether gauze or the newer transparent polyurethane dressings were superior. They made their comparison on the basis of rates of infection, phlebitis, and fall-out, nursing time expended in reinsertion, and cost.

Barbara Tripp, R.N., M.S.N., a clinical nurse specialist in oncology, received funding from the Oncology Nursing Society to study factors contributing to the development of mucositis in patients undergoing chemotherapy with 5-fluorouracil, in order to determine which nursing intervention (allopurinol mouthwash or ice chips) was most effective in treating the condition. Clinical nurse specialist Ms. Droughton designed a study examining the use of a costly new drug to treat xerostomia in head and neck cancer patients. Her research focused on determining the drug's effectiveness, the prevalence and type of side effects, and the characteristics of the patients most likely to benefit from the drug's use.

The Division of Nursing also participated in multi-site and national studies. For example, in the mid-1980s, the Cleveland Clinic participated in the three phases of the Medicus System Corporation's revision of quality monitoring criteria. At the end of the decade, the MICU and P/SICU were part of the Acute Physiology and Chronic Health Evaluation (APACHE) III classification system research study. Objectives of the study included evaluating advanced medical care and new therapies, and collecting information that could be used in treating the intensive care unit patient. As one of eight hospitals selected as Beta Sites for the study, the Clinic Hospital was asked to collect data on 800 intensive care unit admissions. During the early 1990s, patients from the Clinic's cardiovascular intensive care units were enrolled in a study sponsored by the American Association of Critical-Care Nurses "to evaluate the effect of heparinized and nonheparinized flush solutions on the patency of arterial pressure monitoring lines."[109]

Reaching Out

In the early 1980s the Nursing Department had expanded its own mission, and the Foundation's three-part mission, to include a fourth element, outreach to the wider nursing community. The restatement of this goal under Ms.

Coulter's leadership expanded it further: "To act as a resource to the community-at-large on health issues requiring nursing input."[110]

The outreach goal and the other goals of the Division of Nursing were interconnected. When the Cleveland Clinic entered into an agreement with nearby John Hay High School to create a health careers program for students, education and outreach were combined, with an eye toward future patient care. The program, which included the summer employment of students by the Division of Nursing as nursing assistants and unit hostesses, aimed to enhance the educational opportunities of Cleveland students, as well as to promote the training of the future health care work force. Plans for the Cleveland Clinic's Martin Luther King Day celebration in 1993 included a career day for John Hay students, and the awarding of a scholarship.

Reaching out to the wider nursing community, the Cleveland Clinic Department of Nursing had sponsored its first full-scale educational program in the 1960s. In 1967 a one-day "Post-Graduate Course in Nursing" attracted 273 nurses from Ohio, Pennsylvania, Indiana, Michigan, and Illinois. Symposia and seminars on nursing topics, with sessions presented by nurses from within and without the Cleveland Clinic, were held with increasing frequency in subsequent years. These gatherings provided a setting in which Cleveland Clinic nurses could both learn and teach. Frequently, Clinic physicians and members of other disciplines contributed their time and expertise to the symposia, often making joint presentations with nurses.

The "Dimensions in Cardiac Critical Care Nursing" symposium, held annually since 1981, focused on one of the areas in which the Cleveland Clinic was most renowned. It attracted hundreds of nurses from all over the country each year. In 1985 the Department of Orthopaedic/Rheumatology Nursing began holding annual symposia, also attended by nurses from Ohio and beyond. In 1990 the Department of Ambulatory Nursing presented a course designed to prepare nurses in all areas "to meet the challenge of escalating demands in nursing for the 1990s."[111] The first annual "What's Special About Med/Surg Nursing" seminar took place in 1993. In 1994, the Division of Patient Care Operations sponsored five national conferences, including "Nursing Research: Clinical Implications" and "Beyond the '90s: Nursing in the New Millennium." The course, "Beyond the 90s: Preparing for the New Millennium," was planned for 1995 under the direction of Nursing Operations Manager Dolores Wiemels, R.N., B.A., and Hospital Pharmacy Manager David N. Gragg, R.Ph., M.B.A., to include sessions on new developments and trends of interest to both nurses and pharmacists.

The International Nurse Scholar program represented another combination of education and outreach. Cleveland Clinic nurses had hosted visiting colleagues from the area, from across the nation, and from other countries for many years. These nurses were attracted by the international reputation of the Clinic, and eager to learn through observing the facilities and practices in use there. In the 1950s, the Operating Room alone generally received visits from several outside nurses each month. In 1990, at Ms. Coulter's request, Nursing Education director Betty Vasquez outlined a program for International Nurse Scholars, in order to provide a formal structure for them to observe

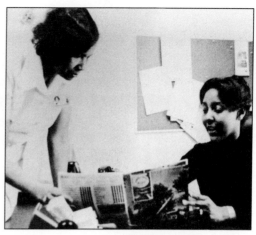

NURSING OUTREACH
For nurses and their co-workers, helping people was part of each day's work. Many Cleveland Clinic nursing employees also participated as volunteers in health-related and other humanitarian causes. In 1977, licensed practical nurse Sarah McCarrell of Clinic Desk 60 (left, with Pamela Bradford, right, of the American Sickle Cell Anemia Association) helped organize a dinner-dance to raise funds for the fight against sickle cell anemia.

the practice of nursing at the Cleveland Clinic, especially in areas like cardio-thoracic, critical care, and operating room nursing, and management. In 1992, the Nursing Division hosted nurse scholars from eight countries: Australia, Brazil, Egypt, Israel, Japan, Norway, Singapore, and Sweden. Ms. Vasquez pointed out that the program "provided many learning opportunities for Clinic nurses as well as establishing a network that reaches from Ecuador to Singapore."[112] Cleveland Clinic nurses shared their skills with international colleagues not only at home, but abroad as well, sometimes partici-pating in interdisciplinary teams with physicians, sometimes accepting invitations to visit and inspect or lecture at hospitals around the world. In 1994, Ms. Coulter and other division members visited locations as distant as Saudi Arabia, Singapore, Turkmenistan, and Argentina.

Other outreach efforts focused on community ser-vice. Many Cleveland Clinic nursing personnel believed that donating their time and money to help others was important. One nursing unit "adopted" a Native Ameri-can baby through a program that matched children and sponsors. Often, especially during the holiday season, nursing personnel collected food, toys, or clothing for hunger centers and sim-ilar agencies. They made pledges during the annual United Way campaign. These were activities that might be shared by people in any workplace. But nurses could also make a special contribution based on their education, expe-rience, and membership in a profession devoted to caring for the sick and pro-moting good health. Community service was a natural extension of their work.

In the 1980s and 1990s some outreach activities were sponsored by the Cleveland Clinic. Others grew out of nurses' involvement in professional orga-nizations or health care associations. Nursing personnel also gave their time to health-related causes on an individual basis.

The Greater Cleveland Volunteer Nurses program, headquartered at the Cleveland Clinic's Nurse on Call office, cooperated with the organization Cleveland Health Care for the Homeless "to perform teaching, counseling and health screening in the City's homeless shelters and outreach centers."[113] Vol-unteer nurses also helped to establish primary health care clinics for home-less persons, provide educational experiences for nursing students, and collect and distribute clothing to area shelters. Charlene Williams, R.N., B.S.N., of Nurse on Call, served as the program's coordinator. The volunteer nurses held bimonthly educational meetings at the Cleveland Clinic. Mem-bers of the Clinic medical staff became involved in the project, and the Divi-sion of Patient Care Operations provided a substantial portion of its funding. During Nurses' Week, Clinic nurses collected money and medical supplies for the primary care clinics.

Cleveland Clinic and association affiliations were combined when the Department of Pediatric Nursing hosted a Children's Health Fair as part of the annual Children and Hospitals Week sponsored by the Association for the Care of Children's Health, an organization in which several Cleveland Clinic nurses were active. Nurses and others presented hands-on learning sessions

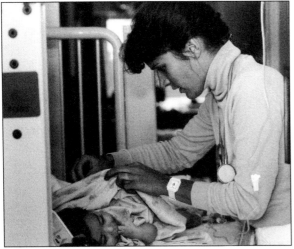

PEDIATRIC NURSING
Although a Hospital pediatrics unit and a Clinic Department of Pediatrics did not open until 1948 and 1951, respectively, Cleveland Clinic nurses had always cared for pediatric patients, and also partici-pated in volunteer activities to pro-mote children's health and welfare.

During the 1950s, many of the Hospital's new practical nurses were assigned to the pediatric floor to give the young patients plenty of care and attention, and did such a good job that some children "didn't want to leave." Beginning in 1959, the Hospital's seventh floor had two pediatric nursing units, one for adolescents and the other for younger children. In 1987, the third floor of the M Building, where the pediatric units were now located, was officially designated the Cleve-land Clinic Children's Hospital.

for children from area elementary schools and day care centers who attended the fair, teaching them about hospitals, health, and fitness. Another program in which pediatric nurses participated gave young renal patients a chance to stay on a ranch.

Pediatric and oncology nurses participated annually in Camp Friendship, sponsored by the state's American Cancer Society (ACS) division. The program gave children with cancer a chance to enjoy summer camp like other children, and to gain confidence in their abilities despite their illness. Volunteer physicians and nurses worked alongside regular counselors, so that campers' regular medical regimens did not have to be interrupted.

Other ACS programs included Daffodil Days and the "Nurse of Hope." Members of the Clinic's Oncology Nursing Task Force helped raise funds for the ACS by organizing the annual sale of flowers at the Clinic. It was both an honor and a responsibility to be chosen as a Nurse of Hope: "The Nurse of Hope program, sponsored by the ACS, has been quite visible at CCF, as many of our nurses have been chosen for that position. Annually, one nurse is selected after an interview process to represent the organization and to function as a public speaker and ambassador of hope."[114] Local chapters each selected a nurse for the position, and from among them a Nurse of Hope was chosen for the state. In 1985 Ann Birkmire, R.N., B.S.N., served as the Ohio Nurse of Hope. Some other area Nurses of Hope or alternates in subsequent years were Cleveland Clinic nurses Cathy Blake, R.N., B.S.N., Amy Weiss, R.N., and Kathleen Jirousek, R.N.

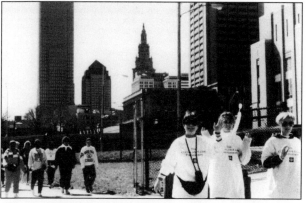

WALKING FOR CURES
As walks, runs, and similar events became popular as a way of raising money for health care causes, Cleveland Clinic nurses quickly became active as participants and sponsors. Annual fund-raisers included the Race for the Cure (breast cancer), for which hundreds of nurses turned out in 1995, the Memory Walk (Alzheimer's disease), and the Swim for Diabetes. Nurses also assisted in collecting and transporting, by motorcycle, teddy bears for hospitalized children during the annual Teddy Bear Ride, organized by local bikers.

Cleveland Clinic psychiatric nurses took their skills out into the community in a variety of ways: speaking to school children, teachers, and counselors; conducting a participative seminar on family communication and problem-solving; volunteering as a Red Cross-certified stress management instructor; and answering the telephone hot line at the Cleveland Rape Crisis Center. In addition, Jane Soposky was appointed to the Cuyahoga County Community Mental Health Board.

Through these activities, and many others, Cleveland Clinic nurses made the connection between work and community, and between professionalism and service, by contributing their knowledge and experience to promote the health and well-being of their fellow citizens.

Beyond the Walls

Ambulatory Nursing was solidly committed to providing patient and family education, and promoting wellness within and beyond the Clinic's walls. "The next way we are going to deliver patient care will be by going out into the community," predicted Director of Ambulatory Nursing Mary Johnson.[115] "Nurse on Call," for which she served as project leader, was a pivotal move in this direction. Implemented in 1991 under the aegis of the Department of Internal Medicine, Nurse on Call was a health information telephone line over which registered nurses answered questions from callers. Besides furnishing information on health-related topics, the nurses triaged calls from patients, helping them to determine if their symptoms warranted a visit to a physician (and referring the caller to a physician if desired), or even an emergency room. They were also able to direct patients to community services and agencies.

During 1994 Nurse on Call handled 97,652 calls, with 130,000 calls projected for 1995. Half of the calls received were for health information. Even though the program was not publicized outside northeastern Ohio, calls came from all 50 states, Canada, Europe, Asia, the Middle East, South America, and the Caribbean. In a way that was both practical and innovative, Clinic nurses were reaching out to the community, and beyond, through the medium of the telephone.

In another response to changing patterns of health care delivery, the Cleveland Clinic in 1988 instituted home health care services as a subsidiary venture. Separate from both the Division of Nursing and the Department of Ambulatory Nursing, Home Care Services was headed by a nurse, Carol Schaffer, R.N., and its contact staff members were available to nursing units to facilitate referrals. The Cleveland Clinic originally contracted with outside agencies to provide nursing and other home care services, but eventually hired its own personnel on a per diem basis.

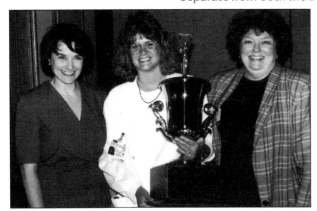

A UNIT APPROACH
The Nursing Division's Patient Satisfaction program approached quality improvement from the unit perspective. Nurse-led teams determined what changes on their own units could increase patient satisfaction. Team members included dietary, housekeeping, and transportation personnel as well as nursing unit staff. Units received recognition for attaining high levels of patient satisfaction, as in the photograph above. Director of Medical-Surgical Nursing Meri Armour (left), Assistant Nurse Manager Sharon Knauss (center), and Nurse Manager Cheryl Lemmerman (right) accept a trophy on behalf of nursing unit H51.

Patient Satisfaction

In some measure, publicity efforts, like promoting media coverage of nursing activities, and marketing programs, like the patient satisfaction project, were also examples of outreach. The patient satisfaction project demonstrated an increasing sensitivity to patient expectations on the part of Cleveland Clinic administrators. They recognized that the complaints of a dissatisfied patient could reverberate in the community, turning prospective patients away. Patients' letters indicated that nursing units and nurses had to be the focus of any effort to attain universally high levels of satisfaction, since modern medical technology was taken for granted. "They write to say how much they appreciate our understanding of their unique needs, that we take the time to talk to them, give them explanations about procedures or routines of care, are willing to bend the rules when necessary, and make provisions for their families when appropriate. Rarely, if ever, do they write expressing how much they valued the new CAT scanner, balloon pump, or modern facilities."[116]

Nurses had always measured patient satisfaction informally. "How are you?" "Is everything all right?" "Can we make you more comfortable?" Questions like these, which in themselves helped to reassure patients that someone cared, might be asked hundreds of times a day, all over the Clinic and Hospital. The formal patient satisfaction program applied the techniques of market research to the process. The Clinic's Marketing Department assisted the Division of Nursing to develop the program as a "care team" approach, with Nursing leading the team. Patients were surveyed to determine their reactions to their hospital stay: what aspects they rated highly, and where improvements were needed. After preliminary studies, the project was piloted in 1991, with G81, G91, G100, H51, H80, and H81 being the first units to participate. It was then expanded to additional units on the way to becoming an institution-wide program. Quarterly scores charted the ongoing progress of each unit in satisfying its patients.

In 1993, the Division of Nursing received a national award sponsored by the Mosby Co., the Patricia Schroeder Award for Innovation in Nursing Care Quality, in recognition of its accomplishments in this area. The phrase "World-Class Care" became a theme and stated goal for the division. Patient satisfaction scores were seen as one way of measuring progress toward that goal.

Nursing Economics

The patient satisfaction program's twofold objective was to affect not only quality of care, but also the institution's bottom line. Throughout the history of the Cleveland Clinic, the connection between nursing and financial health had been clear, from the time when nurses like Emma Barr had coordinated the rapid succession of thyroidectomies on which the Clinic's fortunes were based. In the decade which saw the rise of the prospective payment system and managed care, nurses felt increased pressures to control costs.

In the late twentieth century, operating room time was extremely expensive. Like Miss Barr, Operating Room nursing personnel had to help ensure efficient use of that time by coordinating the arrival of patient and surgeon and reducing the time between procedures. They had to order, store, clean, and prepare expensive equipment and supplies in the most cost-effective way possible. In the ambulatory care setting, patient flow was also a key concern. On the inpatient units, length of stay became especially important after DRGs became the basis of payment.

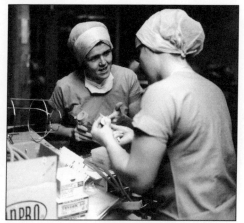

CHECKING SUPPLIES
In 1970, Operating Room nurse Linda Kraus (left) and Assistant Supervisor Patricia Sommer (right) packed supplies for a trip Dr. Turnbull was making to Australia to demonstrate a surgical technique. Ms. Kraus, as head nurse on Dr. Turnbull's service, accompanied him. Organizing supplies, part of the routine work of operating room nursing, has been affected in recent years by substantial growth in the use of disposable items.

A significant development at this time was the increasing use of itemized patient charges. Traditionally, the daily hospital charge paid by the patient included room, board, nursing, and even some of the most commonly used drugs, treatments, and equipment. Over the years, as the quantity and cost of drugs and other items used rose exponentially, hospitals began to charge for them separately. The increased use of disposables contributed to the trend, making it easier to attribute costs to individual patients. At the Clinic Hospital, nursing unit personnel had been given responsibility for seeing that the appropriate charges were made, since medications and supplies were distributed through the units.

In 1989 the division's fiscal coordinator began working out separate charges for dressings and IV starts. The logical extension of charging for specified nursing procedures, which the division continued to investigate, would be to charge for all nursing services, perhaps fixing rates on a unit-by-unit basis, based on patient classification data. Although charging for nursing services might, at first glance, have seemed mercenary, it had reason behind it. Nursing care had always been included in the overall hospital charge. If it were charged as a specific item, Nursing could point out its real contribution to revenue when operating income and expense were calculated. This would set a value on nursing services, making it clear that nursing was not a depreciable asset, like buildings or furniture, to be bundled into a room charge, but an active application of knowledge, skill, judgment, and hard work.

Kaiser and the New Emergency Department

During the 1990s, the Cleveland Clinic was receiving an increasing proportion of its patients through managed care contracts, just as the number of hospital patients covered by insurance had risen during the 1940s and 1950s. The agreement signed with the Cleveland area's Kaiser Foundation health plan in 1992, whereby the Cleveland Clinic would receive hospital patients and tertiary care referrals from Kaiser, meant that the Division of Nursing had to determine how to accommodate these additional patients in the beds available. As the Clinic appeared poised to take on more managed care contracts (with their inherent fiscal constraints) in the mid-1990s, nurses realized that the number of patients to visit Clinic offices, stay on Hospital nursing units, and undergo surgery in the Operating Room would inevitably increase.

Helping to implement the affiliation with Kaiser, to respond to changes in the health care system, and also to fulfill a long-perceived need, the Clinic's new Emergency Department (ED) opened in 1994. "Physicians, nurses, administrators, department heads, engineers and architects" worked together to plan the facility. They made site visits and requested recommendations from all personnel "who would eventually be involved in the new department." Preparation for staffing the ED included new education courses, such as a series of lectures on trauma, "in anticipation of increasing numbers of trauma patient visits," and another series on cardiac topics, "since chest pain is the most frequently encountered complaint." Acting Nurse Manager Linda Shah, R.N., coordinated the move from the old to the new ED on May 10, 1994.[117]

The new department was actually made up of four separate units, including two "complete and independent" emergency units for Clinic and Kaiser patients, as well as the innovative 20-bed Clinical Decision Unit and the Access Clinic. The Access Clinic served as an outpatient clinic where the Internal Medicine Department "could schedule immediate or next day appointments." The Clinical Decision Unit, "a new concept in patient care delivery, was implemented to ensure that Emergency Department patients requiring extended periods of time for diagnosis and/or treatment can be cared for prior to discharge or decision to admit. This new concept required extensive development of protocols, philosophic and all care delivery elements."[118]

Case Management

The financial constraints applied by both public and private third-party payors, the increasing proportion of severely ill patients, and trends within the nursing profession itself which favored giving nurses more accountability for patient outcomes made it necessary to look at new ways of delivering nursing care. A major focus for the Division of Nursing became the implementation of case management, in which nurse case managers tracked the care of individual patients. In the literature, the case manager's responsibilities were described as including ongoing assessment of the patient, "the setting of potential outcomes and evolving plans to meet these outcomes in collaboration with the patient, family, and physician; and...coordination, monitoring, and evaluation" of services to the patient.[119]

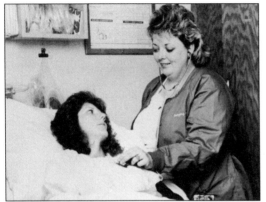

EMERGENCY ROOM NURSING

In the 1950s, the Emergency Room was, literally, a room in the Hospital building. It was open primarily to accommodate Clinic patients between 5 p.m. and 8 a.m. and on weekends. In 1951, the ER had fewer than 1,500 patient visits. Even by the late 1950s, the R.N. covering the room on weekends might care for only one or two patients on some days. In 1968, there were 11,068 emergency visits, three-quarters of them on evenings and weekends. By 1974, the ER had four cubicles, six beds, three treatment rooms, and an ENT room. It was staffed by four R.N.s and three L.P.N.s during the day, and one or two of each during the evening and night shifts. Triage, done by ER nurses, made sure that patients with all manner of symptoms and illnesses were channeled in the proper direction to get appropriate care. In this 1988 photograph, Linda Shah, the ER's assistant head nurse, assesses a patient. In 1994, Ms. Shah coordinated the move to a new four-unit Emergency Department on Carnegie Avenue, designed to accommodate a projected 7,500 patients visits per month.

Case management was considered especially useful in situations where there were many long-term or high-risk cases. Since the Clinic Hospital cared for a large number of high-risk patients with complex problems, this nursing care delivery system seemed particularly appropriate. However, at the time the Division of Nursing began implementing case management, most experience with its use had been in the long-term care rather than the acute care setting, so nurses and administrators at other institutions watched progress at the Cleveland Clinic with interest. The division received frequent inquiries from outside, and its nurses traveled throughout the country and even abroad to give presentations on the subject.

The Division of Nursing began investigating case management for possible use in 1988, and planning pilots in 1989. By the middle of 1990, pilots were in place on several units in the various clinical areas. In 1991, Connie Miller was appointed as the division's project director for case management, and a case management committee had also been formed. Over the following year, the system was extended throughout the Hospital, as all units developed care tracks for their most common DRGs, and more case manager positions were created. A patient brochure explaining case management was written.

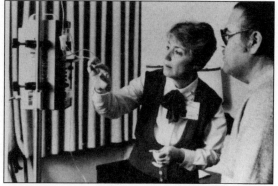

> In the same way as travel agents can help with vacation plans, case managers at the Cleveland Clinic coordinate your care and make sure your recovery is on schedule....
>
> Case managers work with physicians and other medical professionals to set up your anticipated recovery plan, which is called a coordinated care track. Based on our extensive experience we can anticipate how long your hospital stay will be, the tests you will require, the type of physical therapy you will need, and when you should be out of bed and walking. Each day's goals for how you should progress will vary depending on the specific illness or medical problem....
>
> ...While case management standardizes care according to the needs of the typical patient, it allows care to be personalized. The goal is to recognize each patient's personal needs.[120]

TRANSITION CARE
As acute care stays became shorter, patients and their families were apt to feel frightened or overwhelmed when facing sudden discharge from the hospital. In the Hospital's Transition Care Unit, opened in 1986, nurses helped patients make the transition from hospital to home. This was particularly important for Cleveland Clinic patients, many of whom lived out of town or faced complicated medical regimens. Patient and family teaching and support were key activities on the unit. In this photograph, Emily Shea, an ANA-certified family nurse practitioner, and the unit's head nurse, reviews use of the IV pump with a patient.

In 1993, additional coordinated care tracks were developed, and staff nurses became more involved in implementing case management. By the end of 1994, the Clinic Hospital had in use care tracks covering 420 diagnoses and procedures in 190 DRGs. The linkage of care tracks with DRGs, the diagnosis-related groups used to determine Medicare reimbursement, showed the connection between nursing and economics in late twentieth-century America. Both the health of the patient and the finances of the hospital would benefit when the course of care stayed on track.

Innovative Units

The settings in which Cleveland Clinic nurses cared for patients continued to become more diverse over the years: stepdown units, stepup units, short stay and transition care units, and even home care.

The Transition Care Unit that opened in 1986, with Emily Shea, R.N., M.S.N., in charge of nursing services, was a more sophisticated descendant of the old Convalescent Care Units that had been so problematic in the 1950s

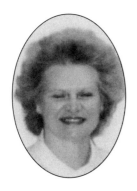

NURSING OPERATIONS
MANAGERS
In 1993, the Hospital's nursing
operations managers were:
(above) Viola Jones, (top row, left
to right) Dee Anne Behrens, Arie
Loretta Prince, Dolores Wiemels,
(lower row) Eleanor Foster, and
Reba Lilley. These registered
nurses, whose position had

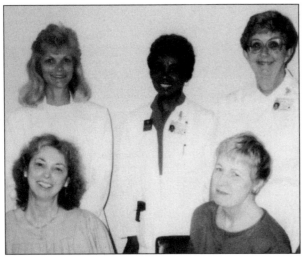

evolved from the traditional role
of nursing supervisor, provided
management support to the Cleveland Clinic Hospital during weekends, holidays, and the evening
and night shifts.

and 1960s. (In between times, an intermediate care area had been opened in the Clinic Inn, with an unexpected result: "Patients in the Clinic Inn are going to the bar and frequently return to the division intoxicated.") Located on the fifth floor of what was now called the Clinic Center Hotel, the new transition care area was a "wellness-focused nursing unit," in which a patient could be joined by a family member, and was assisted by nursing personnel in learning and practicing self-care. "Patients learn to test their health knowledge and develop skills through daily demonstration of self-medication, wound/incision care, trach care, stoma care, home antibiotic therapy infusion, stress reduction, nutritional counseling and activity tolerance. These skills are taught with the lifestyle and values of the patient in mind to increase compliance and positive patient outcomes." Since many of the Clinic's patients came from considerable distances, and could not return frequently for follow-up, it was especially important for patients and families to learn self-care.[121]

The Short Stay, or observation, Unit was planned by the Division of Nursing in conjunction with the Admitting/Registration Department. Opened on M50 in 1990, the new nursing unit would care for patients whose conditions warranted very short periods of hospitalization, and allow for rapid turnover of beds. Innovative in itself, the project also introduced a new feature with potentially broader application: a general health care support worker who would handle nursing assistant, housekeeping, and dietary duties.

The idea of the "patient-centered hospital," or unit, which was gaining the attention of health care administrators nationwide, also involved the cross-training of workers from different departments to perform similar tasks. It shifted the focus of hospital organization away from rigid job descriptions toward the needs of the patient; more ancillary services would be available on the units. Nurses, although not necessarily cross-trained themselves, would have a significant role in directing and coordinating this new work structure on their units. The Division of Nursing began a patient-centered pilot project in 1993. In 1994 the division began piloting a work redesign project on units H70, G100, and G101, as a step toward developing "the most efficient, flexible and cost-effective model for the delivery of patient care."[122]

The Nurse As Expert

From the beginning, Cleveland Clinic nurses were involved in nursing specialty associations, often as charter members. Mary Johnson in ambulatory nursing, Shirley Gullo in oncology nursing, and Maria Zickuhr in post-anesthesia nursing were among the nurses who could look back and remember when each of their respective organizations — the American Academy of Ambulatory Care Nursing (AAACN), the Oncology Nursing Society (ONS), and the American Society of Post Anesthesia Nursing (ASPAN) — had only a handful of members. All three women worked actively to advance the development of their organizations and specialties. For example, Ms. Zickuhr served several terms as chairman of ASPAN's Standards of Nursing Practice Committee.

Ms. Johnson chaired the AAACN Standards Revision Task Force, which in 1993 published nursing standards applicable to all ambulatory environments. Ms. Gullo was the founding president of the Cleveland chapter of the ONS.

Setting standards of practice was one of the most important functions of the specialty associations; providing for certification of individual nurses was another. With the advent of specialty certification, nurses were able to have their expertise in their chosen fields verified by colleagues. Although many of the nurses who did not choose to apply were also highly skilled and knowledgeable, and beyond doubt would have been granted certification had they gone through the process, initials like C.N.O.R. (Certified Nurse - Operating Room) or C.C.R.N. (Certified Critical Care Registered Nurse) following a nurse's name gave immediate notice that she had met certain standards in a given field of practice. Every year, a number of Cleveland Clinic nurses joined the ranks of those who had attained certification. As of 1986, 14 nurses in the Cardiac Nursing Department were certified in critical care nursing; other nursing areas with C.C.R.N. staff members included the various intensive care units and the Post-Anesthesia Care Unit. Nurses who attained certification might then serve as mentors to others. Marilyn Tetonis, R.N., certified in urology, led study sessions that assisted seven more nurses to gain C.U.R.N. (Certified Urological Registered Nurse) status in 1986 alone.

In addition to being certified in a particular clinical specialty, nurses might be certified or examined in a particular procedure, or in the care of a particular type of patient. Such certification or examination might be offered by specialty groups or by physician or other provider associations. Generalist nursing organizations like the ANA and the NLN (National League for Nursing) also gave such exams, as well as general certification or certification in clinical specialties. For example, some Cleveland Clinic nurses were certified in psychiatric and mental health nursing, or as geriatric nurses, by the ANA. In 1988, 16 Cleveland Clinic nurses participated in the pilot achievement test on the care of patients with AIDS given by the NLN. Nurses and also dialysis technicians from the dialysis unit and other areas attained certification in hemodialysis through the Board of Nephrology Examiners for Nurses and Technicians. Enterostomal therapy nurses at the Cleveland Clinic were required to be certified by the Wound, Ostomy, and Continence Nurses Society.

In 1994, 147 R.N.s in the Division of Patient Care Operations held specialty certifications; a number of ambulatory nurses and nurses working in other areas were also certified in specialties. Twenty-four nurses were entitled to use the initials C.N.O.R.; C.C.R.N.s numbered 21; Certified Gerontological Nurses (R.N.C.), 16; Oncology Certified Nurses (O.C.N.), 14; and C.U.R.N.s, 13. Division nurses held certification in 20 additional areas. A number of non-R.N. members of the division were also certified in their areas. They included members of the Pharmacy Department, as well as Certified Registered Central Service Technicians (CRCST) and Emergency Medical Technicians (EMTA).

Technical Skill

Scientific and technical advances in health care necessarily influenced nursing practice at the Cleveland Clinic, as they did in other medical institutions. Nurses everywhere were carrying out procedures their predecessors would never have dreamed of doing.

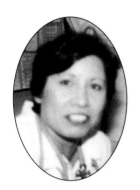

FLOAT NURSING
Hospital and Clinic alike depended on the nurses of their float pools, like registered nurse Barbara Jackson, to supplement permanent unit and departmental staffs. Assigned to different nursing units as needed, they provided staffing flexibility. Float nurses had to be experienced and versatile, able to care for patients in various specialties. Ms. Jackson, a Hospital float nurse, also worked in Nurse on Call, the Clinic's telephone triage and information service, where experience and breadth of knowledge were likewise important.

Intravenous therapy offered a good example of how a "specialist" technical procedure became part of the everyday work of Cleveland Clinic nurses. Until 1958, when the IV nurse team was set up, physicians — usually residents — started intravenous therapy. First IV nurses, and then, under their tutelage, R.N.s on the units handled more and more of the duties relating to IV medication. Of course, staff nurses had always monitored IVs, but they were now also hanging medications, discontinuing IV administration, and even performing venipunctures. In 1975, a nursing policy on IV insertion laid down guidelines: R.N.s who had completed 16 hours of in-service training with the IV team were permitted to start IVs when team nurses were unavailable. L.P.N.s, too, became more involved in IV therapy. By 1983 most of the Hospital's 38 units had L.P.N.s assessing sites, monitoring and adjusting rates, mixing additives, hanging infusions and piggyback medications, changing tubing and dressings, and discontinuing therapy on peripheral lines. In many units, L.P.N.s also performed at least some of these functions on central and other lines. Eventually, L.P.N.s began performing venipunctures as well. (Changes in state regulations later restricted the role of L.P.N.s in IV therapy.)

In the late 1980s, the number of nurses on the IV therapy team was reduced. In the past, the team had responded to routine calls for IV services throughout the Hospital (and also the Clinic). Its mission was now redirected to "complex" IV care and difficult starts. Unit staff R.N.s assumed more responsibility for IV therapy, handling all routine starts on their own units. Many staff R.N.s were already skilled in IV starts and now had the opportunity to use and maintain their skills. A program was set up to ensure that all R.N.s were trained and tested in the procedure. A technical skill that had once been the province of a few nurses was now mandatory for all Hospital staff R.N.s.

Nursing Care: Into the 1990s

Nursing personnel had to become proficient in numerous technically advanced procedures as more seriously ill patients were seen in every setting. Advances in technology and in medical science allowed for more complex and invasive surgical procedures, making it possible for patients with conditions previously considered inoperable to survive longer and sometimes recover. At the Cleveland Clinic Hospital, the number of telemetry beds increased. Patients receiving chemotherapy were admitted to various Hospital units, not only oncology units. Patients on ventilators were now sometimes cared for outside the intensive care units.

Medical advances also created new dilemmas for society and involved health care professionals in ethical issues on a daily basis. The Cleveland Clinic's Ethics Committee, first appointed in 1984, included nurse members, as did the Department of Bioethics. In 1990, the U.S. Congress passed the Patient Self-Determination Act, mandating that hospitals inform patients of their rights to refuse or accept treatment and make advance directives like living wills.

At the same time as Hospital personnel were caring for patients with more complex conditions, DRGs and other fiscal constraints resulted in shorter hospital stays and earlier discharges. Patients in the later stages of illness or postoperative recovery, who in earlier years would have remained in the hospital, were no longer part of the inpatient population. "The acuity level is tenfold what it used to be," declared a Hospital nurse.[123] For instance, a total laryn-gectomy patient, who in the past would have stayed in the hospital for at least two weeks, now stayed for only seven to nine days. At the same time, since laryngectomies were no longer simple removals but often included restorative work as well, the patient would have undergone a more intense surgical proce-dure and would require a higher level of nursing care.

Nursing personnel still had to do the all of the tasks that were part of every admission, including documentation and patient teaching as well as physical care, in a shorter time span. The pace of patient care had accelerated, and was continuing to do so. Here the benefits of case management became clear, as a unit-based case manager was able, using care tracks, to keep a close eye on what each patient needed at what point during the compressed course of the hospital stay.

Ambulatory nurses saw a corresponding rise in the severity of their patients' illnesses, in large part due to the same conjunction of technical advance and fiscal stringency. Pushed by third-party payors, and pulled by the development of new technologies like flexible scopes, which made surgery less traumatic, an increasing number of procedures were done on an outpa-tient basis. As hospitalized patients were discharged earlier, they too received more of their care in the ambulatory setting. Ambulatory nurses increasingly participated in high-tech treatments of episodic illness, as well as in long-term monitoring, evaluation, and promotion of their patients' health.

Sharing the Joy...

By the 1990s, organ transplants had become well-established treatments for certain diseases. Ohio's first lung transplant was performed at the Cleve-land Clinic on February 14, 1990; its first heart-lung transplant followed exactly two years later. In the thirty years following the Clinic's first kidney transplant in 1963, Cleveland Clinic surgeons had performed 1,717 renal, 247 cardiac, 1 heart-kidney, 44 lung, 1 heart-lung, 168 liver, and 14 pancreas transplants. Nurses' key roles in the process, in settings "from critical care to homecare," had also become well-established by this time.[124]

Nurse transplant coordinators were responsible for "orchestrat[ing] the patient's flow through an evaluation process that begins at the initial referral and ends at transplantation."[125] The coordinators educated and encouraged patients, helping them through the gantlet of tests potential organ recipients had to undergo.

Unfortunately, simply completing the tests did not guarantee patients would receive an organ. Some would be judged unable to undergo the proce-dure because of advanced disease, other health problems, or any number of reasons. Other patients would die before a suitable organ could be found; still others would wait for a long, agonizing time. In 1992, national sources listed 515 people waiting for kidney transplants, of whom 151 were Cleveland Clinic patients. "It's easy to become close with patients as they go through the screening process for heart transplantation," observed one of the first heart transplant coordinators. "Both nurses and patients share the disappointment when certain patients are deemed unsuitable candidates. They also share the joy when others are accepted as candidates and put on the waiting list for heart transplantations." Another nurse noted that there were different feelings to be shared with patients at the same moment: "hope for one would mean disappointment and sadness for another."[126]

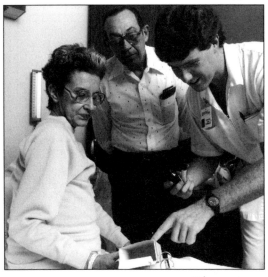

PATIENT EDUCATION
Every patient in the Clinic and Hospital received education from the nursing staff. Nurses cared for patients during illness, and also gave them information they needed to stay well. Here, registered nurse Michael Kelly of the Hospital's weekender staff gives homegoing instructions to a patient and her husband. Although a separate Patient Education Department had opened in 1976, staff nurses continued to provide some patient instruction as well; when the department was phased out in the mid-1990s, the role of staff nurses in patient education was expanded.

Some patients spent the waiting period, or a portion of it, on Clinic Hospital nursing units. Potential liver transplant patients suffering from complications of end-stage liver disease were cared for by the nursing personnel of the MICU. Potential heart transplant patients might be admitted to the Coronary Intensive Care Unit to be monitored and stabilized. For patients with "severe, progressive heart failure," implantation of the HeartMate[R] left ventricular assist device could provide a "bridge" to transplantation.[127] Since this involved modified open heart surgery, patients would recover in the Cardiothoracic Intensive Care Unit (CTICU) before transfer to a telemetry unit. Care of patients in all these areas involved frequent assessment and numerous nursing interventions. The nurse needed to be thoroughly familiar with disease processes and manifestations, as well as with the complex technology used in monitoring and treatment.

When a transplant coordinator received word that a suitable organ was available, the series of events culminating in the surgical procedure was set in motion. The coordinator informed the physicians, nurses, and other members of the transplant and organ procurement teams, and also notified the patient and family. The organ procurement team might have to fly to a distant hospital to obtain the organ (which might turn out not to be suitable after all). The period immediately before surgery could be "the most difficult for the patient, who may experience a myriad of emotions: despair, guilt, excitement, fear, anxiety. During this time the nurse sits and talks with the patient, trying to allay concerns."[128] Meanwhile, in the operating room, nurses and co-workers had gathered supplies and set up tables in preparation for the surgery itself, during which the diseased organ was removed and the donor organ implanted. This would take many hours: 8 to 12 in the case of a liver transplant.

Following surgery, the patient would begin life with the new organ in the appropriate intensive care unit — CTICU for heart, SICU for liver and other transplants. After a few days, if all went well, the patient was stepped down to another nursing unit. Since transplant patients might now be discharged from the hospital less than two weeks after surgery, nursing personnel had to fit many activities into a brief period of time. Nurses cared for the usual needs of a person recovering from major surgery, and the special needs of a transplant recipient, such as monitoring for signs of rejection or infection and treating the side effects of powerful drugs. They also had to prepare the patient, physically, mentally, and emotionally, for the return home, and a new life. "The transplant patient experiences an emotional adjustment during the transplant process. He or she has suffered through a life-threatening illness and a major surgery."[129]

Nursing case managers had a vital role in piloting the patient through the difficult passage from transplant to discharge, seeing that post-surgical care stayed on track, coordinating with other disciplines, assessing the needs of patients and their families, and ensuring that they were prepared to take over their own care at home, with the assistance of home care nurses. Since transplant patients needed "complex, high-tech home infusion therapy" during the weeks after discharge, transplant coordinators and home care coordinators from Cleveland Clinic Home Care Services worked together to develop "a realistic, comprehensive, and safe home-care plan." Home care coordinators helped patients arrange for in-home infusion therapy and supplies. Nursing involvement did not end even here, however. Writing about renal transplant patients, a nurse noted: "Continued close contact among patient, coordinator, and physician is a necessity for the life of the transplanted kidney."[130]

Nursing personnel contributed their clinical skills and emotional support to patients and families during the entire process. In return, patients and families shared their gratitude and joy. One young woman, who had served as a living kidney donor to her husband, wrote:

> The help and care we received from the transplant coordinators have been invaluable, supporting and sustaining. They became our friends and now feel like family. What an incredible job being a nurse. You must have everything: knowledge, timeless energy, great expertise, perfect poise, professionalism, and empathy galore.
>
> ....We are very much looking forward to having children. I look forward to sending the transplant coordinator and transplant team a picture of our first born. I can't think of a better result to all our efforts.[131]

Organ transplantation had become a highly organized and astonishingly successful process, with nursing personnel well-versed in the roles they played. It was nonetheless far from routine, and continued to be an intensely emotional experience for the caregivers involved. A cardiothoracic operating room nurse, in describing the moment at which the new heart began to beat in the chest of the recipient, found it hard to describe her own thoughts: "It is difficult to convey in words the feeling of exhilaration each time one sees this miracle."[132]

A surgical nurse clinician told a moving story of his acquaintance with the Clinic's first heart and kidney transplant recipient. He had met her by chance several months before the operation, while both were taking a moment to watch the sun set from the window of a nursing unit lobby. During the waiting period, the patient's health weakened. "Often I would see her at the window in the lobby surveying the view, [and I would wonder] if she ever thought this would be her last chance." Responding to a cardiac arrest call one evening, he found himself at her bedside. "I stepped forward and took her hand, telling her, 'Don't worry, I'm here and everything is going to be all right. Just try to relax.'" The patient recovered, but the nurse wondered how much longer she would be able to wait. Several days later he relieved a fellow worker in the operating room, where a heart transplant surgery was in progress. Again, seemingly by chance, he was brought together with this special patient. "Dr. Stewart said, 'Pat, hold this' as he made a few more cuts. There I was holding her heart in my hand....It was hard to finish the work with tears in my eyes. However, they were welcome tears of joy — joy for our patient, her new heart, and her new kidney, which she received later that day."[133]

...And the Sadness

Not all patients' stories had a happy ending. Yet nursing personnel could gain satisfaction, if not joy, in working with dying patients. In answer to the question, "How can you work with dying patients all the time?", one nurse shared her wisdom.

> In the process of dying...a lot of living, loving and caring continues. As nurses, we must possess not only technical competency but also share our emotional strength and support with our families and patients....

> Even though it is a sad experience, it can be gratifying. There is much that can be done for the patient and the family members left behind....

> Patients know when they are dying....We must be able to respect patients' decisions to enable them to die with peace and dignity. The actual care for the patient then becomes quite simple, comfort. This element of care comes in many fashions ranging from medications to relaxing visiting hours....

> ...Another focus is family members — talk to them....Also allow them to participate in the care, even if it just means applying a cold compress to the forehead. When the final moment arrives, allow them time...to be alone with the patient or...to be by themselves, so they can gather their thoughts.[134]

Palliative care programs provided a formal structure for giving symptomatic relief and skilled nursing to patients at the end of life, as well as psychological support to them and their families. At the end of 1986, a pilot Palliative Care Consult Service, using an interdisciplinary team of physician, nurse, social worker, and chaplain, began to accept referrals of patients on nursing units G91, G70, G80, and H81. Although the initial focus was on the cancer patient, referrals of patients with diagnoses like end-stage heart disease or AIDS were also accepted, since the palliative care team hoped to extend the program to other patients for whom curative therapies had been exhausted. The pilot project identified a definite need for a palliative care program for Cleveland Clinic patients, even though tertiary care facilities typically concentrated on aggressive treatment rather than palliative care. With the establishment of a permanent program, the Clinic crossed "the traditional boundaries between acute care, skilled nursing care and home care."[135] Another advance came in 1994, when the Horvitz Center opened on M70/71, with special services for patients receiving palliative care.

Nursing the Pulmonary Patient

Respiratory failure, a problem experienced by patients during the last stages of many different illnesses, also called upon the nursing skills and emotional strength of the caregiver. It was "natural for anyone experiencing loss of 'air' to react with fear," especially pulmonary patients who might have reason to fear that a spell of difficulty in breathing would end in death. Moreover, the physiological effects of fear increased the respiratory rate, creating a vicious circle of panic and breathlessness. But the nurse had the ability to break the cycle. "Quiet firm direction, using short phrases to coach breathing efforts, staying with the patient, even getting very close and using one's own respirations to demonstrate 'how to breathe' can assist in decreasing the number of respirations so that each effort, no matter how difficult for the patient, will be the most effective one possible....Positioning for comfort and maximum effectiveness is another essential." Even at the very end, this nurse reminded her colleagues, "there is always something nurses can do. Hand holding, proximity, words of comfort are all important and can make the difference between a sad respiratory death and a terrifying one."[136]

Fortunately, nurses could assist other pulmonary patients to recover. Many such patients were admitted to nursing unit G81. The unit included six rooms with ventilators, the six-bed ResCUnit, and a four-bed stepdown unit, in addition to regular medical-surgical beds. Lung transplant patients, AIDS patients, and laryngectomy patients were among the patients G81 nurses cared for. One of the most challenging tasks they faced was the weaning of ventilator-dependent patients.

Some pulmonary patients had received permanent or temporary tracheostomies. Before discharge, they had to be taught self-care. "While teaching is a challenge, it can also be creative and fun. Our patients include the inner city alcoholic and the truck driver who lives in his truck and requires a suction machine adapted to the cigarette lighter in his cab."[137] Teaching began as soon as the patient arrived on the unit. First, the nurse explained tracheostomy care procedures to the patient and family members as she performed them. Next, the patient began to participate in his own care, learning how to do suctioning, clean the stoma, and change the tracheostomy tube and ties. By the time a patient was ready for discharge, he had learned how to do routine maintenance and simple troubleshooting.

New Ways of Caring

Despite the pervasive influence of technology upon nursing, patient care at its most advanced also included attention to non-physical aspects of care, respect for the basics of nursing, and even a return to treatments that might have seemed outdated.

For instance, most laypersons think of the use of leeches as a repellent and ineffective feature of eighteenth and nineteenth century medicine. However, in a limited number of situations, the old became the new, as leeches came into their own again during the late twentieth century. They proved very effective in draining excess blood after finger reattachment, and their use spread to the treatment of various skin lesions where congestion of blood was a problem. Nurses caring for dermatology patients in the Clinic Hospital were faced with the challenge of getting leeches to stay where they belonged during treatment, since they tended to migrate away from lesions toward healthy tissue — "and they move faster than you would think!" commented a nurse. Phrases like "q 15 minutes leech watch" appeared in nurses' notes, and a leech disposal protocol was written.[138]

The division's skin care program was another example of a component of patient care that, although not outdated, might have seemed too simple to deserve special attention in the "high tech" era. However, wrote Ms. Coulter, the program's success showed that "maintaining skin integrity can have a resounding impact on quality and cost," illustrating "that 'getting back to basics' is not that basic at all."[139]

The non-physical aspects of care included both education and emotional support for patients and families. "High tech, high touch" became a watch-

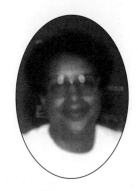

ROBERTA CONNOR
For the Connor sisters, nursing at the Cleveland Clinic was a family tradition. Both licensed practical nurses, Roberta and Rose Connor each spent more than 20 years caring for patients there, mostly on Hospital units.

word for late twentieth-century nursing care.[140] Paradoxically, scientific and technological advances, often viewed as forces tending to remove the nurse from personal contact with the patient, in some cases actually enhanced the holistic care of the patient.

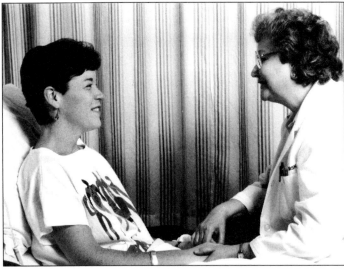

For instance, new anti-emetic drugs allowed Cleveland Clinic oncology nurses to spend less time managing the side effects of chemotherapy, and more time ministering to the emotional needs of cancer patients and their families. In 1985, nurses and social workers joined in organizing the "Second Monday Group," a support group for patients with advanced cancer, and their families and friends. Another innovative intervention was art therapy. Clinical nurse specialist Shirley Gullo developed a program using art as "a powerful tool to help facilitate emotional expression and aid the healing process."[141] The exhibit "Healing Art," presented at the Cleveland Clinic in September 1994, displayed the work of Clinic cancer patients.

A CARING TOUCH

Shirley Gullo, Clinical Nurse Specialist in Oncology, advocated a holistic approach to the care of cancer patients. She began her career at the Cleveland Clinic as a staff nurse in ENT and plastic surgery but soon moved into oncology nursing as a chemotherapy nurse in the Department of Hematology/Oncology. After working as a weekender staff nurse on the Hospital's oncology unit while studying for a master's degree, Ms. Gullo had greater opportunity as a C.N.S. to help cancer patients and their families deal with the emotional and psychosocial implications of their condition. She received numerous awards in recognition of her clinical work and her professional, volunteer, and teaching activities.

Numerous other therapeutic and support groups were created, several by psychiatric nurses, experienced in dealing with patients' emotional and psychological needs. Nurses working in adolescent psychiatry led weekly meetings of the Eating Disorder Group for in- and outpatients with bulimia and anorexia. A support group for family members met at the same time. A nurse and a social worker served as facilitators for the Adolescent Outpatient Group. In another area, the Pain Management Unit, nurses developed and led the Summations Group, which allowed patients to participate in setting their own goals and evaluating their progress. The Renal Transplant Peer Support Group was established in 1988, with nephrology nurses facilitating the weekly meetings of patients who had received or were awaiting or considering a transplant.

For patients with widely varying diagnoses, clinical care and emotional support went hand-in-hand. In the Epilepsy Monitoring Unit, a multidisciplinary team of nurses, physicians, and technicians participated in planning and monitoring "long-term medical therapy, as well as personal support" for patients facing the "lifetime struggle" of dealing with epilepsy. Vascular amputee patients faced a different struggle, that of recovering from surgery and learning to walk with a prosthesis. From nursing personnel they needed "meticulous" skin care, encouragement in performing muscle-strengthening activities, and help in regaining a "positive self-image and sense of control." Providing psychological support, as well as physical care, was also an important responsibility of nurses working with the increasing numbers of AIDS patients.[142]

The Patient Pride℠ program added a new facet to patient care at the Cleveland Clinic. Founded in Phoenix, Arizona, in 1986, Patient Pride was a national, nonprofit organization. Its volunteers visited patients in hospitals and nursing homes, applying light makeup, or perhaps just moisturizer, for those who wished it. The program was based on the idea that "when people look better, they generally feel better," and that increased self-esteem and personal interaction, particularly human touch, could even help speed recovery.[143]

The Division of Nursing piloted Patient Pride at the Clinic Hospital in 1990. This was the first time the program was implemented in a medical institution outside Phoenix. Corinne Hofstetter, retired from the position of Clinic Nursing Supervisor, was hired by Patient Pride to train and direct volunteers to visit female patients. (The Cleveland Clinic had only recently reinstituted formal volunteer programs; unofficial policy had discouraged the use of volunteers for a number of years.) By the end of 1993, Patient Pride volunteers were visiting seven Clinic Hospital units and serving 1,200 patients per year. As other northeastern Ohio hospitals and nursing facilities instituted the program, Ms. Hofstetter assisted them in training volunteers.

Total Commitment

It was also important to consider the patient's family when providing care. Setting hospital visiting hours, for example, involved balancing the patient's need for rest against the need of patient and family to be together. During the 1990s, Clinic Hospital nurses were given more responsibility in setting visiting hours and visitation policies on a unit-by-unit and patient-by-patient basis. In 1991, for example, open visiting hours were instituted within the Cardiac Nursing Department, on units G100-101 and G90. In 1993, the Nursing Executive Council affirmed its support for a policy of flexible visitation, "with each unit determining visitation for the individual patient."[144]

For pediatric patients, especially, family-centered care was a guiding principle at the Cleveland Clinic in all settings. "Ambulatory nurses attempt to involve parents in procedures because parents can distract children with calming and reassuring conversation....The transporting of infants and small children to the operating room can be accomplished via parents' loving arms....In the inpatient hospital units at CCF, parents are encouraged to room with their children."[145] The Pediatric Intensive Care Unit (PICU) had adjacent rooms in which parents could stay overnight.

Before the PICU opened in 1992, high-risk pediatric patients had been cared for in the combined Pediatric-adult Surgical Intensive Care Unit (P/SICU), the Cardiothoracic Intensive Care Unit (G50), and the Pediatric Special Care Unit (PSCU). The PSCU, opened in 1988, had received patients who required close observation but did not need to be in intensive care. The new PICU made it possible to care for both PSCU and ICU patients in a unit specially adapted to the needs of children: "The PICU philosophy maintains that optimal care of children cannot be accomplished without the involvement of their families."[146]

Another program for Cleveland Clinic pediatric patients involved not only families, but also teachers and school classmates. Pediatric oncology nurse clinicians, working with staff from child life, child psychiatry, and social services, offered a school re-entry program for children with cancer. Besides providing information on the child's diagnosis and treatment to the family and educators, the program included a school visit by staff members, in which they met with the child's classmates, helping them "to feel more comfortable around the child with cancer." The overall goal was "to increase the child's self-esteem and return some 'normalcy' into his or her life."[147]

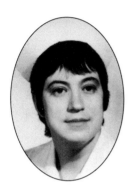

STAFF NURSING
One Cleveland Clinic nurse referred to staff nurses as the "backbone" of nursing. Patients depended on them to provide 24-hour nursing care and therapies ordered by physicians. Beyond this, many staff nurses combined extra activities with their staff nursing roles. For example, registered nurse Susan Horn (above), staff nurse on unit G81, served as a member of the Nursing History Committee and chairman of its Nursing History Book Task Force.

Not all attempts by nurses to meet patients' and families' emotional needs were part of formal programs. Often, nurses were responding to individual, unforeseen situations. In 1993, personnel on orthopaedic nursing unit H71 faced an unusual request: a new mother being admitted for an above-the-knee amputation was breast-feeding her baby, and wished to bring the child into the hospital with her. Staff concerns about caring for a baby on an adult unit gave way to "a second thought...one of total commitment to this patient and her newborn." With the father also staying in the room and caring for the baby, the arrangement worked out wonderfully well, "through the family's strong commitment to each other coupled with the H71 nursing staff's willingness to assist them to the best of their abilities."[148]

Cardiac nurses assisted a mother and child in a tragically different, yet equally moving situation. A young woman was admitted to the Clinic Hospital with an enlarged heart following the birth of her son. The baby, his liver failing, was "fighting for his life" at University Hospitals of Cleveland. When the patient's physician received word that the child would likely live only a few hours longer, nurses made arrangements for the mother "to say good-bye to her son." One nurse accompanied her to University Hospitals, where she held the baby "for the first and last time.... 'It was one of the saddest things I have ever witnessed,'" she later said, with tears in her eyes, to a nurse colleague also caring for the young mother.[149]

That colleague, in telling the story, made an important observation. "While this type of situation is not a daily event, we as nurses know that everything we do, from a smile to cardiopulmonary resuscitation, can affect our patients in ways that are hard to imagine."[150] Nurses supported patients, and served as their advocates, not only in extraordinary situations but throughout the everyday routine of patient care.

The first few hours of a "routine" evening shift for a Cleveland Clinic Hospital unit staff R.N. might go something like this: After receiving the report of the day shift, she began by checking on all her patients. She then took off orders on a transferring patient, made sure her room was ready, and met her when she arrived on the unit. Other duties included removing IVs and going over discharge orders with several departing patients; hanging piggyback IV medications and doing heparin flushes; and working with her L.P.N. partner to check an insulin dosage.

She also, as matter of course, did a number of special things for her patients. She obtained extra meals, for a man who had missed his lunch because of surgery and for the newly-transferred patient. She tracked down a physician to sign an order for another patient's IV to be removed. One patient, barely able to breathe and open his eyes, seemed to have no family or other visitors; she stopped for a few minutes, spoke to him, patted his hand, and adjusted his oxygen more comfortably. She suggested to a physician that a dying man needed more effective pain relief, maybe a morphine drip. She checked with another physician about a "do not intubate" order. A patient remarked that his coffee was cold, and she microwaved it for him. Another patient's wife asked about getting a disability form filled out. The nurse promised to catch the social worker and let her know about it.

A Human Face

The Clinic's reputation in cardiac care and surgery, in particular, had been drawing patients from other states and other countries in growing numbers since at least the 1960s. In 1990, the Clinic's national prestige was further enhanced when U.S. *News and World Report* published its first ranking of "America's best hospitals." The report ranked the Clinic among the top ten hospitals in the country in four medical specialties: cardiology, gastroenterology, neurology, and urology. In following years, the Clinic received a rating among the top ten in additional specialties.

At the international level, Clevelanders had become accustomed to hearing about heads of state, including the kings of Saudi Arabia and Jordan and the presidents of Turkey and Brazil, being treated at the Clinic. (The kings were not the first royalty to visit the Clinic; a queen from a state in western India had come to receive treatment from Dr. Crile, Sr., in 1928.) Private citizens also came from abroad, particularly the Near East and Latin America. Physicians who had visited or studied at the Clinic were an important link in this growing global network. The International Center, formed in 1984, assisted international patients with visas, housing, travel, and financial arrangements, and provided interpreters. Patients from abroad were often admitted to the hospital's "VIP," or "private" medical-surgical nursing unit, G71, but increasingly stayed on other units as well, and received treatment in all outpatient areas.

The Cleveland Clinic's reputation for providing the most advanced medical care available had a drawback. Some people tended to believe that a medical center so large, and so technically proficient, must be impersonal and uncaring as well. From this viewpoint, the Cleveland Clinic appeared as a huge, gleaming, cold machine that operated with precision, but without feeling. Certainly, its size, along with the inevitable complexity of the modern health care system, could be overwhelming. Patients had to find their way through the many buildings and long corridors, fill out bewildering forms in the offices of busy people, undergo batteries of tests, and perhaps end up in a hospital room surrounded by strange machines and changing faces. They had to cope with all this, at the same time they suspected, or knew, that they were very sick, maybe dying. Although much had changed since the era of the founders, the hopes and fears of the patients and families who came to the Clinic remained the same.

Nursing personnel, who were "always there," who spent the most time with patients and families, were able to put a human face on this beautiful, forbidding machine. Mabel Selfe had stated in 1957 that good nursing care made for good public relations. Nursing Operations Chairman Mary Ann Brown, acting as an advocate for patients and their families, made a similar point in 1986.

> Mary Brown reported that a member of the [Advisory] Council would like nursing to discourage families from staying overnight in the ICU lounges by not providing blankets for them and also to discourage the eating of food in the lounges. Mary's response to this was that it would be poor public relations to discourage families from staying overnight and, therefore, nursing would continue to provide blankets for those families wishing to stay. In regard to eating in the lounges, nursing would encourage families to clean up the area after they have eaten.[151]

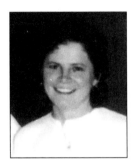

IVANKA ZUZIC
A number of nurses first worked
at the Cleveland Clinic in unit
secretary or nursing unit assistant
positions. Some were motivated
to become R.N.s after spending
some time on the units; others
took nursing unit jobs specifically
to provide income and health care
experience while working toward
their R.N.s. After arriving in the
U.S. as a young woman, Ms. Zuzic
worked as a unit secretary and put
herself through school to become
a registered nurse. She began her
nursing career on Cleveland Clinic
Hospital nursing unit G81.

Cleveland Clinic nurses had added the role of image-maker to a list that already included caregiver, technical expert, leader-manager, recordkeeper, and patient advocate.

Nursing remained the "focal point for patient care," as James Harding had said in 1963. "We do everybody else's jobs," said a nurse 30 years later, partly but not entirely in fun.[152] The nurse was at the center of a network of care and communication, keeping track of the patient's needs according to the physician's orders, the patient's and family's requests, and her own observations. It was her business to monitor those needs and make sure that they were met. This might mean over the course of hours in the operating room, or days on the nursing unit, or years of outpatient visits.

In a sense, case management formalized and extended this, making one nurse accountable for the course of a patient's recovery across shifts, across inter-unit transfers, and even potentially across the gap between hospital and outpatient settings. "A case manager's important role as patient advocate is achieved through integrated and coordinated activities with multiple disciplines, which include medicine, nursing, social service, home care, nutritional services, utilization review, and palliative care," wrote oncology case manager Amy Weiss in 1994.[153]

To Act As A Unit

Cleveland Clinic nurses of the 1990s may have had to spend more time with inanimate objects — by this time including documentation binders, budget worksheets, computer terminals, and Pyxis stations — than their counterparts of 70 or even 20 years before. Nonetheless, health care remained an intensely human industry. Nurses still found both the greatest joys and the greatest problems of their professional lives in their relationships with others. A head nurse expressed the feelings of many fellow caregivers: "The bottom line is the people, both the patients and other nurses."[154]

When asked what they liked about their jobs, Cleveland Clinic nurses most often had answers in one of three areas: interest in the clinical specialty in which they worked; interest in working with patients; and satisfaction with the way in which the staff worked together.

Interest in a clinical specialty and in working with patients often went together. Nurses frequently expressed their satisfaction in terms of contact with a particular type of patient population: "I've...met a diversified patient population from all over the world"; "I enjoy working with pediatric patients"; "I love neuro/neurosurgical patients"; "I enjoy caring for transplant patients. When they occasionally come back to visit us, it is very uplifting to see them." In the Hospital, nursing personnel on units where there were many "repeaters" — patients with long-term illnesses like cancer or AIDS who often returned to the unit — might even become a little bit possessive about "their" patients: no one else, they felt, could care for these patients as well, or care about them as much.[155]

The quality of relationships with co-workers was also very important to nurses. "Current literature reveals that the unit culture is key in staff satisfaction," noted the Nursing Executive Council.[156] As the Cleveland Clinic had grown in size over the years, to the point where it employed approximately ten thousand people, it had become difficult for so many people "to act as a unit" at the institution-wide level. Smaller scale loyalties, to the nursing unit, the surgical service, or the clinical department, became more important in everyday life.

The atmosphere on the unit or within the department could have a tremendous influence on the individual's attitude toward working at the Cleveland Clinic. "We are a very close group on our unit and work as a team well," was a positive comment typical of the way many people felt about their units. On the other hand, some employees felt that poor morale on their units resulted when not everyone took a fair share of a heavy work load. Nursing personnel who felt that they had a supportive nurse manager and co-workers who pitched in to help when needed were much more likely to be satisfied with their own unit and with the Cleveland Clinic in general. Operating room nurses agreed that co-workers' attitudes made all the difference. "I'm really concerned about who's my fellow nurse with me in the room that day....Somebody that you work well with, that's more important than any piece of technology."[157]

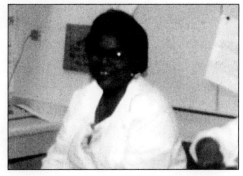

ARLENE WHITE
Ms. White also started out as a unit secretary. After receiving her R.N., she held successive positions of unit staff nurse, assistant head nurse, and head of outpatient Radiation Therapy nursing. She then began studying to become a nurse practitioner.

Relationships with physicians also mattered to nurses. "Physicians on our floor respect and stand behind our comments and standards of care," declared one nurse.[158] However, as in the case of unit morale, some nurses felt more positive than others. To advance the working relationship between the two groups, the Nurse/Physician Collaboration Committee was set up. In 1991 a resident mentoring program, "Partners in Care," began matching new residents with nurse mentors. The nurses helped introduce the residents to their units or areas, establishing communication from the very beginning of the young physician's contact with Cleveland Clinic nursing. Other initiatives, including a series of forums called "Can We Talk?", were also directed at promoting dialogue between physicians and nurses. The Division of Nursing established the Nightingale Award for Physician Collaboration to recognize "the unique ability of a physician to collaborate with nurses toward the goal of excellence in patient care in a professional and positive manner."[159] The award was given annually to a Clinic physician, beginning with an honorary presentation to Dr. Loop in 1992.

Different Identities

Unit culture was important to nurses on the inpatient nursing units, in the surgical suites, and in the outpatient clinics. However, these three areas did not have identical cultures. The more regular work schedule in both Ambulatory and Operating Room Nursing was an obvious difference, as was the difference in numbers. Some nurses who had worked in both Clinic and Hospital settings felt that Ambulatory Nursing was more relaxed, less pressured, even a "break" from the Hospital's hectic pace. Others dissented strongly, pointing to the wide variety of treatments and procedures carried out in the ambulatory setting. Well children, chronic headache sufferers, lung transplant recipients experiencing rejection — by the mid-1990s, all were cared for on an outpatient basis when possible.

Even within a single Clinic department, nurses put into practice a wide variety of nursing skills. For instance, the outpatient Colorectal Surgery Department was considered a highly technical area, in which nursing personnel had to work with many different instruments. But nurses also did a great deal of patient teaching. They stayed with patients during long procedures. They made sure that patients who had undergone sedation met discharge criteria. One nurse had a ready reply for people who asked her how she could work in such an area. She pointed out the great difference that new surgical procedures could make in allowing colorectal patients to return to normal lives, with the help of care, support, and teaching given by nurses. "My patients," she said, "get better."[160]

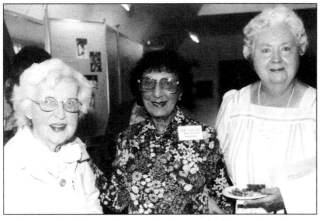

SPANNING THE DECADES
Registered nurse Mary Cooper (left) came to the Cleveland Clinic from St. Vincent Charity Hospital in 1933, and was employed in Clinic Nursing until her retirement in 1966. She worked at Desk 30 (ENT) and Desk 80 (Rheumatology, Hematology, and Internal Medicine). With her in the photograph are fellow retirees Victoria Asadorian (center), whose career as a Clinic laboratory technician began in 1922, and Elizabeth Minnick (right). Betty Minnick, a Pittsburgh native and a 1954 graduate of Cleveland's Central School of Practical Nursing, worked in the Clinic's Department of General Surgery from 1957 to 1983. In 1990, the institution's Clinical Excellence Award for L.P.N.s was named in her honor.

Unlike the Hospital, the Clinic did not hire new graduates, but required at least a year of hospital experience. In the Clinic setting, nurses had to function independently from the very beginning. "I look for the seasoned R.N., who doesn't have to be told, who instinctively moves to do things," said one Clinic nurse manager.[161] Unit culture in the Clinic also differed from the inpatient floors in that Clinic nurses worked with physicians throughout the day, every day. Physicians had their offices in the Clinic. On the nursing units, they were occasional visitors. Clinic nurses had much more contact with staff physicians, while Hospital unit nurses more often worked with residents. Besides the Clinic Nursing staff of nearly 200 members, Ambulatory Nursing continued to have administrative responsibility for departmental assistants. By the mid-1990s, there were approximately 150 nurse clinicians who worked with physicians in both Hospital and Clinic settings.

The Department of Surgical Services also had its own identity. Operating room nurses, although part of the Division of Nursing, felt separate in some ways. The doors physically isolating the operating suites from the rest of the Hospital symbolized this separation. The intense, and sometimes tense, atmosphere of the operating room, relieved by kidding and joking among the members of the operative team, fostered camaraderie. Operating room nurses often identified more strongly with team members from other disciplines than with nurses working in other care settings. Like Clinic nurses, they worked closely with members of the medical staff, and praised the willingness of Clinic surgeons to share their knowledge. "One of the things that I always appreciated and still do is that if you were interested as a nurse you could learn as much as you wanted to....They wanted us to learn the anatomy, and to know what was going on....You can still ask questions and get answers." Operating room nurses, too, valued "seasoned" colleagues: "It's always nice to have a nurse in the room that you know you don't have to keep saying, well, did you send for this, did you call for this, did you do this, did you do that...It makes the job together so much better and it makes the whole day easier."[162]

Bridging the Gap

Cleveland Clinic nurses were aware of the real and imaginary barriers that divided their own ranks. Unit cohesion was good in that it gave nursing personnel a focus, an identification, and even an occupational "home" within the hugely expanded "hotel for the sick." However, too much insularity could impede cooperation. "I think we should bridge the gaps between departments," said a Clinic nurse. "Departments should be more flexible using personnel."[163] Another nurse, addressing a more general issue within the profession, regretted the distinctions made between nurses of differing educational background.

The big gap among nurses at the Cleveland Clinic had traditionally been between Clinic and Hospital Nursing. During the 1970s, efforts had been made to bring the two areas closer together. Nurses continued to build bridges between Clinic and Hospital Nursing during the 1980s and 1990s. Nurses who worked in the same clinical areas began to set up specialty groups within the institution, where they could meet with their colleagues from other departments and care settings and exchange information. The Oncology Nursing Task Force was one example of this. The Orthopaedic/Rheumatology Nursing Forum, organized in 1986, included representatives from Hospital orthopaedic units, Operating Room Nursing, several Clinic areas, and departmental assistants. The purpose of the Neurology Nursing Group, formed in 1989, was "to ensure that formal structures and informal networks link neurology nurses with Ambulatory Nursing and the Division of Nursing to more effectively meet patient care needs."[164]

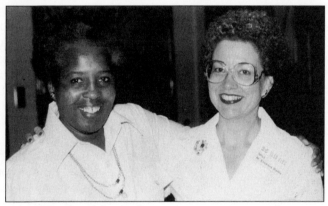

TRANA DANIELS AND ELEANOR REILLY
As of 1995, these two individuals, in different nursing roles, and different departments, had each contributed for more than 35 years to patient care at The Cleveland Clinic Foundation. Licensed practical nurse Trana Daniels (left) came to work on the Hospital's pediatric floor in 1957. After a number of years in the Hospital, she transferred to the Pediatrics Department in the outpatient Clinic. She worked there in Ambulatory Nursing until her retirement in 1995. Eleanor Reilly (right), a registered nurse, also began in the Hospital Nursing Department, but left it when Central Supply, which she headed, became a separate department in 1965. This photograph, taken at the 25 Year Club Dinner in 1983, shows Ms. Daniels, a 1982 member, congratulating new member Ms. Reilly.

Under the leadership of Ms. Coulter and Ms. Johnson, cooperation between the two areas continued to advance. Ms. Johnson had long supported a collaborative approach to patient care, among nurses and among other disciplines, and in 1990 she joined the Nursing Management Group as a voting member. There was now a formal link at the policy-making level between Hospital and Clinic Nursing, although the two areas remained administratively separate.

Ambulatory Nursing and the Division of Nursing made additional moves to dovetail their operations in the 1990s. Ambulatory Nursing Manager Susan Paschke, R.N., M.S.N., in charge of coordinating quality assurance for Clinic Nursing, and Ms. Atkins, responsible for quality assurance in the Division of Nursing, worked together in matters relating to patient education and patient discharge. Clinic nurses assisted Hospital Nursing by helping patients begin to fill out the Nursing Admission Assessment form, because it was "the right thing to do by patients," and promoted collaboration between the two areas. Clinic and Hospital Nursing implemented automated order entry in tandem, and nurses from both areas participated in the resident mentoring program. Ambulatory Nursing sent a representative to the division's Policy and Procedure Committee as of 1992. By the middle of 1993, salary scales for Ambulatory Nursing personnel had been brought into parity with those of Hospital Nursing, signaling positive "recognition of Ambulatory Nursing practice."[165]

A Higher Profile

Nurses and their co-workers helped patients and families to negotiate the health care system. But nursing personnel, too, needed help and support to deal with the hectic pace and inherent stress of their work. In 1985, Ms. Danielsen had stated that one of the Nursing Department's goals should be: "Support and retention of caregivers."[166] "Support" could mean supplying necessary workplace resources: enough personnel, the right equipment, good liaison with other departments. It also meant giving intellectual and moral support, so that the caregiver would have the inner resources to be able to give, in turn, to her patients.

During the 1980s and 1990s, ongoing efforts were made by nurses to promote cohesiveness and professional pride, create an increased awareness of nursing's role within the Cleveland Clinic, and raise the profile of nursing in the community. In 1991, the Nursing Image Committee was charged with "position[ing] Cleveland Clinic Nursing as the highest quality patient care in the market," and creating a positive image of the Cleveland Clinic among the nursing public, as well as a positive image of nurses among the general public.[167] A task force on business and professional attire addressed the question of image at its most literal; it selected uniforms for unit secretaries, and worked on revising uniform and dress code policies for all division personnel.

The Nursing History Committee traced the contribution of nurses to the Cleveland Clinic over time, and made preparations for the institution to host the annual meeting of the American Association for the History of Nursing in 1996 — the first time the organization would be meeting in a non-academic setting. The Nursing Publications Committee oversaw the production of the division's semiannual publication, *Cleveland Clinic Nurse*, and also had responsibility for submitting articles to the monthly *Greater Cleveland Nursing News* and generally publicizing Cleveland Clinic nurses in the electronic and print media.

Annual events also focused attention on the achievements and contributions of nursing personnel. Especially during National Nurses' Week in May, Cleveland Clinic nurses celebrated their role and accomplishments. A program including speakers, seminars, receptions, and luncheons was scheduled throughout the week. All nursing personnel — R.N.s, L.P.N.s, assistants, and secretaries — were invited to participate in the event.

As of 1990, a central feature of Nurses' Week at the Cleveland Clinic was the presentation of the annual Excellence in Nursing awards to selected nursing personnel. Two committees chose award recipients from among each years' nominees. The first awards, all named after past and present Cleveland Clinic nursing employees, were the Emma Barr Award for Clinical Excellence (to an R.N.), the Elizabeth Minnick Award for Clinical Excellence (to an L.P.N.), the Edward E. Rogers Award for Nursing Unit Assistant Excellence, the Karen Bourquin Award for Unit Secretary Excellence, the Abbie Porter Leadership Award, and the Poinsetta Jeffery Humanitarian Award.

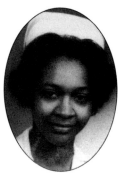

POINSETTA JEFFERY
A practical nursing graduate of the Jane Addams Vocational High School, Ms. Jeffery received her license and began work at Cleveland's Mt. Sinai Hospital in 1963. In 1973 she came to the Cleveland Clinic, where she worked as an L.P.N. for 15 years, mostly on the Hospital's orthopaedic nursing unit. Described as "at peace with herself" and "committed to nursing care," she drew an immediate response from patients. "Her patients raved about her," co-workers recalled. Her illness and death in 1988 cut short her nursing career, but the memory of her cooperative attitude and, above all, her kindness to patients, remained vivid. In 1990, when the Division of Nursing created its Nursing Excellence Awards program to honor employees for excellence in patient care, the humanitarian award was named in her honor.

The first presentation of the Nursing Unit Excellence Award and the first honorary presentation of the Nightingale Physician Collaboration Award took place in 1992. The Hannah Boland Award for Pediatric Clinical Excellence was added in 1993, and the Ambulatory Nursing Unit Excellence Award in 1994. The first presentation of the Sharon J. Coulter Patient Support Service Collaboration Award, to recognize the contributions of employees outside the nursing and medical staffs, was scheduled for 1995. Plans for the future included obtaining corporate support for additional awards.

The excellence of Cleveland Clinic nurses was also recognized publicly by the wider nursing community and the wider Cleveland community. Peer recognition accorded to Cleveland Clinic nurses at the national level included the naming of Gayle Whitman as a Fellow of the American Academy of Nursing and the selection of Betty Bush as Operating Room Manager of the Year. One form of lay recognition for area nurses came during *The Cleveland Plain Dealer*'s annual "Best of the Best" contest, instituted in 1993. In a special section, the newspaper featured profiles of nurses judged most outstanding on the basis of nominations received from the community. Pediatric nurse Kathleen Jirousek won the top honor in the first year of the contest, and Cleveland Clinic nurses were among the finalists in each of the succeeding years.

Public awards praising nurses' skills and compassion reflected private tributes. Notes of appreciation sent by Cleveland Clinic patients and their families arrived in every mail delivery. They were posted on nurses' bulletin boards throughout the institution, and served as ongoing recognition for Cleveland Clinic nursing personnel of every job description in every setting — recognition that spoke directly from heart to heart.

Moving On

By the mid-1990s, the Ambulatory Nursing Department had 200 members. There were also 150 nurse clinicians. Each day, nearly 3,500 ambulatory patients visited the Clinic. Nursing personnel in the Division of Patient Care Operations numbered 2,400. The Cleveland Clinic Hospital had 1,000 beds, and admitted more than 40,000 patients each year, with more than 120 operations performed each day. The Emergency Department recorded 400 visits per day. In all of these settings, nurses and their co-workers provided care.

Nursing at the Cleveland Clinic had changed greatly in the quarter century since 1970. In that year, the Nursing Department was made up of 650 employees, who worked in a 610-bed hospital. Clinic Nursing had eighty employees. During the next dozen years, the Hospital Nursing Department was decentralized, recentralized, and expanded to include Operating Room nursing. This renewed department gained division status in 1987, and then became the core of the new Division of Patient Care Operations in 1993. Ties between the division and Ambulatory Nursing grew closer.

Changes in nursing practice overshadowed these changes in structure, however. Most obviously, the positions filled by nurses and nursing personnel at the Cleveland Clinic had grown tremendously in number and diversity, both inside and outside the traditional nursing departments. Innovations in medical science and technology, as well as in health care delivery and finance systems, also affected nursing practice, bringing both pressures and

THE DIVISION
OF PATIENT CARE
OPERATIONS

At the beginning of 1995, the division, under the direction of its chairman, had seven departments, including the new Women's and Children's Services area, headed by Karen Westmeyer, and the Pharmacy, headed by Bruce McWhinney. A reorganization at mid-year created a management structure with three Vice-Chairs/Directors, Marlene Donnelly and Gayle Whitman for Nursing, and Lois Bock for Surgical Services; and Directors of Pharmacy and Operational Redesign, Mr. McWhinney and Diana Settevendemie. The chairman's responsibility was expanded to include Patient Care Support Operations, directed by Dale Goodrich.

opportunities. Nurses took less for granted. Through means as diverse as nursing research and market research, certification and documentation, they turned a keener eye to examining their own role, as members of a profession without whose aid the primary mission of the Cleveland Clinic, "better care of the sick," could not be accomplished.

In 1990, the Division of Nursing had chosen Virginia Henderson's definition of nursing to define its own endeavors: "Nursing is primarily helping the individual, sick or well, in performance of activities contributing to health or its recovery (or to a peaceful death) that she or he would perform unaided had she or he the strength, will, or knowledge. It is likewise the unique contribution of nursing to help people to be independent of such assistance as soon as possible."[168] As the new millennium approached, Cleveland Clinic nurses prepared to incorporate more changes into their practice. It was true that change was a constant. But it was also true that some things remained the same. "Care of the sick"; "nursing care"; "patient care"; "care delivery"; "managed care"; "wellness-focused care": whatever the technologies, the settings, or the individuals involved, nursing's "unique contribution" continued to be, as always, care.

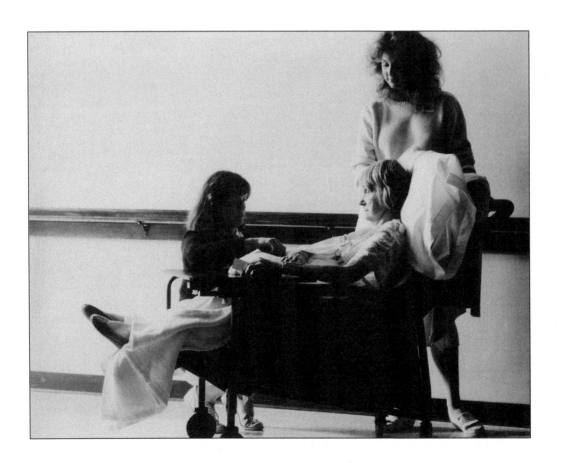

Conclusion

Nursing Then and Now

The history of nursing at the Cleveland Clinic spanned most of the twentieth century. Measured in years, this is not an especially long period of time. It was, however, a period of great change for the field of health care as well as for society in general. Over the course of the twentieth century, the Cleveland Clinic established itself as one of the country's preeminent health care institutions. At the same time, advances in medicine, pharmacology, and psychology combined with changes in the nursing profession itself to create a new health care world. Amid the changes, however, some of the fundamental skills and responsibilities of nurses remained the same.

Florence Nightingale had stressed that a nurse must be a careful observer of her patient's condition. Isabel Hampton Robb had pointed out the crucial role of good nursing judgment. Nurses had always used sight and touch to monitor their patients. They could see whether a patient was flushed or pale, and feel if the skin was moist or dry, hot or cold. Nurses had also always extended their own senses with whatever instruments were available at the time, of which the simple glass thermometer was one of the most basic.

In the late twentieth century, cardiac nurses, for example, used very sophisticated technology, including EKGs and arterial lines, to monitor their patients. They were in fact performing one of the same activities as nurses throughout history: observing the patient and using nursing judgment to determine when medical or nursing intervention might be necessary. "Without their aid" the CICUs and other ICUs would have been of little use. It took nurses to transform rooms full of expensive equipment into intensive *care* units.

Tending to the emotional and psychological needs of patients and including their families in care and teaching are now considered integral to nursing practice. However, nurses had always done this on an informal basis. During the First World War, Lakeside Unit nurses communicated by letter with patients' distant families, and put on an elaborate Christmas celebration to boost the spirits of wounded, homesick soldiers. In the 1920s, Clinic nurses acted as "mommies" toward little Madeleine Bebout during her prolonged stay at the Diabetic House. By the 1950s, helping hospitalized children to feel loved and secure was formally recognized as part of nursing care, and was the responsibility of the first L.P.N.s on the Hospital's pediatric floor. In more recent years, programs from art therapy for cancer patients to family-centered care for children in all settings have focused on patients' inner lives and emotional well-being.

The expert nurse had been valued throughout the Cleveland Clinic's history. In the early years, a Clinic physician had cited the ability of the Hospital's graduate nurses to act "practically automatically" in any situation as a great advantage for patient care at the institution. In the 1990s, a nurse manager used very similar words in describing the ideal Clinic nurse: someone able to move "instinctively" to do what was needed.

Patients, too, valued their nurses. During the First World War, an account of Lakeside Unit nurses' extraordinary service brought cheers from an audience of Clevelanders, especially when they heard the familiar names of nurses who had cared for them. In the 1920s, a Cleveland Clinic patient commended the nursing staff's willingness "to go the full length of their ability" to give care that was more than routine. In the 1990s, Cleveland Clinic nurses, nominated by their patients, were always among the finalists named in a tribute to the "best of the best" Cleveland-area nurses.

Great Variety

Like changes over time, the great variety of roles filled by Cleveland Clinic nursing personnel at a given moment, whether 70 years ago or today, could disguise similarity of purpose. This was something that affected the course of my research. Over many months, I had talked with Cleveland Clinic nurses, active and retired; I had observed today's nurses at work; and I had read about their predecessors. I very soon gave up on trying to depict a "typical Cleveland Clinic nurse." Even though I knew I was seeing some common characteristic among these nurses, I could not pinpoint what it was. The variety of the work they did was far more apparent.

In the early years, job descriptions within the Nursing Department itself were relatively few: orderly, ward maid, general staff nurse, head nurse, operating room nurse, plus a few nurse administrator positions. But even then, nurses also worked in many areas outside the Nursing Department. Most medical departments in the Clinic employed one or more nurses. Other nurses served in positions like nurse anesthetist, X-ray technician, receptionist, and purchasing agent. The Hospital superintendent was a nurse.

In those years, employees of the entire Cleveland Clinic numbered in the hundreds. Today, Hospital Nursing alone employs 2,400 individuals: R.N.s, L.P.N.s, operating room and patient care technicians, nursing unit assistants, and unit and administrative secretaries. Ambulatory Nursing and other departments employ hundreds more. Nurses work in areas ranging from pediatrics to geriatrics, from cardiac rehabilitation to palliative care. They serve as transplant coordinators, nurse midwives, nurse researchers, post-anesthesia nurses, case managers, ethicists, enterostomal therapy nurses, and in many other positions.

Diversity among the individuals filling these roles is also great. Women and men of many ethnic backgrounds work as nurses and in many support positions to care for the Cleveland Clinic's patients. Some are single, some married; some have children, others do not. Educational backgrounds also vary, as do ages and levels of experience. Some nurses are recent graduates; some have worked at other institutions; some have spent many years at the Cleveland Clinic. Others have come to nursing as a second or third career.

Still hoping to find a common thread, I asked people about their reasons for entering nursing. No two gave exactly the same answer. "Ever since I can remember, I wanted to be a nurse." "I had a mid-life crisis." "I was living out my mother's dream, she wanted me to be a nurse." "I wanted to be a nurse but my mother thought I would never make it because I was afraid of blood." "I couldn't afford to go to college." "My father was a doctor." "My mother was a medical secretary." "My cousin was a nurse, and I wanted to be like her, she was so kind, and so warm, and caring." "No one in my family was ever a nurse or a doctor as far as I know." "When I was little I used to take care of kittens and other animals on our farm when they were hurt." "I just like to help people."

Good Will and Confidence

Yet there was, in fact, an underlying similarity. Individuals who gave these very different answers all appeared to have found personal as well as professional fulfillment in the practice of nursing. Nurses often mentioned "autonomy of practice" as an outstanding feature of nursing at the Cleveland Clinic. Nurses who valued autonomy necessarily had confidence in their own abilities.

A book chapter written by two Cleveland Clinic nurses finally gave the answer that had been eluding me. Tracing the "becoming" of a nurse through several stages of career development, the authors observed that self-confidence formed the basis on which future career growth depended. "As the novice nurse seeks out new experiences and values the challenge of complicated procedures or difficult interpersonal interactions, control over the environment lends itself to mastery over self-doubt and insecurity. An autonomous nurse accepts with pride his or her own abilities and exudes a feeling of good will and confidence in dealings with others."[1]

"Good will and confidence in dealings with others": it was exactly this, I realized, that had impressed me as an almost universal trait of Cleveland Clinic nurses long before I had read the phrase itself. Other words often used to describe desirable qualities of nurses are "competence" and "compassion." These three qualities — competence, confidence, and compassion — are interdependent. Nurses can be confident when they are competent; and out of self-confidence develops that "good will in dealing with others," a good will that embraces compassion.

I had fully expected to find that Cleveland Clinic nurses would be competent, and more than competent — no surprises there. Meeting high standards of expertise, they also worked to advance those standards, and to share their expertise with the profession at large. I had taken it for granted, in addition, that Cleveland Clinic nurses and all nurses were compassionate, or at least gave the outward impression of being so. It is often assumed that in a large referral center like the Cleveland Clinic, technical virtuosity tends to replace warmth and humanity. Nonetheless, I sensed a compassion that was genuine, not pretended, forced, or sentimental, in the actions and attitudes of Cleveland Clinic nursing personnel.

This is not to say that Cleveland Clinic nursing employees always smile; never complain about doctors, patients, or each other; never make flippant remarks or irreverent jokes among themselves; and never think about leaving for another job. It is also not to say that each person is continually reaching toward new levels of excellence. Like everyone else, nurses and their co-workers get tired or annoyed or discouraged.

Unity in Diversity

Some problems stem from the fact that individuals approach nursing differently, and have always done so. Historians have pointed to divisions within the profession, between "traditionalists" and "professionalizers," between "professionalizers" and "worker-nurses," or between "worker-nurses" and "rationalizers."[2] The history of nursing at the Cleveland Clinic reflected similar divisions over time. Although all nurses agreed that their goal was giving the best possible patient care, they had different notions of how this could be accomplished: through concentration on the job at hand, through use of management techniques, through professional development.

This diversity of outlook can be a strength, rather than a source of conflict, when nurses look at their differing interests as complementary rather than opposed. A large institution like the Cleveland Clinic is particularly well-placed to take advantage of the different attitudes and talents among its nursing personnel. It needs nurses with high levels of technical skill to meet the demands of an internationally known tertiary care center. It needs nurses interested in research and writing to examine practice issues and communicate advances to the wider nursing community. It needs managers to meet the challenges of organizing a large work force and coping with financial constraints. It needs nursing personnel of all job descriptions who can act "practically automatically" to help people, who can empathize with the fears and hopes of patients and families, who know the value of a kind word, a gentle touch, a sympathetic ear, and who are strong enough to lend support to others.

The establishment of the Cleveland Clinic's Nursing Excellence Awards in 1990, at the opening of the last decade of the twentieth century, was perhaps a good omen for the future. The awards symbolized the possibility of creating a new unity out of diversity, among nursing employees from varied backgrounds with different skills and outlooks. The annual awards ceremony celebrated the contributions of all members of the nursing team. Ambulatory nursing, Hospital unit nursing, and Operating Room nursing; R.N.s, L.P.N.s, patient care technicians, nursing assistants, and unit secretaries: all were included.

More than any other single award, the Poinsetta Jeffery Humanitarian Award recognized the contribution that individuals could make, in their relationships with each other, with members of other disciplines, and above all with patients and their families. Open to all, this award affirmed a traditional belief: the belief that in nursing, character mattered. Nursing employees working in different jobs had different education and training, and different skills, all needed; but a humanitarian outlook, confined to no job description, gave nursing its heart.

This humanitarian bent has animated Cleveland Clinic nursing from the beginning. Born, strangely enough, of war, it survived disaster and Depression. It also survived success and prosperity. The past does not predict the future. There have been many changes over the past 75 years, and it does, indeed, seem that the pace of change has quickened, and will continue to do so. Some things, however, do not change. It is impossible to say exactly what instruments, medications, and treatment modalities will be in use at the Cleveland Clinic 10, 25, or 75 years from now. It is impossible to say how care delivery will be organized, or what nursing practice will look like. But it is impossible to imagine that nursing care will not be given in the same spirit of good will and confidence, based on competence and embracing compassion.

Notes

In lieu of a separate bibliography, a full citation is given here at the first mention of each source. Taken together, the published works, manuscript collections, and archival record groups cited comprise a complete bibliography of the sources used.

Chapter One

1. Marion Blankenhorn, "Dr. Eisenbrey," typescript, 1933, George W. Crile Papers, Container 3, Folder 3, Western Reserve Historical Society Library, Cleveland, Ohio. Citations to the Crile Papers refer to a chronological sequence of material assembled by Dr. Crile's wife, Grace McBride Crile, to aid her in producing his autobiography. The sequence includes Dr. Crile's own letters and diary entries; complete or excerpted letters, diary entries, and other writings of individuals associated with Dr. Crile; and newspaper clippings and other published items. Many of the unpublished items appear in the form of typewritten transcriptions.

2. Amy F. Rowland diary, 25 May 1917, Crile Papers, Container 3, Folder 6.

3. Philip A. Von Blon, "Lakeside Unit Set for Next Allied Smash," *Cleveland Plain Dealer*, 30 May 1917, scrapbook, Base Hospital No. 4 Papers, Stanley A. Ferguson Archives of University Hospitals of Cleveland, Ohio.

4. "First Force for Oversea [sic] Duty," undated news clipping, scrapbook, Base Hospital No. 4 Papers.

5. "Fifty Years Ago: Mud, Tears, War," *Cleveland Press*, 4 May 1967, scrapbook, Base Hospital No. 4 Papers.

6. Susan M. Reverby, *Ordered to Care: the Dilemma of American Nursing*, 1850-1945 (New York: Cambridge University Press, 1987), 80-82.

7. Philip A. Kalisch and Beatrice J. Kalisch, *The Advance of American Nursing*, 2d ed. (Boston: Little Brown and Company, 1986), 51, 72.

8. Blankenhorn, "Dr. Eisenbrey," 1933, Crile Papers.

9. "American Ambulance - Aftermath," bound typescript, vol. 1, p. 229, Cleveland Clinic Foundation Archives (hereafter referred to as "Clinic Archives"), A93-04, Box 6; and unidentified news clipping, 12 October 1918, Crile Papers, Container 11, Folder 2.

10. "American Ambulance - Aftermath," vol. 2, p. 46, Clinic Archives, A93-04, Box 6.

11. William Edgar Lower diary, 11 June 1917, Crile Papers, Container 4, Folder 3.

12. Minutes of the Professional Council, AEF Base Hospital Unit No. 4 serving at BEF General Hospital No. 9, 27 May 1917, Crile Papers, Container 3, Folder 7.

13. Ibid., 4 June 1917, Container 4, Folder 1.

14. Ibid.

15. "Crile Hastens Work on City's Hospital Unit," *Cleveland Leader*, 1 May 1917; and Professional Council minutes, 10 July 1917, Crile Papers, Container 3, Folder 5, and Container 5, Folder 1.

16. Reverby, *Ordered to Care*, 161; Kalisch and Kalisch, *Advance of American Nursing*, 345-348; and Samuel Mather to G. W. Crile, 27 September 1918, Crile Papers, Container 11, Folder 2.

17. Rowland diary, 25 May 1917, Crile Papers, Container 3, Folder 7.

18. Professional Council minutes, 4 June 1917, Crile Papers, Container 4, Folder 1.

19. Order signed by the Major/Director-in-Chief of AEF Base Hospital Unit No. 4, 1 June 1917, Crile Papers, Container 4, Folder 1.

20. Minutes of the Professional Council, 4 June 1917, Crile Papers, Container 4, Folder 1.

21. Ibid., 22 June 1917, Container 4, Folder 5.

22. Rowland diary, 23 September 1917, Crile Papers, Container 6, Folder 3.

23. A. Rowland, undated typescript; and Arvilla Walkinshaw to Grace Crile, 17 March 1918, Crile Papers, Container 1, Folder 3, and Container 8, Folder 5.

24. Orders No. 271, AEF Base Hospital Unit No. 4, 28 September 1918; and Ida F. Preston to A. Rowland, 14 October 1918, Crile Papers, Container 11, Folders 2 and 3.

25. Professional Council minutes, 22 June 1917, Crile Papers, Container 4, Folder 5; and news clipping from *Nursing Times*, 2 June 1917, scrapbook, Base Hospital No. 4 Papers.

26. Professional Council minutes, 4 June 1917, Crile Papers, Container 4, Folder 1.

27. A. Walkinshaw to Grace Crile, 17 March 1918, Crile Papers, Container 8, Folder 5.

28. U.S. Army Regulation 142-1/2, in Orders No. 148, AEF Base Hospital Unit No. 4, 10 October 1917, Crile Papers, Container 6, Folder 5.

29. Rowland diary, 26 September 1917, Crile Papers, Container 6, Folder 3.

30. G. W. Crile to Franklin Martin, 2 January 1918, Crile Papers, Container 7, Folder 5.

31. Professional Council minutes, 27 June 1917, Crile Papers, Container 4, Folder 6.

32. Rowland diary, 12 August 1917, Crile Papers, Container 5, Folder 7.

33. Marie Shields, news clipping, *Cleveland Press*, [1918], scrapbook, Base Hospital No. 4 Papers. Mrs. Shields wrote a short series of articles, apparently revised to conform to newspaper style, for the *Press* after her return to Cleveland during the summer of 1918.

34. Professional Council minutes, 4 July 1917, Crile Papers, Container 4, Folder 7.

35. Lower diary, 11 June 1917, Crile Papers, Container 4, Folder 3.

36. Ibid., 1 June 1917, Container 4, Folder 1.

37. Henry D. Piercy, "History of the Lakeside Unit of World War I," part 3, *Ohio State Medical Journal* 58 (July 1962): 762; and I. Preston diary, 24 July 1917, Crile Papers, Container 5, Folder 2.

38. Preston diary, 24 July 1917; I. Preston to A. Rowland, 19 March 1918; and G. W. Crile to Grace Crile, 16 April 1918, Crile Papers, Container 8, Folder 5, and Container 9, Folder 2.

39. S. Mather to G. W. Crile, 23 July 1918; and G. W. Crile to S. Mather, 15 August 1918, Crile Papers, Container 10, Folders 4 and 5.

40. I. Preston to W. E. Lower, 5 October 1918; and to A. Rowland, 14 November 1918, Crile Papers, Container 11, Folders 3 and 4.

41. Harriet Leete to G. W. Crile, 19 September 1917, Crile Papers, Container 6, Folder 3.

42. Professional Council minutes, 20 September 1917, Crile Papers, Container 6, Folder 3.

43. Rowland diary, 23 September 1917, Crile Papers, Container 6, Folder 3.

44. G. W. Crile diary, 20 July 1917, Crile Papers, Container 5, Folder 2.

45. M. Shields, news clipping, *Cleveland Press*, [1918], and "Lakeside Hospital Unit Meets Today," news clipping, May 1937, scrapbook, Base Hospital No. 4 Papers.

46. Dorothy Barney diary, 21 July 1917, Crile Papers, Container 5, Folder 2.

47. Ibid.

48. Rowland diary, 12 August 1917, Crile Papers, Container 5, Folder 7.

49. Lower diary, 29 June and summary of 9-30 June 1917, Crile Papers, Container 4, Folder 6.

50. Ibid., 22 July 1917, Container 5, Folder 2.

51. Ibid., 25 July 1917, Container 5, Folder 3.

52. Ibid., 30 July 1917, and summary of Third Battle of Ypres, Container 5, Folder 3.

53. Ibid., summary of Third Battle of Ypres.

54. G. W. Crile diary, summary of 31 July-5 August, and 25 August 1917, Crile Papers, Container 5, Folder 4, and Container 6, Folder 1.

55. Lower diary, 2 August 1917, Crile Papers, Container 5, Folder 4.

56. Ibid., 1 August 1917.

57. W. E. Lower, "Treatment of the Slightly Wounded," Crile Papers, Container 7, Folder 3.

58. Preston diary, 18 August 1917, Crile Papers, Container 5, Folder 7.

59. Lower diary, 11 June 1917, Crile Papers, Container 4, Folder 3.

60. Henry Sanford to G. W. Crile, 2 August 1917, Crile Papers, Container 5, Folder 4.

61. Lower diary, 16 June 1917, Crile Papers, Container 4, Folder 4.

62. Rowland diary, 15 September 1917, Crile Papers, Container 6, Folder 2.

63. Preston diary, 19 September 1917, Crile Papers, Container 6, Folder 3.

64. Rowland diary, 20 September 1917, Crile Papers, Container 6, Folder 3.

65. "Now It's Nurse Who Wins Fame for Cleveland Unit," undated news clipping, scrapbook, Base Hospital No. 4 Papers.

66. H. Sanford letter, 29 June 1917, Crile Papers, Container 4, Folder 6.

67. I. Preston to Grace Crile, 21 October 1918, Crile Papers, Container 11, Folder 3.

68. Rowland diary, 20 June 1917, Crile Papers, Container 4, Folder 5.

69. I. Preston to Mabel Lower, 29 July 1917; and A. Walkinshaw to Grace Crile, 17 March 1918, Crile Papers, Container 5, Folder 3, and Container 8, Folder 5.

70. Grace Allison's report as quoted in "What Lakeside and Chicago Units Are Doing at the Front," undated news clipping, scrapbook, Base Hospital No. 4 Papers; and I. Preston to Miss Decker, December 1917, Crile Papers, Container 7, Folder 4.

71. Minnie Strobel to her mother and sister, series of letters dating from October-December 1917, published in the Massillon, Ohio, *Evening Independent*, 29 January 1918, Crile Papers, Container 8, Folder 1.

72. Grace Allison to Grace Crile, 16 January 1918, Crile Papers, Container 8, Folder 1.

73. H. Sanford letter, June 13, 1917, Crile Papers, Container 4, Folder 3; and M. Strobel, as in above note 71.

74. H. Sanford letter, June 13, 1917, Crile Papers, Container 4, Folder 3.

75. M. Strobel to her brother, [31 March 1918], "Letters from 'Over There': Swamped with Wounded, Says Lakeside Nurse," published in unidentified newspaper, scrapbook, Base Hospital No. 4 Papers.

76. I. Preston to W. E. Lower, 5 October 1918, Crile Papers, Container 11, Folder 3.

77. "Mrs. Mabel Marcy Recalls 1917 Yule Season in War-Torn France," Conneaut, Ohio, *News-Herald*, 19 December 1963, scrapbook, Base Hospital No. 4 Papers.

78. H. Sanford letter, June 13, 1917, Crile Papers, Container 4, Folder 3.

79. M. Shields, "How the Wounded Help Cure the Wounded," *Cleveland Press*, n.d., scrapbook, Base Hospital No. 4 Papers.

80. G. W. Crile diary, 22 October 1918, Crile Papers, Container 11, Folder 3.

81. Lower diary, 14 June 1917, Crile Papers, Container 4, Folder 3.

82. Lyn MacDonald, *They Called It Passchendaele* (London: Michael Joseph, 1978), 127.

83. G. W. Crile diary, summary of February 1918, Crile Papers, Container 8, Folder 3.

84. Grace Crile, ed., *George Crile: An Autobiography* (Philadelphia: J. B. Lippincott Company, 1947), 301; and Blankenhorn, "Dr. Eisenbrey," 1933. The historical role of the nurse as "the physician's hand" is examined in Barbara Melosh's study by that name, *"The Physician's Hand": Work Culture and Conflict in American Nursing* (Philadelphia: Temple University Press, 1982).

85. Kalisch and Kalisch, *Advance of American Nursing*, 56, quoting Florence Nightingale in Richard Quain, ed., *A Dictionary of Medicine*.

86. Lower diary, 13 July 1917, Crile Papers, Container 5, Folder 1.

87. M. Shields, news clipping, *Cleveland Press*, [1918], scrapbook, Base Hospital No. 4 Papers; and M. Strobel, as in above note 71.

88. Professional Council minutes, 30 July 1917, Crile Papers, Container 5, Folder 3.

89. G. W. Crile diary, summary of February 1918, Crile Papers, Container 8, Folder 3.

90. "Mrs. Mabel Marcy," 19 December 1963, scrapbook, Base Hospital No. 4 Papers.

91. Ibid.

92. G. W. Crile to S. Mather, 4 January 1918, Crile Papers, Container 7, Folder 5.

93. M. Strobel, as in above note 71.

94. Lower diary, 16 December 1917, Crile Papers, Container 7, Folder 4.

95. M. Strobel, as in above note 71; Josephine Cunningham to Grace Crile, 10 January 1918, Crile Papers, Container 7, Folder 5. Reverby, *Ordered to Care*, examines the idea of the nurse as a "daughter" in the civilian hospital; see for example p. 130.

96. M. Strobel, as in above note 71.

97. Ibid.

98. Lower diary, 25 December 1917, Crile Papers, Container 7, Folder 4.

99. Lower diary, 30 March 1918, Crile Papers, Container 8, Folder 6.

100. I. Preston to A. Rowland, 2 April 1918, Crile Papers, Container 9, Folder 1.

101. M. Strobel, as in above note 75.

102. Unidentified enlisted man, possibly to A. Rowland, 5 April 1918, Crile Papers, Container 9, Folder 1.

103. Lower diary, 27 March 1918, Crile Papers, Container 8, Folder 6.

104. Preston diary, 26 March 1918, Crile Papers, Container 8, Folder 6.

105. J. Cunningham to Grace Crile, 10 January 1918, Crile Papers, Container 7, Folder 5.

106. G. W. Crile to A. Rowland, 16 August 1917, Crile Papers, Container 5, Folder 7.

107. I. Preston to W. E. Lower, 10 June 1918, Crile Papers, Container 10, Folder 1; and "Cleveland Nurse Is Decorated by King," undated news clipping, and "Crile, Gilchrist and Three Nurses Are Cited for Valor," *Plain Dealer*, 29 December 1917, scrapbook, Base Hospital No. 4 Papers.

108. "Lauds Nurses' Bravery," news clipping with dateline 11 April 1918; and G. W. Crile to Margaret Crile, 30 June 1918, Crile Papers, Container 9, Folder 1, and Container 10, Folder 2.

109. Col. Herbert Bruce, quoted in typescript account of meeting, [June 22, 1918], Crile Papers, Container 10, Folder 2.

110. I. Preston to A. Rowland, 16 August 1918, Crile Papers, Container 10, Folder 5.

111. Lt. Col. Corser, quoted in G. W. Crile summary notes on Lakeside Unit's service, Container 1, Folder 4.

112. "Lakeside Unit Meets," May 1937, scrapbook, Base Hospital No. 4 Papers.

113. G. W. Crile diary, 28 September 1918, Crile Papers, Container 11, Folder 2.

114. Ibid., 17 October 1918; and W. E. Lower to G. W. Crile, 23 October 1918, Crile Papers, Container 11, Folder 3.

115. I. Preston to Grace Crile, 21 October 1918, Crile Papers, Container 11, Folder 3. This nurse was attached to the unit on a temporary basis only, so the Lakeside Unit officially recorded no war dead among its members.

116. G. W. Crile diary, 31 October 1918, Crile Papers, Container 11, Folder 3; and Lt. Col. Corser, as in above note 111.

117. "Mrs. Mabel Marcy," 19 December 1963, scrapbook, Base Hospital No. 4 Papers.

118. News clipping, *Cleveland Press*, 11 November 1964, biographical file, Constance Hanna, *Cleveland Press* Collection, Cleveland State University Archives.

119. G. W. Crile summary notes on Lakeside Unit's service; and I. Preston to Grace Crile, 22 December 1918, Crile Papers, Container 1, Folder 4, and Container 12, Folder 2.

120. Frank E. Bunts, summary report on the Lakeside Unit, Crile Papers, Container 12, Folder 3. Dr. Bunts assumed command of the Lakeside Unit in August 1918.

121. "Violets and Lilies for War Heroines," news clipping, [10 April 1919], Crile Papers, Container 12, Folder 5.

122. "Lakeside Unit Girls Are Home," news clipping, [10 April 1919], Crile Papers, Container 12, Folder 5.

123. "Violets and Lilies"; and "Bravery Disclaimed by Lakeside Nurses," news clipping, 10 April 1919, Crile Papers, Container 12, Folder 5.

124. News clipping, *Cleveland Plain Dealer*, 10 April 1919, Crile Papers, Container 12, Folder 5.

125. G. Allison, as in above note 70.

126. Edith Fuller to A. Rowland, 8 December 1918, Crile Papers, Container 12, Folder 1.

Chapter Two

1. M. L. Roberts, "Samson and Delilah Revisited: The Politics of Women's Fashions in 1920s France," *American Historical Review* 98 (June 1993): 678-682; and Antoine Prost, "Public and Private Spheres in France," in A *History of Private Life*, trans. Arthur Goldhammer and ed. Philippe Ariès and Georges Duby, vol. 5, *Riddles of Identity in Modern Times*, ed. A. Prost and Gérard Vincent (Cambridge, Massachusetts: The Belknap Press, 1991), 88.

2. David D. Van Tassel and John J. Grabowski, eds., *Encyclopedia of Cleveland History* (Blooming-ton: University of Indiana Press, 1987), xliv.

3. Ibid., xxxii.

4. Ibid., 520, 522.

5. Paul Starr, *The Social Transformation of American Medicine* (New York: Basic Books, Inc., 1982), 73-75.

6. James H. and Mary Jane Rodabaugh, *Nursing in Ohio: A History* (Columbus, Ohio: The Ohio State Nurses' Association, 1951), 98.

7. Grace Crile to G. ("Barney") Crile, Jr., 23 April 1931, Crile Papers, Container 24, Folder 1. "First" may mean first in Cleveland. According to Rodabaugh and Rodabaugh (op. cit., p. 234), the National Cash Register Company of Dayton was probably the first Ohio company to hire an industrial nurse, in 1901, while the Cleveland Hardware Company's program started in 1907.

8. Bertha E. Melcher to Alexander T. Bunts, 22 September 1958, Bunts Family Papers, Alexander T. Bunts, Box 4, Folder 129, Historical Division of the Cleveland Medical Library Association (Allen Memorial Medical Library), Cleveland, Ohio.

9. Ibid.

10. Ibid.

11. Ibid.

12. News clipping, *Cleveland News*, 11 March 1926, Crile Papers, Container 18, Folder 1.

13. "How the School of Nursing of Charity Hospital Began," *St. Vincent Charity Hospital News* 1, no. 4 (1928), Bunts Family Papers, Frank E. Bunts, Box 1, Folder 32.

14. Frank E. Bunts, address to Lutheran Hospital nursing school graduating class, ca. 1920s, and "The Nurse," address to Grace Hospital (Conneaut, Ohio) nursing school graduating class, 3 October 1913, Bunts Papers, Box 1, Folder 32.

15. F. Bunts, "The Nurse," 3 October 1913, Bunts Papers.

16. F. Bunts, address to Lutheran Hospital class, ca. 1920s, Bunts Papers.

17. F. Bunts, "A Discussion on the Present Status of Nursing," [ca. 1920s], Bunts Papers, Box 1, Folder 32.

18. F. Bunts, unidentified address to a nursing school graduating class, n.d., Bunts Papers, Box 1, Folder 32.

19. F. Bunts, "Present Status of Nursing," [ca. 1920s], Bunts Papers.

20. F. Bunts, address to the St. Barnabas Society of Nurses at the annual Florence Nightingale Memorial Service held at Trinity Cathedral of the Episcopal Diocese of Cleveland, 12 May 1921, and "Present Status of Nursing," [ca. 1920s], Bunts Papers, Box 1, Folder 32.

21. G. W. Crile, "Evolution Since the War," typescript dated October 1924, Crile Papers, Container 16, Folder 4.

22. G. W. Crile to Margaret Crile, 1 June 1918, Crile Papers, Container 10, Folder 1.

23. Grace Crile to Dr. H. L. Foss, 10 April 1935, Crile Papers, Container 28, Folder 1.

24. A. Rowland, undated typescript, Crile Papers, Container 1, Folder 3.

25. John Phillips, "Treatment of Pneumonia," from paperbound volume of lectures on therapeutics, n.d., p. 15, John Phillips Family Papers, Container 1, Folder 18, Western Reserve Historical Society.

26. Ibid., 18.

27. Ibid., 17.

28. Isabel Hampton Robb, "Address of Mrs. Hunter Robb at Dedicatory Exercises," in Lakeside Hospital Annual Report (1898), 96. All Lakeside Hospital Annual Reports cited are held in the Ferguson Archives of University Hospitals of Cleveland.

29. Lakeside Hospital was first known as Cleveland City Hospital and also, informally, as the Wilson Street Hospital. For clarity's sake, the name Lakeside Hospital is used throughout here. Lakeside later became the largest of the member hospitals of University Hospitals of Cleveland. Lakeside was incorporated in 1866 and began admitting patients in 1868.

30. Lakeside Hospital Annual Report (1899), 104.

31. Jo Ann Ashley, *Hospitals, Paternalism, and the Role of the Nurse* (New York: Teachers College Press, 1976), 21.

32. Lakeside Hospital Annual Report (1899), 35-36.

33. Starr, *American Medicine*, 117, 121; and G. H. Fitzgerald to Grace Crile, 27 September 1943, Crile Papers, Container 36, Folder 3.

34. Lakeside Hospital Annual Report (1898), 97.

35. Lakeside Hospital Annual Report (1910), 17.

36. Lakeside Hospital Annual Report (1898), 11-12.

37. Reverby, *Ordered to Care*, 105-109.

38. G. Crile, *Autobiography*, 195, 199.

39. A *50 Year Retrospective of the American Association of Nurse Anesthetists* (Chicago: AANA, 1981), 5, citing Virginia Thatcher, *History of Anesthesia*.

40. Patricia Ann Quinn, *History of the University Hospitals of Cleveland School of Anesthesia, 1911-1954*, p. 3, citing *Ohio State Medical Journal* 12 (October 1916): 679; and typescript excerpts from Agatha C. Hodgins, "A Narrative of Endeavor," 31 October 1925; both in School of Anesthesia Records, Ferguson Archives of University Hospitals of Cleveland.

41. Earlier pioneering efforts in nurse anesthesia took place, most notably, at St. Mary's Hospital in Rochester, Minnesota. See Virginia Thatcher, *History of Anesthesia: with Emphasis on the Nurse Specialist* (Philadelphia: Lippincott, 1953), for an account of the field's development.

42. S. Mather to G. W. Crile, 19 March 1918, Crile Papers, Container 8, Folder 5.

43. Shattuck W. Hartwell, Jr., ed., *To Act As A Unit: The Story of the Cleveland Clinic* (Philadelphia: W. B. Saunders Company, 1985), 8-9.

44. Ibid., 8; and G. W. Crile to Grace Crile, 16 June 1917, Crile Papers, Container 4, Folder 4.

45. Grace Crile to G. W. Crile, 3 March 1918, Crile Papers, Container 8, Folder 4.

46. W. E. Lower to G. W. Crile, 23 October 1918, Crile Papers, Container 11, Folder 3; and W. E. Lower, typescript account of the founding of the Clinic, Clinic Archives, 33-H, Box 1, Folder 2.

47. G. W. Crile diary, summary entry "Return from France," late 1919, Crile Papers, Container 13, Folder 1. See Mark Gottlieb, *The Lives of University Hospitals of Cleveland: The 125-Year Evolution of an Academic Medical Center* (Cleveland, Ohio: Wilson Street Press, 1991), Chapters 4-6, for an alternative, more detailed account of events at Lakeside Hospital in relation to the founding of the Cleveland Clinic.

48. Howard Dittrick, "The Origin of the Cleveland Clinic," reprinted from the *Ohio State Archaeological and Historical Society Quarterly*, [1947], 17, in Clinic Archives, 33-H, Box 1, Folder 4; and Lower typescript on the Clinic's founding, Clinic Archives, 33-H, Box 1, Folder 2.

49. G. W. Crile diary, summary entry "Evolution Since the War," October 1924, Crile Papers, Container 16, Folder 4.

50. Legal documents and correspondence, Clinic Archives, 33-LA, Box 1, Folder 13; and Amy F. Rowland, *Cleveland Clinic Foundation* (Cleveland, Ohio: The William Feather Company, 1938), 19. The possibility that Mrs. Oxley owned or at least held title to the property is supported by the fact that the homes bore her name, in the same way that proprietary hospitals and nursing homes often bore the names of their proprietors.

51. John Phillips, address at the opening of the Clinic Hospital, 14 June 1924, "Archives" volume, Clinic Archives, 33-B, Box 1.

52. Hartwell, *To Act As A Unit*, 14, 82; and account book, Crile Papers, Box 1, Folder 1.

53. John Hammond Bradshaw, "A Visit to the Cleveland Clinic (Crile's) Hospital," typescript of letter submitted to the *Journal of the Medical Society of New Jersey* (March 1926), Crile Papers, Container 18, Folder 1.

54. Ibid.

55. Ibid.; and W. H. Bowen, excerpts from paper "The Mayo and Crile Clinics: with Special Reference to Thyroid Surgery," [1923], Crile Papers, Container 14, Folder 4. Thyroid operations were performed more often on women than on men, so many sources refer to patients in the feminine.

56. Bowen, "Mayo and Crile Clinics," Crile Papers, Container 14, Folder 4.

57. Bradshaw, "Visit to the Cleveland Clinic," Crile Papers, Container 18, Folder 1.

58. Ibid.

59. Evarts A. Graham, obituary for Dr. Crile, *Year Book of the American Philosophical Society* (1943), 380-383, Crile Papers, Container 1, Folder 1.

60. News clipping, 5 March 1923, Crile Papers, Container 14, Folder 4.

61. Florence Kempf to G. W. Crile, 21 September 1939, Crile Papers, Container 32, Folder 4. For additional detail on the difficulties that large numbers of thyroid surgery cases caused Lakeside Hospital nurses, see Margene O. Faddis, *The History of the Frances Payne Bolton School of Nursing* (Cleveland: Western Reserve University Press, 1948), 97-98.

62. George Crile, Jr., and William L. Proudfit, "The Supporting Cast, 1921-1940," typescript, Clinic Archives, 3-PR20, Employees.

63. G. W. Crile diary, summary entry "Evolution Since the War," October 1924, Crile papers, Container 16, Folder 4.

64. Information from the following sources was collated to determine which Clinic nurses had graduated from or worked at Lakeside Hospital: Nursing Historical Files and Lakeside Hospital Annual Reports, Ferguson Archives of University Hospitals of Cleveland; and Cleveland Clinic personnel rosters and annual meeting programs, Clinic Archives, 3-PR20, Employees, and 3-VA. The numbers arrived at are a minimum rather than a maximum, since complete records have not survived.

65. Agatha Hodgins to G. W. Crile, 24 January 1934, Crile Papers, Container 26, Folder 4.

66. Lakeside Hospital Annual Report (1924), 68.

67. Bradshaw, "Visit to the Cleveland Clinic," Crile Papers, Container 18, Folder 1.

68. W. B. Hamby, "The Cleveland Clinic," typescript, [1929], Crile Papers, Container 1, Folder 1.

69. The Lakeside Hospital Training School for Nurses was merged into Western Reserve University's new School of Nursing in 1924.

70. John Phillips, in transcript of proceedings at annual meeting, p. 5-6, "Archives" volume, Clinic Archives, 33-B, Box 1.

71. News clipping, *Cleveland Plain Dealer*, 24 June 1924, "Archives" volume, Clinic Archives, 33-B, Box 1; and Hartwell, *To Act As A Unit*, 17.

72. John L. Wray letter, 10 August 1928, Crile Papers, Container 20, Folder 4.

73. G. W. Crile diary, summary of 1925, Crile Papers, Container 17, Folder 3.

74. Statements of Clinic employees to disaster investigators, vol. 3, p. 1924, Clinic Archives, 33-D, Box 2.

75. Information on personnel and salaries in this and the following paragraphs is from memo, M. M. Fennell to E. C. Daoust, 20 February 1946, and Clinic annual meeting program, 1922, Clinic Archives, 3-PR20, Employees, and 3-VA.

76. Reverby, *Ordered to Care*, 106-107; and minutes of subcommittee on special duty nursing of the Cleveland Central Committee on Nursing, [1927], Nursing Historical Files, Ferguson Archives of University Hospitals of Cleveland.

77. Cleveland Clinic Hospital patient brochure, [1926], Crile Papers, Container 18, Folder 2.

78. Brochure, Official Registry for Nurses, District No. 4 of the Ohio State Nurses' Association, [1920s], Flora E. Short Papers, Historical Division of the Cleveland Medical Library Association (Allen Memorial Medical Library).

79. Minutes of subcommittee on special duty nursing, [1927], Nursing Historical Files, Ferguson Archives.

80. All information on Miss Short is from the Flora E. Short Papers. The file includes a complete log of her private duty calls from a career spanning the years 1921-1956.

81. Call log, Flora E. Short Papers; and William Ganson Rose, *Cleveland: The Making of a City* (Cleveland, Ohio: The World Publishing Company, 1950), 798, 891.

82. Lakeside Unit Women's Newsletter, 1929, Crile Papers, Container 37, Folder 1.

83. News clipping, *Cleveland Plain Dealer*, 19 May 1929, Crile Papers, Container 40, Folder 3.

84. Statements of Clinic employees to disaster investigators, vol. 3, p. 1916, Clinic Archives, 33-D.

85. Ibid., 1919-1920.

86. Ibid., 1917.

87. Ibid., 1921; and Lakeside Unit Women's Newsletter, 1929, Crile Papers.

88. Lakeside Unit Women's Newsletter, 1929, Crile Papers.

89. Ibid.

90. Statements of Clinic employees to disaster investigators, vol. 2, p. 1257, Clinic Archives, 33-D.

91. Lakeside Unit Women's Newsletter, 1929, Crile Papers.

92. Statements of Clinic employees to disaster investigators, vol. 2, pp. 1331-1332, Clinic Archives, 33-D.

93. News clipping, [*Cleveland News*, 19 May 1929], Crile Papers, Container 40, Folder 3. Newspaper reporters, like the general public, tended to refer to any uniformed female health worker as a "nurse," so that any statement regarding an unidentified nurse must be treated with caution.

94. William J. Engel, "Memories of the Founding of the Board of Governors in the Early Years at the Cleveland Clinic," typescript, Clinic Archives, 33-H, Box 1, Folder 8; and G. W. Crile to Franklin Martin, 31 May 1929, Crile Papers, Container 37, Folder 1.

95. News clippings, *Cleveland Press*, 16 May 1929, and [*Cleveland Plain Dealer*], 18 May 1929, Crile Papers, Container 40, Folders 1 and 3.

96. Henry John, reminiscences of the disaster, 1955, Clinic Archives, 33-D, Box 1, Folder 11.

97. G. W. Crile to Franklin Martin, 31 May 1929, Crile Papers, Container 37, Folder 1.

98. G. W. Crile, notes on conference regarding settlement, 1 July 1932, Crile Papers, Container 25, Folder 2.

99. News clipping, *Cleveland Plain Dealer*, 25 July 1932, Crile Papers, Container 25, Folder 2; and "Crile Claims," *Time*, 8 August 1932, 30, Clinic Archives, 33-D, Box 3, Folder 20.

100. "Disaster Account," 10 January 1940, Crile Papers, Container 33, Folder 1.

101. "Goiter," *Time*, 29 May 1933, Crile Papers, Container 25, Folder 6.

102. Board of Trustees to employees of the Cleveland Clinic, 19 January 1933, Clinic Archives, 1-GC.

103. Donald M. Glover, editor of the *Bulletin* of the Academy of Medicine of Cleveland, to Elizabeth P. August, General Secretary of the Ohio State Nurses' Association, 22 March 1932; and E. August to all district associations of the OSNA, 29 January 1934, Greater Cleveland Nurses' Association Records, Container 6, Folder 17, Western Reserve Historical Society. The letter from Dr. Glover to Miss August is part of an exchange of correspondence regarding his article, "Cutting the Cost," published in the *Bulletin* 58 (March 1932): 12.

104. Grace Crile to G. Crile, Jr., April 1931, Crile Papers, Container 24, Folder 1.

105. Letter to G. W. Crile, 27 March 1932, Crile Papers, Container 24, Folder 1.

106. "City Health Department's Nurses Demand Pay Raise," *Cleveland Plain Dealer*, 14 February 1936, subject file, Nurses, *Cleveland Press* Collection.

107. "Nurses Prefer Cash to Board," *Cleveland Press*, 27 February 1937, subject file, Nurses, *Cleveland Press* Collection.

108. Cleveland Clinic Hospital Annual Report, 1937, Clinic Archives, 12-AR, Box 1. All Cleveland Clinic Hospital Annual Reports cited are held in the Cleveland Clinic Archives. At this time, the title "Director of Nursing" comes into use, replacing "Superintendent of Nurses." Documents from the 1950s discuss the role of floor supervisor as a recent innovation. Miss Jones' title of floor supervisor in the 1930s indicates that the position existed earlier but fell into disuse in the interim.

109. Ibid.; and Kalisch and Kalisch, *Advance of American Nursing*, 547.

110. Cleveland Clinic Hospital Annual Report, 1938, 12-AR, Box 1. Some of the Clinic Hospital's patients had been covered by private insurance before this time, but none of these companies, singly or collectively, had the impact of the Blues plans.

111. Cleveland Clinic Hospital Annual Report, 1939, 12-AR, Box 1.

112. Ibid.

113. Cleveland Clinic Hospital Annual Report, 1940, 12-AR, Box 1.

Chapter Three

1. Cleveland Clinic Foundation *Bulletin*, No. 34, 8 June 1936, Crile Papers, Container 28, Folder 5.

2. G. W. Crile, "To All Members of Professional Staff, Clinic and Hospital Employees," memo, [1936], Crile Papers, Container 28, Folder 4.

3. Cleveland Clinic Foundation Administrative Board minutes, 3 March 1936, Clinic Archives, 1-TV, Box 1, Folder 6.

4. Van Tassel and Grabowski, *Encyclopedia of Cleveland History*, 241-2, 522, 672.

5. Rodabaugh and Rodabaugh, *Nursing in Ohio*, 205, 221.

6. News clipping, *Cleveland News*, 15 July 1941, subject file, Nurses, *Cleveland Press* Collection.

7. Unlike their counterparts of WWI, nurses during WWII had military rank: "relative" rank at first, with lower status than male officers, and then regular rank by the end of the war. See Vern and Bonnie Bullough, *The Care of the Sick: The Emergence of Modern Nursing* (New York: Prodist, 1978), 178-179, for more detail.

8. Grace Crile diary, 27 May 1941, Crile Papers, Container 34, Folder 2.

9. G. W. Crile to Ross T. McIntire, 31 December 1941, Crile Papers, Container 34, Folder 6.

10. Grace Crile to Elisabeth Crisler, 27 February 1942, Crile Papers, Container 35, Folder 1.

11. News clipping, *Cleveland Press*, 18 August 1945, subject file, Nurses, *Cleveland Press* Collection.

12. Barney Crile to Thomas Jones, 13 November 1942, Crile Papers, Container 35, Folder 4.

13. Cleveland Clinic Hospital Annual Reports, 1940 and 1944, Clinic Archives, 12-AR, Box 1. The 1940 figure included supervisory staff; the 1944 figure probably did as well, but this is not entirely clear.

14. Personal communication/oral history. See Preface, xvi, xvii, regarding this form of citation.

15. Cleveland Clinic Hospital Annual Report, 1942, 12-AR, Box 1.

16. Cleveland Clinic Hospital Annual Report, 1944, 12-AR. Box 1.

17. Cleveland Clinic Hospital Annual Report, 1940, 12-AR, Box 1.

18. Cleveland Clinic Hospital Annual Reports, 1942 and 1943, 12-AR, Box 1.

19. Ibid.

20. Administrative Board, Attachment to agenda, 26 December 1941, Clinic Archives, 1-TV, Box 2, Folder 1.

21. Cleveland Clinic Hospital Annual Report, 1942, 12-AR, Box 1.

22. Cleveland Clinic Hospital Annual Report, 1944, 12-AR, Box 1.

23. Monthly "call reports" on private duty nurses called from the Central Registry/Bureau of Nursing Services appear at intervals in the Board minutes of the Greater Cleveland Nurses' Association, (OSNA District No. 4), Greater Cleveland Nurses' Association Records (hereafter referred to as GCNA Records), Western Reserve Historical Society.

24. Board of Trustees minutes, 12 June 1942, GCNA Records, Container 2, Folder 1.

25. Ibid.

26. Ibid.

27. Board of Trustees minutes, 18 February 1943, GCNA Records, Container 2, Folder 1.

28. Cleveland Clinic Hospital Annual Report, 1943, 12-AR, Box 1.

29. General Secretary's Report, 12 January 1945, GCNA Records, Container 2, Folder 3.

30. Financial Secretary's Report, 17 May 1943, GCNA Records, Container 2, Folder 1.

31. Cleveland Clinic Hospital Annual Report, 1944, 12-AR, Box 1.

32. See Rodabaugh and Rodabaugh, 215-216, for the number of student nurses enrolled in Ohio schools before, during, and after the Cadet Nurse Corps program.

33. General Secretary's Report, 12 January 1945, GCNA Records, Container 2, Folder 3.

34. Ibid.

35. Harold Burton to Jack Burns of the Cleveland Building and Construction Trades Council, 9 February 1945, and Frances Payne Bolton to J. Burns, 31 January 1945, GCNA Records, Container 6, Folder 18.

36. Administrative Board minutes, 25 October 1945, Clinic Archives, 1-TV, Box 2, Folder 5.

37. Joint meeting of District No. 4 Board of Trustees, Cleveland Central Committee on Nursing, and Cleveland Office of Civilian Defense Committee on Nursing, minutes, 28 April 1942, GCNA Records, Container 1, Folder 22.

38. News clipping, *Cleveland Press*, 8 August 1942, subject file, Nurses, *Cleveland Press* Collection.

39. Administrative Board minutes, 4 February, 11 March, and 8 May 1942, Clinic Archives, 1-TV, Box 2, Folder 2.

40. Edward C. Daoust, memo, "Information for the Administrative Board," ca. 1 February 1943, Clinic Archives, 1-TV, Box 2, Folder 3.

41. Administrative Board minutes, 2 March 1944, Clinic Archives, 1-TV, Box 2, Folder 4.

42. Financial Secretary's Report, 17 May 1943, and General Secretary's Report, 17 September 1943, GCNA Records, Container 2, Folders 1 and 2.

43. Administrative Board minutes, 22 February 1945, Clinic Archives, 1-TV, Box 2, Folder 5.

44. Ibid.

45. Ibid.

46. Ibid., 17 May 1945.

47. Ibid., 4 June 1943, Folder 3.

48. Ibid., 19 August 1943; and "Memorandum of Some Things to Consider in Connection with the Surgical Nursing Service," [September 1943], Clinic Archives, Box 2, Folder 3.

49. Abbie Porter to E. Daoust, 18 December 1944, Clinic Archives, 1-TV, Box 4, Folder 4.

50. Administrative Board minutes, 1 March 1943, Clinic Archives, 1-TV, Box 2, Folder 3.

51. John C. Davis, "Hospitals Meet Emergencies of War," *Cleveland Plain Dealer*, 8 December 1942, Crile Papers, Container 35, Folder 4.

52. Grace Crile to one of her children, [11] December 1939, Crile Papers, Container 32, Folder 6.

53. Grace Crile diary, April 1941, Crile Papers, Container 34, Folder 1.

54. Josephine Belfield to G. Crile, Jr., 11 January 1943, Crile Papers, Container 35, Folder 5.

55. J. Belfield to Grace Crile, 10 January 1943, Crile Papers, Container 36, Folder 2. The fact that Mrs. Belfield, a private duty nurse, said she was expressing the feelings of "every nurse in the Cleveland Clinic Hospital" shows how much private duty nurses were integrated into the nursing service there.

56. Bullough and Bullough, *Care of the Sick*, 186; and Rodabaugh and Rodabaugh, *Nursing in Ohio*, 236.

57. Cleveland Clinic Hospital Annual Report, 1945, 12-AR, Box 1.

58. Administrative Board minutes, 29 January 1943, Clinic Archives, 1-TV, Box 2, Folder 3.

59. Ibid., 1 March 1943.

60. Cleveland Clinic Hospital Annual Report, 1943, 12-AR, Box 1.

61. Cleveland Clinic Hospital Annual Report, 1942, 12-AR, Box 1.

62. Administrative Board minutes, 30 July 1946; and E. Daoust to surgical department heads, 22 January 1946, Clinic Archives, 1-TV, Box 2, Folder 6.

63. Cleveland Clinic Hospital Annual Report, 1945, 12-AR, Box 1.

64. Ibid.; and Administrative Board minutes, 9 May and 4 June 1946, Clinic Archives, 1-TV, Box 2, Folder 6.

65. Administrative Board minutes, 26 November 1946, Clinic Archives, 1-TV, Box 2, Folder 6.

66. Ibid., 1 April 1947, Folder 7.

67. A. Porter to Hospital nursing staff, 25 March 1947, Clinic Archives, Box 2, Folder 7.

68. Cleveland Clinic Hospital Annual Report, 1947, 12-AR, Box 1; and Administrative Board minutes, 27 May 1947, Clinic Archives, 1-TV, Box 2, Folder 7.

69. Administrative Board minutes, 12 October 1944, Clinic Archives, 1-TV, Box 2, Folder 4.

70. Cleveland Clinic Hospital Annual Reports, 1947 and 1948, 12-AR, Box 1.

71. Cleveland Clinic Hospital Annual Report, 1948, 12-AR, Box 1.

72. Cleveland Clinic Hospital Annual Report, 1951, 12-AR, Box 2. The 1953 statistics for nurses and aides do not include Operating Room personnel, since the Operating Room had become a separate department by this time.

73. See above note 19. No in-house statistics are available; the Bureau figures underreport the actual number of private duty cases since not all calls were made through the Bureau.

74. Committee to Study Private Duty Nursing, report to Board of Trustees, 12 September 1946, GCNA Records, Container 2, Folder 4.

75. General Secretary's Report, 13 September 1946, GCNA Records, Container 2, Folder 4.

76. Cleveland Clinic Hospital Annual Report, 1947, 12-AR, Box 1.

77. Board of Trustees minutes, 15 February 1937, GCNA Records, Container 1, Folder 19.

78. See Kalisch and Kalisch, 551-553, 579-582, regarding declining enrollment rates, and demographic factors that affected nursing.

79. Private Duty Committee report, 11 October 1946, GCNA Records, Container 2, Folder 4; and Elizabeth K. Bidwell, "Changing Frontiers in Private Duty Nursing," *The Trained Nurse* 56 (March 1941): 190.

80. Excerpt from Board of Trustees series, 23 June 1924, History file, GCNA Records, Container 1, Folder 3.

81. Ibid., 24 May 1943, Container 2, Folder 1.

82. Ibid., 11 June 1937, Container 1, Folder 19.

83. Mildred S. Steibel, Board Secretary, District No. 4, to presidents of all OSNA districts, 3 February 1949, GCNA Records, Container 6, Folder 19.

84. Cleveland Clinic Hospital Annual Report, 1951, 12-AR, Box 2.

85. Rodabaugh and Rodabaugh, *Nursing in Ohio*, 200. Melosh, in *"The Physician's Hand,"* 159, cites national statistics on nurses employed in hospitals as "nearly half" in 1940, and "a decisive majority" by the end of WWII.

86. See notes 19 and 65 above. Commercial registries also furnished private duty nurses, but the overall numbers were still declining.

87. Cleveland Clinic Hospital Annual Report, 1952, 12-AR, Box 2.

88. Board of Trustees minutes, 31 July 1958, GCNA Records, Container 2, Folder 16.

89. "Special care units" is used here as a broader term to include both recovery rooms and intensive care units; use of the term also emphasizes that these units were caring for patients who would formerly have had private duty "special" nurses.

90. Melosh, *"The Physician's Hand,"* 187, and Kalisch and Kalisch, *Advance of American Nursing*, 729. See these sources for more detailed information on the development of recovery rooms and intensive care units in the United States.

91. Cleveland Clinic Hospital Annual Report, 1948, 12-AR, Box 1.

92. Ibid.

93. Cleveland Clinic Hospital Annual Report, 1949, 12-AR, Box 1.

94. Cleveland Clinic Hospital Annual Report, 1948, 12-AR, Box 1.

95. Melosh, *"The Physician's Hand,"* 163. "Laymen" is used here to mean individuals without background in nursing, medicine, or other "hands-on" health care fields; it is used in the masculine since management was overwhelmingly a men's occupation at the time.

96. Cleveland Clinic Hospital Annual Report, 1949, 12-AR, Box 1.

97. Cleveland Clinic Hospital Annual Report, 1944, 12-AR, Box 1.

98. Administrative Board minutes, 19 October 1944, Clinic Archives, 1-TV, Box 2, Folder 4.

99. Cleveland Clinic Hospital Annual Report, 1945, 12-AR, Box 1.

100. Administrative Board minutes, 29 January 1946, Clinic Archives, 1-TV, Box 2, Folder 6.

101. G. Crile, Jr., and W. Proudfit, "Supporting Cast," Clinic Archives, 3-PR20, Employees.

102. Cleveland Clinic Hospital Annual Report, 1952, 12-AR, Box 2.

103. Cleveland Clinic Hospital Annual Report, 1951, 12-AR, Box 2.

Chapter Four

1. News clipping, *Cleveland Press*, 30 May 1956, subject file, Nurses, *Cleveland Press* Collection. See Preface, xiv, for an explanation of the variable use of the abbreviation "R.N." and abbreviations designating advanced degrees in the text.

2. Cleveland Clinic Hospital Annual Report, 1963, 12-AR, Box 3. Physical therapists had actually been employed by the Clinic since at least the 1930s.

3. Cleveland Clinic Hospital Annual Report, 1956, 12-AR, Box 2.

4. Cleveland Clinic Hospital Annual Report, 1951, 12-AR, Box 2.

5. Personal communication/oral history.

6. Personal communication/oral history.

7. Some management and other support functions were handled by the Foundation as a whole, and so do not appear as part of the Hospital's organization chart. For instance, the Personnel Department was a Foundation-wide department; the Hospital did not have its own personnel officer.

8. Cleveland Clinic Hospital Annual Report, 1952, 12-AR, Box 2.

9. Cleveland Clinic Hospital Annual Report, 1953, 12-AR, Box 2.

10. No figures were available for the 1950s, but the Nursing Department's share of the Hospital budget was put at over 30 percent in the 1964 Annual Report.

11. Cleveland Clinic Hospital Annual Reports, 1945 and 1948, 12-AR, Box 1.

12. Cleveland Clinic Hospital Annual Report, 1951, 12-AR, Box 2.

13. Cleveland Clinic Hospital Annual Report, 1953, 12-AR, Box 2.

14. Ibid.

15. See Hartwell, *To Act As A Unit*, 133-138, for more on the Bunts Institute.

16. St. John College closed in 1975, and its nursing program was transferred to Ursuline College in the Cleveland suburb of Pepper Pike.

17. Cleveland Clinic Hospital Annual Report, 1959, 12-AR, Box 2.

18. Cleveland Clinic Hospital Annual Report, 1960, 12-AR, Box 2.

19. Cleveland Clinic Hospital Annual Reports, 1959 and 1968, 12-AR, Boxes 2 and 3.

20. Cleveland Clinic Hospital Annual Report, 1964, 12-AR, Box 3.

21. Cleveland Clinic Hospital Annual Reports, 1966 and 1970, 12-AR, Boxes 3 and 4.

22. Personal communication/oral history; and nurse recruitment brochure, attached to Cleveland Clinic Hospital Annual Report, 1969, 12-AR, Box 4.

23. Cleveland Clinic Hospital Annual Reports, 1957 and 1959, 12-AR, Box 2.

24. Cleveland Clinic Hospital Annual Report, 1957, 12-AR, Box 2; and "The Girls from St. John's," *Cleveland Clinic Newsletter*, March 1958, Clinic Archives, 3-AC, Box 1.

25. Cleveland Clinic Hospital Annual Report, 1963, 12-AR, Box 3.

26. Cleveland Clinic Hospital Annual Report, 1964, 12-AR, Box 3.

27. Cleveland Clinic Hospital Annual Report, 1966, 12-AR, Box 3.

28. "Licensed registered nurses" is actually a redundancy, since registered nurses are licensed by definition. The Clinic's official policy on employing unlicensed nurses is unclear for earlier years; it is likely that no formal policy existed. There is evidence that at least up into the 1930s or 1940s, non-registered nurses were sometimes employed. The GCNA Records indicate that this was true at the Cleveland Clinic Hospital in the 1920s, and one employee stated that even in later years, the designation "R.N." was not put on nurses' name badges because some nurses were not registered. Annual reports began referring to practical nurses as "L.P.N.s" about 1960.

29. Cleveland Clinic Hospital Annual Report, 1956, 12-AR, Box 2; and personal communication/oral history.

30. Cleveland Clinic Hospital Annual Report, 1964, 12-AR, Box 3.

31. Cleveland Clinic Hospital Annual Reports, 1958 and 1959, 12-AR, Box 2.

32. Cleveland Clinic Hospital Annual Report, 1968, 12-AR, Box 3.

33. Cleveland Clinic Hospital Annual Report, 1959, 12-AR, Box 2.

34. Personal communication/oral history.

35. Pat Sommer, "Is There a Place for the R.N. in Surgery?", *Under Your Cap* 2 (May 1970), Clinic Archives, 3-DN1.

36. Ibid.; and personal communication/oral history.

37. Cleveland Clinic Hospital Annual Report, 1953, 12-AR, Box 2.

38. Cleveland Clinic Hospital Annual Report, 1955, 12-AR, Box 2.

39. Cleveland Clinic Hospital Annual Report, 1958, 12-AR, Box 2.

40. Cleveland Clinic Hospital Annual Report, 1961, 12-AR, Box 3.

41. Personal communication/oral history. Most of the information in this section on outpatient Clinic nursing came from interviews with Miss Hofstetter and other Clinic nurses, or from written responses to an "oral" history questionnaire that was distributed to employee and retiree nursing personnel.

42. "The Challenge, Privilege and Responsibility of Nursing at the Cleveland Clinic," part 2, *Cleveland Clinic Newsletter*, December 1960, Clinic Archives, 3-AC, Box 1.

43. Personal communication/oral history.

44. Ibid.

45. Response to "oral" history questionnaire.

46. Response to "oral" history questionnaire.

47. Ibid.

48. Personal communications/oral histories. The assignment of services to rooms did not, of course, remain absolutely unchanged over decades. The most notable alteration came when cardiothoracic surgery moved to the separate sixth floor unit in 1967.

49. Ibid.

50. Ibid.

51. Cleveland Clinic Hospital Annual Report, 1958, 12-AR, Box 2.

52. Cleveland Clinic Hospital Annual Report, 1956, 12-AR, Box 2.

53. Cleveland Clinic Hospital Annual Report, 1957, 12-AR, Box 2. For more on the PPC model, see Melosh, *"The Physician's Hand,"* 186.

54. Cleveland Clinic Hospital Annual Report, 1956, 12-AR, Box 2.

55. General Secretary's Report, 15 February 1957, GCNA Records, Container 2, Folder 15.

56. Board of Trustees minutes, 17 May 1957, GCNA Records, Container 2, Folder 15; and Cleveland Clinic Hospital Annual Report, 1956, 12-AR, Box 2.

57. Letter to Board of Trustees from Private Duty Section, 8 January 1958, GCNA Records, Container 2, Folder 16.

58. Melosh, *"The Physician's Hand,"* 187.

59. Cleveland Clinic Hospital Annual Report, 1960, 12-AR, Box 2.

60. Cleveland Clinic Hospital Annual Report, 1964, 12-AR, Box 3.

61. Ibid.

62. Personal communications/oral histories. By the mid- to late 1960s, the Constant Care Units were being more frequently referred to as "intensive care units" or "ICUs."

63. Ibid.

64. Ibid.

65. Ibid.

66. Ibid.

67. Cleveland Clinic Hospital Annual Report, 1965, 12-AR, Box 3; Cresap, McCormick and Paget, "Cleveland Clinic Hospital: A Study of the Nursing Services," November 1965 (hereafter referred to as "Cresap study"), cover letter to James Harding and Introduction, Clinic Archives.

68. Cresap study, III-1, 2.

69. Cleveland Clinic Hospital Annual Report, 1954, 12-AR, Box 2.

70. Cleveland Clinic Hospital Annual Report, 1966, 12-AR, Box 3.

71. Cresap study, III-9, 10.

72. Cleveland Clinic Hospital Annual Report, 1965, 12-AR, Box 3.

73. Cleveland Clinic Hospital Annual Report, 1968, 12-AR, Box 3.

74. Cleveland Clinic Hospital Annual Report, 1957, 12-AR, Box 2.

75. Cresap study, II-3.

76. Ibid.

77. Cleveland Clinic Hospital Annual Reports, 1960 and 1969, 12-AR, Boxes 2 and 4.

78. Jan L. Lee, "A History of Care Modalities in Nursing," in *Managing Nursing Care: Promise and Pitfalls*, ed. Kathleen Kelly, vol. 5 of *Series on Nursing Administration* (St. Louis: Mosby, 1993), 28; and Cleveland Clinic Hospital Annual Report, 1954, 12-AR, Box 2.

79. Cresap study, II-9.

80. Ibid., II-10.

81. Ibid., III-11, 32.

82. Ibid., II-13.

83. Ibid., II-15.

84. Ibid., III-16, 19.

85. Cleveland Clinic Hospital Annual Report, 1967, 12-AR, Box 3.

86. Cleveland Clinic Hospital Annual Report, 1969, 12-AR, Box 4.

87. Cleveland Clinic Hospital Annual Report, 1967, 12-AR, Box 3.

88. Nancy L. Burkle, "Perioperative Nursing — A Diverse Challenge," *Essence of Nursing* 5 (Winter 1987): 12, Clinic Archives, 3-DN1.

89. Personal communications/oral histories.

90. Ibid.

91. Ibid.

92. Ibid.

93. Ibid.

94. Ibid.

95. Ibid.

96. Alexa McCubbin, "Rigid Instrument Containers: A Bacterial Barrier Technology in Packaging Instrumentation," presented at a meeting of the Association of Operating Room Nurses, 26 March 1986; and personal communication/oral history.

97. Personal communications/oral histories.

98. Ibid.

99. Cresap study, III-22.

100. G. Crile, Jr., and W. Proudfit, "Supporting Cast," Clinic Archives, 3-PR20, Employees.

101. Cleveland Clinic Hospital Annual Reports, 1958 and 1967, 12-AR, Boxes 2 and 3.

102. Cleveland Clinic Hospital Annual Report, 1943, 12-AR, Box 1; and Administrative Board minutes, 16 November 1944, Clinic Archives, 1-TV, Box 2, Folder 4.

103. Cleveland Clinic Hospital Annual Report, 1942, 12-AR, Box 1.

104. Cleveland Clinic Hospital Annual Report, 1950, 12-AR, Box 2.

105. Membership in the ANA was through the local and state organizations. Therefore, a Cleveland nurse had to join the District in order to become a member of the OSNA and the ANA (see pp. 80 and 107). See Sandra Beth Lewenson, *Taking Charge: Nursing, Suffrage, and Feminism in America, 1873-1920* (New York: Garland Publishing, Inc., 1993), 104-120, for a concise history of the NACGN.

106. News clippings, *Cleveland Plain Dealer*, 11 August 1954, and *Cleveland Press*, 24 June 1955, subject file, Nurses, *Cleveland Press* Collection.

107. Personal communications/oral histories.

108. The librarian was actually an employee of the Cleveland Public Library stationed part-time at the Clinic.

109. Cleveland Clinic Hospital Annual Reports, 1955 and 1962, 12-AR, Boxes 2 and 3.

110. Cleveland Clinic Hospital Annual Report, 1967, 12-AR, Box 3.

111. Cleveland Clinic Hospital Annual Report, 1959, 12-AR, Box 2.

112. Cleveland Clinic Hospital Annual Report, 1967, 12-AR, Box 3.

113. Cleveland Clinic Hospital Annual Reports, 1968 and 1970, 12-AR, Boxes 3 and 4.

114. Cleveland Clinic Hospital Annual Report, 1967, 12-AR, Box 3.

115. Ibid.

116. Cleveland Clinic Hospital Annual Report, 1969, 12-AR, Box 4.

117. Cleveland Clinic Hospital Annual Report, 1968, 12-AR, Box 3.

118. Ibid.

119. Cleveland Clinic Hospital Annual Reports, 1968 and 1969, 12-AR, Boxes 3 and 4.

120. Cleveland Clinic Hospital Annual Report, 1970, and Division of Patient Care Services Annual Report, 1971, Clinic Archives, 12-AR, Box 4, and 3-DA, Box 2, Folder 1.

121. Cleveland Clinic Hospital Annual Reports, 1963 and 1969, 12-AR, Boxes 3 and 4.

122. Cleveland Clinic Hospital Annual Report, 1967, 12-AR, Box 3.

123. Ibid.

124. Cleveland Clinic Hospital Annual Report, 1956, 12-AR, Box 2.

125. Cleveland Clinic Hospital Annual Report, 1957, 12-AR, Box 2.

126. Cleveland Clinic Hospital Annual Report, 1969, 12-AR, Box 4.

127. Cleveland Clinic Hospital Annual Report, 1957, 12-AR, Box 2.

128. Ibid.

129. Cleveland Clinic Hospital Annual Report, 1966, 12-AR, Box 3.

130. Cleveland Clinic Hospital Annual Report, 1960, 12-AR, Box 2.

131. Cleveland Clinic Hospital Annual Report, 1965, 12-AR, Box 3.

132. Cleveland Clinic Hospital Annual Reports, 1965 and 1969, 12-AR, Boxes 3 and 4.

133. "A Personal View," *Cleveland Clinic Newsletter*, November 1970, Clinic Archives, 3-AC, Box 1.

134. Cleveland Clinic Hospital Annual Report, 1964, 12-AR, Box 3.

135. Cleveland Clinic Hospital Annual Report, 1970, 12-AR, Box 4.

136. Cleveland Clinic Hospital Annual Report, 1964, 12-AR, Box 3.

137. "Unique Surgical Heart Unit Opens," *Cleveland Clinic Newsletter*, December 1967, Clinic Archives, 3-AC, Box 1.

138. Ibid.

139. Cleveland Clinic Hospital Annual Reports, 1967 and 1968, 12-AR, Box 3.

140. Cleveland Clinic Hospital Annual Report, 1968, 12-AR, Box 3.

141. Cleveland Clinic Hospital Annual Reports, 1969 and 1970, 12-AR, Box 4.

142. Cleveland Clinic Hospital Annual Report, 1969, 12-AR, Box 4.

143. Response to "oral" history questionnaire; and Cleveland Clinic Hospital Annual Reports, 1967 and 1968, 12-AR, Box 3.

Chapter Five

1. Hartwell, *To Act As A Unit*, 53.

2. Van Tassel and Grabowski, *Encyclopedia of Cleveland History*, li-liii.

3. Ibid., l, lv, 522.

4. Division of Patient Care Services Annual Report, 1971, Clinic Archives, 3-DA, Box 2, Folder 1. The Division of Patient Care Services of the 1970s should not be confused with the Division of Patient Care Operations, created in 1993.

5. Ibid.

6. Personal communication/oral history.

7. Patient Care Services Annual Report, 1972, Clinic Archives, 3-DA, Box 2, Folder 2.

8. Ibid.

9. Ibid.

10. Ibid.

11. Ibid.

12. Head Nurse Committee minutes, 3 October 1972, Clinic Archives, 3-DN15.

13. Ibid., 5 December 1972.

14. Ibid., 1 May 1973.

15. Patient Care Services Annual Report, 1972, Clinic Archives, 3-DA, Box 2, Folder 2.

16. Ibid.

17. Ibid.

18. Ibid.

19. *The Clinic News*, September 1977, Clinic Archives, 3-AC, Box 3.

20. Cleveland Clinic Hospital Annual Report, 1970, 12-AR, Box 4.

21. Patient Care Services Annual Report, 1973 and 1976, Clinic Archives, 3-DA, Box 2, Folders 3 and 6; Nursing Directors minutes, 28 November 1972, Clinic Archives, A85-03, Box 1.

22. Nursing Division minutes, 3 June 1981, Clinic Archives, A85-03, Box 4. Although Nursing was a department rather than a division at this time, some records dating from 1980-1981 use the word "division" in place of "department."

23. Response to "oral" history questionnaire.

24. Personal communication/oral history.

25. Nursing Directors minutes, 6 January 1972, Clinic Archives, A85-03, Box 1.

26. Patient Care Services Annual Report, 1976, Clinic Archives, 3-DA, Box 2, Folder 6.

27. Nursing Directors minutes, 16 June 1973, Clinic Archives, A85-03, Box 1.

28. Jacalyn R. Golden, "Who Are Advanced Practice Nurses?", *Cleveland Clinic Nurse* 2 (May 1994): 6, Clinic Archives, 3-DN1. All issues of the Department/Division of Nursing/Patient Care Operations publications *Memo to Nursing Staff* (cited as *Memo*), *Essence of Nursing* (cited as *Essence*), and *Cleveland Clinic Nurse* (cited as *CCN*) cited here are held by the Cleveland Clinic Archives.

29. Nursing Directors minutes, 6 December 1972, Clinic Archives, A85-03, Box 1.

30. Patient Care Services Annual Report, 1976, Clinic Archives, 3-DA, Box 2, Folder 6.

31. Cleveland Clinic Hospital Division of Nursing Annual Report, 1980, Clinic Archives, A88-09.

32. Cleveland Clinic Hospital Annual Report, 1955, 12-AR. Miss Nightingale believed that, ideally, nurses should commit their observations to memory; however, she encouraged nurses to write notes as an aid to memory if necessary.

33. Nursing Directors minutes, 18 October 1972, Clinic Archives, A85-03, Box 1.

34. Nursing Audit Committee minutes, 27 July 1973, Clinic Archives, A85-03, Box 1.

35. Nursing Directors minutes, 12 July 1973, Clinic Archives, A85-03, Box 1.

36. Nursing Directors minutes, 28 February 1979, Clinic Archives, A85-03, Box 2.

37. Nursing Division Annual Report, 1980, Clinic Archives, A88-09.

38. Executive Head Nurse Board minutes, 8 January 1980, attachment, Clinic Archives, 3-DN15.

39. Department of Nursing report, Goals and Objectives for 1983, Clinic Archives, A88-09.

40. Nursing Operations Group, 22 June 1982, attachment, Clinic Archives, 3-DN15, Box 1.

41. Ibid.

42. Ibid.

43. Department of Nursing report, Missions, Goals, and Objectives for 1985; and Department of Nursing Annual Report, 1986, Clinic Archives, A88-09.

44. Department of Nursing Annual Report, 1986, Clinic Archives, A88-09.

45. Nursing Division minutes, 11 February 1981, Cleveland Clinic Archives, A85-03, Box 4.

46. Department of Nursing Annual Report, 1986, A88-09.

47. After this major move, various nursing units continued to be moved from one geographical area to another. No attempt has been made in the text to trace the movements of each unit over the years.

48. Personal communication/oral history.

49. Response to "oral" history questionnaire; personal communication/oral history.

50. Personal communication/oral history.

51. Personal communication/oral history.

52. Personal communication/oral history.

53. Personal communication/oral history

54. Ibid.

55. Nancy L. Burkle, "Perioperative Nursing: A Diverse Challenge," *Essence of Nursing* 5 (Winter 1987): 12; 3-DN1.

56. Arlene A. Gorczycki, "TCI: Caring Nurses Meet The Challenge," *Essence* 6 (Summer 1988): 10; 3-DN1.

57. Connie Krug and Sandy Ausmundson, "A New Look for Outpatient Surgery," *Essence* 6 (Fall 1988): 3; 3-DN1.

58. Helen Raggets and Dorothy Martin, "PreCare: The Perioperative Holding Area," *Essence* 6 (Fall 1988): 2; 3-DN1.

59. Geraldine Tanks and Roberta Stokes, "Nurse to Nurse Consultation: A Case for M82," Cleveland Clinic *Memo to Nursing Staff* 5 (August 1986): 4; and Doreen Dever, "Collaborating with Social Services," *Memo* 5 (August 1986): 5; 3-DN1.

60. Kelly McNulty, "Kids and Kidneys," *Memo* 5 (August 1986): 1; 3-DN1.

61. Eva Fitzgerald, "Reflections of a Mother," *CCN* 1 (May 1993): 26; 3-DN1.

62. Donna Graneto, "New Drug Fights Renal Transplantation Rejection," *Memo* 5 (August 1986): 7; 3-DN1.

63. Ellen Liljeberg, "Liver Transplantation in Children: Implementing a Patient Program," *Essence* 5 (Spring 1987): 5; 3-DN1.

64. Ibid., 5, 10.

65. Ibid., 10.

66. Joan Booth, Suzanne Moodry, and Val Rossos, "Overview: Heart Transplantation," *Memo* 6 (September 1986): 4-5; 3-DN1.

67. Barb Williams, "Cardiac Nursing: New Challenges," *Memo* 6 (September 1986): 1, 6; 3-DN1.

68. Marcy Diethorn, "Cardiac Telemetry Units: A New Challenge," *Essence* 5 (Winter 1987): 2; 3-DN1.

69. Dianna Howaniak, "Cardiotomy Autotransfusion," *Memo* 6 (September 1986): 4; 3-DN1.

70. Ibid.

71. Kimberly Brown, "Cardiac Interventional Nursing," *Memo* 7 (Winter/Spring 1989): 2; 3-DN1.

72. Shawn Ulreich, "Through the Years: The Oncology Nursing Task Force," *Essence* 7 (Winter/Spring 1989): 9; 3-DN1.

73. Jan Faehnrich, "The Expanded Role of the Nurse in Cancer Care," *Essence* 5 (Fall 1987): 11; 3-DN1.

74. Ann Bachnich, "Hematology-Oncology Nurses Develop Mouth-Care Protocol," *Essence* 5 (Fall 1987): 1; 3-DN1.

75. Sue Sanders, "Mouth Care for Oncology Patients," *Memo* 4 (October 1986): 4; 3-DN1.

76. Bachnich, "Hematology-Oncology Nurses," 2.

77. Antje Horwitz, "Adult Leukemia: Nursing Implications for M70/M71," *Essence* 7 (Winter/Spring 1989): 12; 3-DN1.

78. Catherine Fox, "Demand for Outpatient and Home Delivery of Chemotherapy Steadily Grows," *Essence* 7 (Winter/Spring 1989): 10; 3-DN1.

79. Mary Ansberry, "Interleukin-II and Nursing Implications," *Essence* 7 (Winter/Spring 1989): 13; 3-DN1.

80. Sharon J. Coulter, Deborah M. Nadzam, and Amy Yehoda Caslow, "New Leadership: A Chance to Analyze Resource Allocation," *Nursing Administration Quarterly* 13 (Fall 1988): 20.

81. "Nursing at The Cleveland Clinic Foundation: A Tradition of Excellence," recruitment brochure, [1992], Clinic Archives, 3-DN1.

82. Personal communication/oral history.

83. Nursing Executive Council minutes, 29 October 1991, attachment, Clinic Archives, 3-DN15.

84. Nursing Management Group minutes, 4 October 1989, attachment, Clinic Archives, 3-DN15.

85. Nursing Executive Council minutes, 25 September 1991, attachment, Clinic Archives, 3-DN15.

86. "Nursing at The Cleveland Clinic Foundation," [1992].

87. Nursing Executive Council, 15 July 1992, attachment, Clinic Archives, 3-DN15.

88. Ann Hadlock, "Spirit of Ownership," *Essence* 7 (Summer 1989): 11; 3-DN1.

89. The presentations and publications listed in this and the following paragraphs are a sample, based on available information.

90. "Professional Activities and Achievements," *Essence* 6 (Fall 1988): 10; 3-DN1.

91. Gayle R. Whitman, "Shock," in *Clinical Reference for Critical-Care Nursing*, 3d ed., ed. Marguerite Kinney, Donna R. Packa, and Sandra B. Dunbar (St. Louis: Mosby, 1993), 133.

92. Janine Stone, Doris Samstag, Laurie S. Canala, and Nancy L. Burkle, "Overview of the Circulating Nurse's Activities," in *The Role of the Circulator Series* (Garden Grove, California: MEDCOM, Inc., 1994), 1.

93. Gregory B. Collins, Kathleen Weiss, Dennis Cozzens, Jan Thorpe, Margaret Kotz, and Joseph W. Janesz, "A Multidisciplinary Approach to the Treatment of Drug and Alcohol Addiction", in *Comprehensive Handbook of Drug and Alcohol Addiction*, ed. Norman S. Miller (1991), 994.

94. Karen Mae Smith and Christine A. Wynd, "Factors Influencing Postoperative Urinary Retention in the Patient Undergoing Orthopedic Surgical Procedures: A Pilot Study," *CCN* 1 (September 1993): 19; 3-DN1.

95. Kimberly Brown, JoAnne Hughes-Morscher, Ellen Montague, Michelle Casedonte, Marion Piedmonte, and Gayle Whitman, "An Analysis of Bleeding and Vascular Complications in Percutaneous Coronary Interventional Patients," *CCN* 2 (May 1994): 30-31; 3-DN1.

96. "Nursing at the Cleveland Clinic Foundation," [1992].

97. Department of Nursing Annual Report, 1986, attachment, Clinic Archives, A88-09.

98. Nursing Executive Council minutes, 19 February 1991, attachment, Clinic Archives, 3-DN15; Division of Nursing Annual Report, 1992, Clinic Archives, 3-DN10.

99. "The Nursing Education and Research Fund," brochure, Cleveland Clinic Archives, 3-DN.

100. Nursing Executive Council minutes, 4 October 1989, Clinic Archives, 3-DN15.

101. Betsy Antenucci Kuhn and Linda J. Lewicki, "Clinical Practice Guidelines: Pressure Ulcers in Adults"; and Karen A. Gelliarth, "The Unit Based Skin Care Nurse Model," *CCN* 2 (October 1994): 40, 11; 3-DN1.

102. "Skin Care Task Force Uncovers Interesting Facts," *Greater Cleveland Nursing News* 1 (September 1991): 5.

103. Gelliarth, "Unit Based Skin Care Nurse," 11.

104. Ibid.

105. Ibid., 12.

106. Lorraine Mion, personal communication and written notes. This section, "Focusing on Outcomes," makes extensive use of information provided by Dr. Mion.

107. Ibid.

108. Ibid.

109. Kathleen A. Tripepi-Bova, "The Effects of Heparinized and Nonheparinized Flush Solution on the Patency of Arterial Pressure Monitoring Lines," *CCN* 1 (September 1993): 18; 3-DN1.

110. "Nursing at the Cleveland Clinic Foundation," [1992].

111. "Competent - Creative - Confident: Nurses of the Nineties," brochure, Clinic Archives, 3-DN22.

112. Elizabeth F. Vasquez, "Cleveland Clinic Nurses Influence Patient Care Around the World," *Greater Cleveland Nursing News* 1 (September 1991): 15.

113. Charlene Williams to Sharon Coulter, 30 September 1995, Cleveland Clinic Division of Patient Care Operations office files.

114. Shawn Ulreich, "Oncology Nursing Task Force," *Memo* 4 (October 1986): 8; 3-DN1.

115. Personal communication/oral history.

116. Sharon J. Coulter, P. Mardeen Atkins, Dawn Bailey, Mary Ellen Blatt, Lori Blashford, and Sandra Shumway, "Patient Satisfaction: A QI Pilot Project," in *Improving Quality and Performance: Concepts, Programs, and Techniques*, ed. Patricia Schroeder (St. Louis: Mosby, 1994), 105.

117. Debbie Charnley, Nina M. Fielden, and Linda Shah, "Evolution of a New Emergency Service at The Cleveland Clinic Foundation," typescript, Cleveland Clinic Division of Patient Care Operations.

118. Ibid.; and Division of Patient Care Operations Annual Report, 1994, Division office files.

119. Karen Zander, "The Impact of Managing Care on the Role of a Nurse," in *Managing Nursing Care: Promise and Pitfalls*, ed. Kathleen Kelly, vol. 5 of *Series on Nursing Administration* (St. Louis: Mosby, 1993), 76.

120. Nursing Executive Council, 13 May 1992, attachment, Clinic Archives, 3-DN15.

121. Nursing Directors minutes, 7 November 1972, Clinic Archives, A85-03, Box 1; Transition Care Program Fact Sheet and Mission Statement, typescript, 1991, Clinic Archives, 3-DN11.

122. Division of Patient Care Operations Annual Report, 1994, Division office files.

123. Personal communication/oral history.

124. Roberta Stokes, "From the Editor," *CCN* 1 (May 1993): 5; 3-DN1.

125. Mary Lee Matyk, "From Dialysis to Transplantation and Beyond: The Role of the Transplant Coordinator," *CCN* 1 (May 1993): 10; 3-DN1.

126. Ibid., citing Lifebanc; Patrick J. Ginley III, "Heart Transplant: A Gift of Life," and Fitzgerald, "Reflections," *CCN* 1 (May 1993): 21, 26; 3-DN1.

127. Nancy M. Albert and Hal E. Augsburger, "Dilated Cardiomyopathy: Caring for the Critically Ill Patient—Home Dobutamine to Heart Mate[R]," *CCN* 1 (May 1993): 17, 19; 3-DN1.

128. Renee Bennett and Diane McCormick, "Heart Transplantation: A New Beginning," *CCN* 1 (May 1993): 23; 3-DN1. The description in this paragraph is a basic outline; procedures for different organs vary somewhat.

129. Susan I. Wilson, "Postoperative Care of the Liver Transplant Recipient," *CCN* 1 (May 1993): 33; 3-DN1.

130. Patricia Adler and Patti Dock, "Home Care Coordination of the Transplant Patient," and Matyk, "From Dialysis to Transplantation," *CCN* 1 (May 1993): 36, 11; 3-DN1.

131. Matyk, "From Dialysis to Transplantation," 11.

132. Bennett and McCormick, "Heart Transplantation," 23.

133. Ginley, "Heart Transplant," 22.

134. Sheila Smith, "Caring for the Dying Patient," *Memo* 4 (October 1986): 13-14; 3-DN1.

135. Jan Didich, "Palliative Care in a Tertiary Care Facility," *Essence* 5 (Fall 1987): 13; 3-DN1.

136. Carla Breth-Kupec, "Respiratory Failure: Fear Compounded," *Essence* 7 (Summer 1989): 5; 3-DN1.

137. Kate Leavy, "Homegoing Teaching: Tracheostomy Care," *Essence* 7 (Summer 1989): 1; 3-DN1.

138. Personal communication/oral history.

139. Sharon J. Coulter, "Chairman's Message," *CCN* 2 (October 1994): 3; 3-DN1.

140. Vicki L. Fisher and Dorothy J. Hamilton, "High Tech, High Touch," *Essence* 7 (Winter/Spring 1989): 3; 3-DN1.

141. Shirley M. Gullo, "Healing Art: Communicating the Cancer Experience Through Art," *CCN* 2 (October 1994): 28; 3-DN1.

142. Benita Cole, "A Collaborative Approach for Nursing Care in the Epilepsy Monitoring Unit," *Essence* 7 (Summer 1989): 4; and Patricia Holbrook, "The Vascular Amputee Patient," *Essence* 5 (Winter 1987): 15; 3-DN1.

143. "Your Part in Restoring Patient Pride^SM," brochure, [ca. 1993].

144. Nursing Executive Council minutes, 19 May 1993, Clinic Archives, 3-DN15.

145. Kathleen McCue, Lynne Aron, Kathleen T. Jirousek, Deborah L. Long, and Connie Moze, "Management of Stress and Anxiety in Children in Health Care Settings," *CCN* 1 (September 1993): 11-12; 3-DN1.

146. Eileen Griffin and Joan Holden, "Pediatric Intensive Care Unit: One Year and Growing," *CCN* 1 (September 1993): 16; 3-DN1.

147. Donna Cupp and Faye Kleinbaum, "School Re-entry in the Child with Cancer," *CCN* 1 (September 1993): 21; 3-DN1.

148. Sharon Plona, "Orthopaedic Nursing: An Unexpected Family Challenge," *CCN* 2 (May 1994): 20-21; 3-DN1.

149. Ellen M. Swenton, "Nursing: One Step Beyond," *CCN* 2 (October 1994): 26; 3-DN1.

150. Ibid., 27.

151. Nursing Operations Group minutes, 2 September 1986, Cleveland Clinic Archives, A88-09.

152. Personal communication/oral history.

153. Amy Weiss, "The Changing Design of Nursing Practice," CCN 2 (May 1994): 1; 3-DN1.

154. Robert J. Van Kirk, "Nursing for a Change...of Life," *Essence* 7 (Winter/Spring 1989): 1; 3-DN1.

155. Nursing Executive Council, 21 July 1993, attachment, Clinic Archives, 3-DN15; personal communication/oral history.

156. Nursing Executive Council, 6 November 1991, Clinic Archives, 3-DN15.

157. Nursing Executive Council, 21 July 1993, attachment, Clinic Archives, 3-DN15; personal communication/oral history.

158. Nursing Executive Council, 3 November 1993, attachment, Clinic Archives, 3-DN15.

159. "Nursing Excellence Awards," brochure, 1995, Division of Patient Care Operations office files.

160. Personal communication/oral history.

161. Personal communication/oral history.

162. Personal communication/oral history.

163. Personal communication/oral history.

164. Cathie Olsen and Cathy Ceccio, "Neurology Nursing Group Forms," *Essence* 7 (Summer 1989): 3; 3-DN1.

165. Ambulatory Clinic Nursing minutes, 14-15 June, 1993, Ambulatory Nursing office files.

166. Nursing Operations Group minutes, 10 September 1985, Clinic Archives, A88-09.

167. Nursing Executive Council minutes, 16 October 1991, Clinic Archives, 3-DN15.

168. Ibid., 18 December 1990, 20 November 1991, Clinic Archives, 3-DN15.

Conclusion

1. Doris M. Modly and Kathleen Weiss, "Why Nurses Leave Nursing," in *Managing the Nursing Shortage: A Guide to Recruitment and Retention*, ed. Terence F. Moore and Earl A. Simendinger (Rockville, Maryland: Aspen, 1989), 54.

2. Reverby, *Ordered to Care*, 122; and Melosh, *"The Physician's Hand,"* 22, 209.

Photograph Credits

The source from which each photograph or other illustration was obtained is listed here with grateful acknowledgment for their use.

Stanley A. Ferguson Archives of University Hospitals of Cleveland: 7, 8, 16, 17, 19, 20, 22, 23, 24, 26, 36, 37, 42, 44, 46, 48, 53 (top), 61, 64, 80, 84, 100, 101; *Paul Hamilton*: 72, 121; *Bill Graber*: 75, 103, 132; *Elizabeth Hartman*: 98 (lower), 151; *Central School of Practical Nursing*: 105, 113, 117, 128, 129; *Historical Division of the Cleveland Medical Library Association (Allen Memorial Medical Library)*: 109; *Corinne Hofstetter*: 153, 154; *Cleveland Press Collection at Cleveland State University Archives*: 87, 155; *Karen Westmeyer*: 166 (left and lower); *Susan Richards*: 201; *Karen Bourquin*: 203; *Alexa McCubbin*: 204; *Mardi Atkins*: 206; *Linda Solar*: 215; *Susan Horn*: 218, 233, 245, 252, 257, 260, 262, 263; *Sharon Coulter*: 227, 230; *Division of Patient Care Operations*: 246; *Dolores Wiemels*: 250.

All other illustrations are from the collections of The Cleveland Clinic Foundation Archives, or from photographers Tom Merce and Tony Buck in the Division of Marketing and Managed Care.

Index

Italics indicate an illustration with its accompanying text; **boldface** indicates textual information in sidebars or elsewhere outside the main body of the text. An *f* following a page number shows that the subject is further treated on the following page(s). If a term is not used along with a place or institutional name, it is understood to be in the context of the Cleveland Clinic or its department/division of nursing. Names of the main individuals in photographs are indexed if they have been identified, except for large group shots, where for space reasons names are not given. All initials indicating degrees or titles after names have been dropped.

Without Whose Aid

was composed in the ITC Novarese type face;
printed by sheet-fed offset on 70-pound Hammermill Regalia,
Lustre finish, Olde Porcelain paper;
Smyth sewn and bound over .095 binder's boards
in Holliston Roxite Green Linen cloth;
with 70-pound Simpson Sundance, Maize endpapers,
and wrapped with dustjackets printed in six colors and varnished
on 60-pound gloss cover stock by Lorain Printing Company;
Color separations by Pinnacle Graphics & Imaging;
Book Design and Production by JoAnne Porras
Department of Graphic Services
Cleveland Clinic Foundation

Susan R. Pacheco RN 3/85
Bernadine Koproski RN 8/71
Nancy L. Bean RN 4/94
Kimberly Hilton U.S. 7/94
Susan Berg Koger RN 8/87
Joan C. Bacon LPN 2/9/71
Sandra Spirko RN 4/89
Joan E. Cleppe LPN/CVT 2/17/75
Holly L. Sufaljko RN 11/88
Marci Molnar, RN, NM 7/89
Laurie A. Faulkner — April '82
Melinda Rogers RN — December 94
Stacey Decker RN 12/93
Elsie D. Cayayan RN 6/5/88
Anita M. Maliski RN 1977
Mary Bunn Richardson RN 6-24-91
Tricia Nolder RN 4-18-94
Susan Loboda RN 10-93
Mary V. Stillman RN 10/80
Susan Stem RN, CCRN 9/86
Teresa Kuzma RN 12/3/83
Janice Thomas RN 6/90
Bonnie J. Hensler RN 6/89
Louise Gillian Ra 3/4/94
Kathleen J. Headling NUA 1/17/94
Lillian L. Johnson RN 3/85
Robin P. Sharp RN 10-5-87
Sheree B. Jimenez RN 7-15-91
Terri Lynn Gonzales RN 2/91
Lisa M. Dubenstyn RN 11/87
Farley M. Lee RN 9/76
Mattie Adams NUA 9/72
Jean M. Bartley RN 4/90
Margie Clowero Lpn 10/4/71
Karen M. Trout RN 12-12-94
Eleanor M. Foster RN 8-15-65
Janice M. Dobbis 4-25-94 NM
Robert Carlen RN 8/5/92
Ruby Proa LPN 10-14-67
Suzanne Moody R.N. 6-19-77
Sally Mulka Administrative Secretary 5/30/75
Irice Beans Administrative Sec. 5/21/91
Loretta A. Planowsky, R.N. MSN 9/27
Linda A. Shell RN, CEN nurse manager 9/3/72
Pearl J. Prata LPN 1/30/67
Mary E. Harris LPN 3/4/68
Pamela Welch RN 5/20/82
Mary Craig RN MSN MBA 3.11.94
Nina M. Fielder MSN, RN 1/4/88
Jandyn Madden 10-12-81
D. Harrison 10/15/90
Claire L. Parker 8/21/78
Gracelia King 11-15-93
Susan Null RN 5-1-88
Rebecca Maynard RN 6/10/89
John Bresley 4/20/67
Grace Ann Steere 3-14-95
Frances Eden 6.23.80
Anna Maria Amicucci RN 4-27-91
Sandra M. Lupario RN TNCC 3-14-95
Susan Gaffney RRT 6-13-94
Cathryn A. Kupas RN, BSN 3-87
Roselyn Edwards RN 2-10-86
Andrea McFarland RN, BSN, BA 6-19-89
Elizabeth Akeupe RN, BSN, CEN 5/11/94
Dena Drake Larson RN, BSN 7/15/91
Germaine M. Smith, Secy 4/25/94
Beverly J. Michel RN 9/12/95
Alyce Hymel RN 1-23-94
Betty Carenie RN 5/81

Wanda J. Russell US 4-12-93
Tracy Gaeylor 2/27/95
Julie Gorden 8/5/91
Kathleen R. McArdren RN BSN CEN
David H. Jame RN CEN 3-28-15
Betsy Vargo RN 6-89
Kimberly Oh 7-94
Robbie Browning 8.22.94 U.C.
Gail Gall RN 3-94
Sandra R. Prentura RN-TNCC/ACLS 9/94
Joannet Villegas RN 3/29/94
Deborah L. Chazalez 12/91
Nancy Stetter Kemp RN 1/88
Lisa D. Cole 7/93
Laurel St. John 4/92
Deborah D. Daniel R.N. 8-3-92
Kimberly D. Smith 7-13-93
Lori Hoffman Hogg RN NS OCN 2/13/95
Patsy Val. US 08-04-86 G62
Gail A. Mill RRT 7-6-93
Jennifer L. Zito, RRT 11-1-93
Martha Bemer 7/15/91
John Kimball RRT 9-4-90
Lynnee Skrtz 3.15.82
John Atkin 5/20/98 Unit Sec
Karen A. Schrejder RN 2-21-94
Anne C. Haffney 9-15-80
Victoria Hilson May 9, 1994
Lynne Cattanzio RN 9/86
Marie Vision 6/13-77
Mary B. Bell 11-5-81
Billie Jo Wortman 11-90
Nancy Steele 4-87
Colleen Kiltane 10/84
Diana Conner 4/92
Diana Birele 1/95
Alexis Wolfman 1/10/74
Debbie (Nichols) Mastri RN 8/30/20
Corinne Hostetter 2/28/57
Susan R. Haas RN 7/5/83
Sandra Shumway RN 9/10/84
Frederick K. Kautzenhein 4/13/84
Diane Everet Grabowski April 1993
JoAnne Porras 6-27-93
Joseph R. Jance RN 1/10/94
Brenda J. Raiter RN 11/29/93
Michele Jablunski RN 8/88
Jean Morgar 3/92
Susan P. Wilson 7/87
Jean Campara 1/81
Richard Moorehead 7/25/94
Kathleen C. Surace 5/87
Sarah C. Mutschleiner 6/90
Kimberly Bingaman 5/91
Michelle Carm Roach 8/87
Mary J. Moore 8/87
Mary J. Posey RN, BSN, CNOR 12/67
Karen K. Harold RN 9/69
Lynnia H. Lewis RN 3/80
Lois A. Bock, R.N. 6/77
Doris Samotag, RN, BSN, CNOR 4/25/79
James C. Barton, R.N. 3/7/94
Annette H. Picozel, R.N. 10/8/62
Deborah J. Ensberger RN, MSN, CRM 11/6/78
Shirley C. Johnson 10-15-73
Judith Blast 6-15-81
Susan M. Stephens 2-14-77
Cynthia Marie Morgan Chervino 8/30/93
Mary H. Soave RN 9/19/94
Jane R. Budman RN 4/6/94
Kimberly Nye RN 6/3/91
Amy Poree RN 6/91

Dawn Bailey RN 6/15/81
Lavon Wiggins N.U.A. 8-23-93
Cynthia A. Wittig RN 5/26/87
Kathleen G. Opaskar RN 12/78
Norma L. Hogue / US 1/24/74
Ryan R. Rex PCT 9/01/94
Marilyn C. Sahonter RN 9/86
Oscar T. Dejelo RN 4/20/92
Karen Cain RN 10/17/94
Katherine M. Sibula, RN 4-12-93
Danielle Prosski RN 8-26-91
Sandy Roberts, US 9-88
Sally Pratt RN MSN 2-18-91
LaVonne Williams RN 3-1-87
Amy M. Strawer RN 11-1-93
Roberta Thurston RN 1981-
Alicia A. Hayk RN 5/87
Chrisce RN 2/10/86
Mary M. Casey RN 5/88
John C. Aaron RN 6/72
Kate Sandstrom RN 1/87
Diana E. Edwards 6/9/86 NUA
Dana Glickeman 11/87 U.S.
James G. Symon RN 1/95
Monica Weber RN 7/81 + 3/92
Diana Rinkard 9/16/91
Jane Rudzitis 2/81
Anne L. Gurafovac, RNC 6.24.74
Cindy L. Phil RN 2-21-94
Josette M. Snyder RN MSN 14/5/84
Peggy Van Kirk 7/17/78
Kathleen R. Palmieri 7/12
Joanne A. Bsone RN NM 7/84
August P. Withers, NUA 7/7/86
Eva B. Scopo 9/18/18
Denise Smith RN BSN 6-20-94
M. Anastasia Dusolcki RN BSN 6-20-94
Sandy Piruitz, RN 9/11/89
Wendy Thyer, secretary 10/20/86
Sheila Pittman RN 1/4/93
Annie M. Shiller, RN 6/1/76
Sharlene A. Donelly RN 9-9-74
Cheryl Roch-Waldon RN Sept. 1980
Sarah H. Dunn RN Jan. 94
Violet L. Boisfieri Feb 71
Crystal Ann Kalas RN 6-3-91
Lisa C. McBride RN Nov. 93
Karen B. Schrock RN Aug 8, 1994
Nancy Recophal RN Aug, 1994
Jane O. Mesereau RN Jan 29, 1979
Andrea (Mussy) Sules RN 2-13-95
Carol McDonald RN 8 Aug 94
Kim Litton Schroeder RN
Maureen Barry RN 10/94
Hope R. Kucinski RN 8/20/94
Sally Mvdolo RN 11-93
Kelly Nickas RN 1-18-93
Dianna Joyce Malik RN 7-64
Reba J. Kelley RN 3-64
Anne Roskowski, RN 3/86
Catherine L. Scheide, RN 11-93
Christine M. Bennett RN 2-89
Peggy L. George RN BSN 5-27-80
Laura J. Bennett, RN, BSN 12-1-80
Diane McCormick RN, 3-74
Karen A. Bontin 5/22/64
Claudia Strank MSN RNC 1/89
Kathleen Boone MSN, RN, CCRN 3/94
Jocelyn R. Collen BSN, CRNP 7/88
Nancy Ridgway MSN, RNC 7/94